Gender, Racial, and Socioeconomic Issues in Perioperative Medicine

Editors

KATHERINE T. FORKIN
LAUREN K. DUNN
EDWARD C. NEMERGUT

ANESTHESIOLOGY CLINICS

www.anesthesiology.theclinics.com

Consulting Editor
LEE A. FLEISHER

June 2020 • Volume 38 • Number 2

ELSEVIER

1600 John F. Kennedy Boulevard • Suite 1800 • Philadelphia, Pennsylvania, 19103-2899

http://www.theclinics.com

ANESTHESIOLOGY CLINICS Volume 38, Number 2
June 2020 ISSN 1932-2275, ISBN-13: 978-0-323-71287-3

Editor: Colleen Dietzler
Developmental Editor: Kristen Helm

Anesthesiology Clinics (ISSN 1932-2275) is published quarterly by Elsevier Inc., 360 Park Avenue South, New York, NY 10010-1710. Months of issue are March, June, September, and December. Periodicals postage paid at New York, NY and at additional mailing offices. Subscription prices are $100.00 per year (US student/resident), $364.00 per year (US individuals), $446.00 per year (Canadian individuals), $728.00 per year (US institutions), $920.00 per year (Canadian institutions), $100.00 per year (Canadian student/resident), $225.00 per year (foreign student/resident), $474.00 per year (foreign individuals), and $920.00 per year (foreign institutions). To receive student and resident rate, orders must be accompanied by name of affiliated institution, date of term, and the *signature* of program/residency coordinator on institutions letterhead. Orders will be billed at individual rate until proof of status is received. Foreign air speed delivery is included in all *Clinics'* subscription prices. All prices are subject to change without notice. POSTMASTER: Send address changes to *Anesthesiology Clinics,* Elsevier Health Sciences Division, Subscription Customer Service, 3251 Riverport Lane, Maryland Heights, MO 63043. Customer Service (orders, claims, online, change of address): Elsevier Health Sciences Division, Subscription Customer Service, 3251 Riverport Lane, Maryland Heights, MO 63043. **Tel:1-800-654-2452 (U.S. and Canada); 314-447-8871 (outside U.S. and Canada). Fax: 314-447-8029. E-mail: journalscustomerservice-usa@elsevier.com (for print support); journalsonlinesupport-usa@elsevier.com (for online support).**

Reprints. For copies of 100 or more of articles in this publication, please contact the Commercial Reprints Department, Elsevier Inc., 360 Park Avenue South, New York, NY 10010-1710. Tel.: 212-633-3874; Fax: 212-633-3820; E-mail: reprints@elsevier.com.

Anesthesiology Clinics, is also published in Spanish by McGraw-Hill Inter-americana Editores S. A., P.O. Box 5-237, 06500 Mexico D. F., Mexico.

Anesthesiology Clinics, is covered in *MEDLINE/PubMed (Index Medicus), Current Contents/Clinical Medicine, Excerpta Medica, ISI/BIOMED*, and *Chemical Abstracts*.

Contributors

CONSULTING EDITOR

LEE A. FLEISHER, MD, FACC, FAHA
Robert D. Dripps Professor and Chair of Anesthesiology and Critical Care, Professor of Medicine, Perelman School of Medicine, University of Pennsylvania, Philadelphia, Pennsylvania, USA

EDITORS

KATHERINE T. FORKIN, MD
Assistant Professor, Department of Anesthesiology, University of Virginia Health System, Charlottesville, Virginia, USA

LAUREN K. DUNN, MD, PhD
Assistant Professor, Department of Anesthesiology, University of Virginia Health System, Charlottesville, Virginia, USA

EDWARD C. NEMERGUT, MD
Frederic A. Berry Professor of Anesthesiology, Professor of Neurosurgery, Department of Anesthesiology, University of Virginia Health System, Charlottesville, Virginia, USA

AUTHORS

ANOUSHKA AFONSO, MD
Department of Anesthesiology and Critical Care Medicine, Memorial Sloan Kettering Cancer Center, New York, New York, USA

ANNE ELIZABETH BAETZEL, MD
University of Michigan, CS Mott Children's Hospital, Ann Arbor, Michigan, USA

MARIAM BATAKJI, MD
Critical Care Fellow, University of Virginia Health System, Charlottesville, Virginia, USA

ALLISON J. BECHTEL, MD
Assistant Professor, Department of Anesthesiology, University of Virginia Health, Charlottesville, Virginia, USA

HONORIO T. BENZON, MD
Professor, Department of Anesthesiology, Northwestern University Feinberg School of Medicine, Chicago, Illinois, USA

JEANNA BLITZ, MD
Associate Professor of Anesthesiology, Director of Preoperative Anesthesia and Surgery Screening (PASS) Clinic, Director of the Perioperative Medicine Fellowship, Duke University School of Medicine, Durham, North Carolina, USA

ALBERTO A. CASTRO BIGALLI, MSc
East Carolina University Brody School of Medicine, Greenville, North Carolina, USA

JAIME DALY, MD
Department of Anesthesia, Critical Care and Pain Medicine, Obstetric Anesthesia Fellowship Associate Program Director, Massachusetts General Hospital, Instructor in Anaesthesia, Harvard Medical School, Boston, Massachusetts, USA

NICOLE DOBIJA, MD
University of Michigan, CS Mott Children's Hospital, Ann Arbor, Michigan, USA

GREGORY W. FISCHER, MD
Department of Anesthesiology and Critical Care Medicine, Memorial Sloan Kettering Cancer Center, New York, New York, USA

PAMELA FLOOD, MD, MA
Professor, Department of Anesthesiology, Perioperative, and Pain Medicine, Stanford University School of Medicine, Stanford, California, USA

ERICA GABRIELLE FOLDY, PhD
Associate Professor of Public and Nonprofit Management, Wagner School of Public Service, New York University, New York, New York, USA

KRISTINA L. GOFF, MD
Assistant Professor of Anesthesiology and Critical Care Medicine, The University of Texas Southwestern Medical Center, Dallas, Texas, USA

KARIM HEBISHI, MD
Departments of Internal Medicine and Psychiatry, Vidant Medical Center, East Carolina University Brody School of Medicine, Greenville, North Carolina, USA

EBONY J. HILTON, MD
Associate Professor of Anesthesiology and Critical Care Medicine, University of Virginia Health System, Charlottesville, Virginia, USA

ASHLEE HOLMAN, MD
University of Michigan, CS Mott Children's Hospital, Ann Arbor, Michigan, USA

JULIE L. HUFFMYER, MD
Associate Professor, Department of Anesthesiology, Residency Program Director, University of Virginia Health, Charlottesville, Virginia, USA

JALEESA JACKSON, MD
Department of Anesthesia, Critical Care and Pain Medicine, Pain Medicine Fellow, Massachusetts General Hospital, Clinical Fellow in Anaesthesia, Harvard Medical School, Boston, Massachusetts, USA

ABBAS M. KHAN, MD
The MORZAK Collaborative, Greenville, North Carolina, USA

AMANDA M. KLEIMAN, MD
Assistant Professor, Department of Anesthesiology, University of Virginia Health System, Charlottesville, Virginia, USA

NATALIE KOZLOV, MD
Assistant Professor, Department of Anesthesiology, Northwestern University Feinberg School of Medicine, Chicago, Illinois, USA

ALBERT HYUKJAE KWON, MD
Clinical Fellow in Pain Medicine, Department of Anesthesiology, Perioperative, and Pain Medicine, Stanford University School of Medicine, Stanford, California, USA

ELIZABETH M.S. LANGE, MD
Assistant Professor, Department of Anesthesiology, Northwestern University Feinberg School of Medicine, Chicago, Illinois, USA

CHOY R. LEWIS, MD
Assistant Professor, Department of Anesthesiology, Northwestern University Feinberg School of Medicine, Chicago, Illinois, USA

NADIA LUNARDI, MD, PhD
Assistant Professor of Anesthesiology and Critical Care Medicine, University of Virginia Health System, Charlottesville, Virginia, USA

TATIANA LUTZKER, MD
Assistant Professor, Department of Anesthesiology and Critical Care Medicine, The George Washington University Medical Center, Washington, DC, USA

ANDREW C. MILLER, MD
Department of Emergency Medicine, Vidant Medical Center, East Carolina University Brody School of Medicine, The MORZAK Collaborative, Greenville, North Carolina, USA

REBECCA D. MINEHART, MD, MSHPEd
Director, Obstetric Anesthesia Fellowship Program, Assistant Professor of Anaesthesia, Harvard Medical School, Massachusetts General Hospital, Department of Anesthesia, Critical Care and Pain Medicine, Massachusetts General Hospital, Boston, Massachusetts, USA

OLUBUKOLA OLUGBENGA NAFIU, MD, FRCA, MS
Nationwide Children's Hospital, Columbus, Ohio, USA

SURAJ PATEL, MD
PGY-4/CA-3 Resident Physician, Department of Anesthesiology and Critical Care Medicine, The George Washington University Medical Center, Washington, DC, USA

PAUL IRVIN REYNOLDS, MD
University of Michigan, CS Mott Children's Hospital, Ann Arbor, Michigan, USA

ELLEN W. RICHTER, MD
Assistant Professor, Department of Anesthesiology, Emory University School of Medicine, Atlanta, Georgia, USA

DOROTHEA S. ROSENBERGER, MD, PhD
Professor of Anesthesiology and Critical Care Medicine, University of Utah School of Medicine, Salt Lake City, Utah, USA

ROSHNI SREEDHARAN, MD
Assistant Professor of Anesthesiology and Critical Care Medicine, Case Western Reserve University School of Medicine, Cleveland, Ohio, USA

BOBBIEJEAN SWEITZER, MD, FACP
Professor of Anesthesiology, Associate Chair, Perioperative Clinical Practice, Northwestern University Feinberg School of Medicine, Chicago, Illinois, USA

JENNA SWISHER, MD
Assistant Professor of Anesthesiology, Northwestern University Feinberg School of Medicine, Chicago, Illinois, USA

PALOMA TOLEDO, MD, MPH
Assistant Professor, Department of Anesthesiology, Center for Health Services and Outcomes Research, Northwestern University Feinberg School of Medicine, Chicago, Illinois, USA

LUIS E. TOLLINCHE, MD
Department of Anesthesiology and Critical Care Medicine, Memorial Sloan Kettering Cancer Center, New York, New York, USA

AMIR VAHEDIAN-AZIMI, PhD
Trauma Research Center, Nursing Faculty, Baqiyatallah University of Medical Sciences, Tehran, Iran

CHRISTIAN VAN ROOYEN, MD
Department of Anesthesiology and Critical Care Medicine, Memorial Sloan Kettering Cancer Center, New York, New York, USA

ANITA N. VINCENT, MD
Assistant Professor, Department of Anesthesiology and Critical Care Medicine, The George Washington University Medical Center, Washington, DC, USA

SUSAN M. WALTERS, MD
PGY-4/CA-3 Resident Physician, Department of Anesthesiology, University of Virginia Health System, Charlottesville, Virginia, USA

CINDY B. YEOH, MD
Department of Anesthesiology and Critical Care Medicine, Memorial Sloan Kettering Cancer Center, New York, New York, USA

Contents

Foreword: Gender, Racial, and Socioeconomic Issues in Perioperative Medicine xiii

Lee A. Fleisher

Preface: Gender, Racial, and Socioeconomic Issues in Perioperative Medicine xv

Katherine T. Forkin, Lauren K. Dunn, and Edward C. Nemergut

Special Considerations Related to Race, Sex, Gender, and Socioeconomic Status in the Preoperative Evaluation: Part 1: Race, History of Incarceration, and Health Literacy 247

Jeanna Blitz, Jenna Swisher, and BobbieJean Sweitzer

Patients anticipating surgery and anesthesia often need preoperative care to reduce risk and facilitate services on the day of surgery. Preparing patients often requires extensive evaluation and coordination of care. Vulnerable, marginalized, and disenfranchised populations have special concerns, limitations, and needs. These patients may have unidentified or poorly managed comorbidities. Underrepresented minorities and transgender patients may avoid or have limited access to health care. Homelessness, limited health literacy, and incarceration hinder perioperative optimization initiatives. Identifying patients who will benefit from additional resource allocation and knowledge of their special challenges is vital to reducing disparities in health and health care.

Special Considerations Related to Race, Sex, Gender, and Socioeconomic Status in the Preoperative Evaluation: Part 2: Sex Considerations and Homeless Patients 263

Jenna Swisher, Jeanna Blitz, and BobbieJean Sweitzer

Patients anticipating surgery and anesthesia often need preoperative care to lower risk and facilitate services on the day of surgery. Preparing patients often requires extensive evaluation and coordination of care. Vulnerable, marginalized, and disenfranchised populations have special concerns, limitations, and needs. These patients may have unidentified or poorly managed comorbidities. Underrepresented minorities and transgender patients may avoid or have limited access to health care. Homelessness, limited health literacy, and incarceration hinder perioperative optimization initiatives. Identifying patients who will benefit from additional resource allocation and knowledge of their special challenges are vital to reducing disparities in health and health care.

Racial Differences in Pregnancy-Related Morbidity and Mortality 279

Rebecca D. Minehart, Jaleesa Jackson, and Jaime Daly

Racism in the United States has deep roots that affect maternal health, particularly through pervasive inequalities among black women compared with white. Anesthesiologists are optimally positioned to maintain vigilance for these disparities in maternal care, and to intervene with their unique acute critical care skills and knowledge. As leaders in patient safety, anesthesiologists should drive hospitals and practices to develop and implement national bundles for patient safety, as well as using team-based training practices designed to improve hospitals that care for racially diverse mothers.

Perioperative Considerations Regarding Sex in Solid Organ Transplantation **297**

Susan M. Walters, Ellen W. Richter, Tatiana Lutzker, Suraj Patel, Anita N. Vincent, and Amanda M. Kleiman

Sex plays a role in all stages of the organ transplant process, including listing, sex/size matching of organs, complications, graft survival, and mortality. Sex-related differences in organ transplantation are likely multifactorial related to biological and social characteristics. More information is needed to determine how sex-related differences can lead to improved outcomes for future donors and recipients of solid organs. This article provides an overview on the impact of sex on various types of solid organ transplant, including kidney, pancreas, liver, lung, and heart transplants.

Considerations for Transgender Patients Perioperatively **311**

Luis E. Tollinche, Christian Van Rooyen, Anoushka Afonso, Gregory W. Fischer, and Cindy B. Yeoh

With a shift in the cultural, political, and social climate surrounding gender and gender identity, an increase in the acceptance and visibility of transgender individuals is expected. Anesthesiologists are thus more likely to encounter transgender and gender nonconforming patients in the perioperative setting. Anesthesiologists need to acquire an in-depth understanding of the transgender patient's medical and psychosocial needs. A thoughtful approach throughout the entirety of the perioperative period is key to the successful management of the transgender patient. This review provides anesthesiologists with a culturally relevant and evidence-based approach to transgender patients during the preoperative, intraoperative, and postoperative periods.

Racial Disparities in Pediatric Anesthesia **327**

Anne Elizabeth Baetzel, Ashlee Holman, Nicole Dobija, Paul Irvin Reynolds, and Olubukola Olugbenga Nafiu

Racial disparities in health care have been extensively documented. Although race is a recognized determinant of the incidence and outcome of disease, few studies have examined the role of race in the delivery of pediatric perianesthesia care. Whereas racial differences in health outcomes may not be easy to modify, disparities in health care delivery are modifiable. The authors examined literature to determine whether racial disparities exist in the delivery of pediatric anesthesia. They explored putative contributors to disparities at the provider, patient, and systems level and propose ideas to address potential causes of disparities in the practice of pediatric anesthesia.

Genetics and Gender in Acute Pain and Perioperative Opioid Analgesia **341**

Albert Hyukjae Kwon and Pamela Flood

Experimental and clinical acute pain research in relation to biological sex and genetics started in the 1980s. Research methods became more powerful and sensitive with the advancement in affordable gene sequencing methods and high-throughput genetic assays. Decades of research has identified several potential pharmaceutical targets, providing insights into future research direction, and understanding of acute pain and opioid analgesic effects in the clinical setting. However, there is insufficient evidence to make generalized recommendations for using genetic tests for clinical practice of acute pain management.

The Flaw of Medicine: Addressing Racial and Gender Disparities in Critical Care **357**

Ebony J. Hilton, Kristina L. Goff, Roshni Sreedharan, Nadia Lunardi, Mariam Batakji, and Dorothea S. Rosenberger

The age of modern medicine has ushered in remarkable advances and with them increased longevity of life. The questions are, however: Has everyone benefited from these developments equally? and Do all lives truly matter? The presence of gender and racial health disparities indicates that there is work still left to be done. The first target of intervention may well be the medical establishment itself. The literature presented in this article identifies potential targets for interventions and future areas of exploration.

Two Sides of the Same Coin: Addressing Racial and Gender Disparities Among Physicians and the Impact on the Community They Serve **369**

Ebony J. Hilton, Nadia Lunardi, Roshni Sreedharan, Kristina L. Goff, Mariam Batakji, and Dorothea S. Rosenberger

The influence of historical cultural norms is evident when analyzing the physician demographics in the United States. To this day, there exists a paucity in diversity as it pertains to gender balance and ethnicity. This phenomenon is particularly concerning when studies support the notion that race and gender concordance are associated with improved outcomes. The literature presented in this article identifies potential targets for interventions on how to attract, train, and retain minority physicians.

Ethical Issues Confronting Muslim Patients in Perioperative and Critical Care Environments: A Survey of Islamic Jurisprudence **379**

Andrew C. Miller, Abba M. Khan, Karim Hebishi, Alberto A. Castro Bigalli, and Amir Vahedian-Azimi

Ethical dilemmas may arise when medical management conflicts with a patient's values, culture, religion, or legal considerations. Many Muslims encounter ethical dilemmas as patients in perioperative and critical care settings. This article discusses the fundamentals of Islamic jurisprudence and how this may affect hospitalized patients in terms of cleanliness and prayer in the setting of stoma and urinary catheters, fasting, transfusion, transplants, xenografts and animal-based medications, do-not-resuscitate orders, and postmortem examinations. Provider familiarity with how such situations may affect Muslim patients is important to navigate potential conflict and to deliver competent care.

Gender Differences in Postoperative Outcomes After Cardiac Surgery **403**

Allison J. Bechtel and Julie L. Huffmyer

Women presenting for cardiac surgery tend to be older and have hypertension, diabetes, and overweight or underweight body mass index than men.

Despite improvements in surgical techniques and medications, women have increased risk for morbidity and mortality after multiple types of cardiac surgery. Women presenting for transcatheter aortic valve replacement are older and frailer than men, and have increased risk of intraoperative complications, but lower mortality at mid- and long-term ranges compared with men. Adherence to recovery and rehabilitation from cardiac surgery is challenging for women. Solutions should focus on increased family support, and use of group exercise and activities.

Role of Gender and Race in Patient-Reported Outcomes and Satisfaction **417**

Natalie Kozlov and Honorio T. Benzon

The role of gender, race, and socioeconomic status in outcomes and satisfaction are reflected in patient-reported outcomes using measurement tools representing outcome domains. These domains include pain relief, physical and emotional functioning, adverse events, participant disposition, and patient satisfaction. Measurement tools exist for each of the outcomes in both acute and chronic pain. Patients with lower economic status have greater difficulty accessing care, are involved less in shared decision-making process, and are less satisfied with their care. Blacks, Hispanics, and Asians also have increased difficulty in accessing good quality care. Women have inferior outcomes after medical and surgical interventions.

Effects of Gender and Race/Ethnicity on Perioperative Team Performance **433**

Rebecca D. Minehart and Erica Gabrielle Foldy

We judge each other every day using demographic characteristics (such as gender and race/ethnicity), and these social identities shape our lives in profound ways. The impacts of demographic diversity in perioperative teams are poorly understood, and mixed results are reported in other team-based work settings. Drawing from decades' worth of organizational behavior literature, the authors propose a model of critical factors related to interplays between diversity, communication, and conflict, all which take place in a hierarchical environment influenced by power differences. Evidence-based recommendations are provided, aimed at maximizing benefits of diversity in perioperative teams while minimizing negative consequences.

Women and Underrepresented Minorities in Academic Anesthesiology **449**

Paloma Toledo, Choy R. Lewis, and Elizabeth M.S. Lange

The demographics of the United States is changing with 51% of the population being female, and 32% of the population identifying as an underrepresented minority (URM, ie, African American/black, Hispanic/Latino, American Indian/Alaska Native, Native Hawaiian/Pacific Islander). Women and URMs have been historically underrepresented in medicine and in academic anesthesiology. This article provides an overview of the current status of women and URM faculty in academic anesthesiology and provides a framework for academic advancement. Throughout the text, the terms woman/women are used, as opposed to female, as the terms woman/women refer to gender, and female refers to biological sex.

ANESTHESIOLOGY CLINICS

FORTHCOMING ISSUES

September 2020
Pediatric Anesthesia
Alison Perate and Vanessa Olbrecht, *Editors*

December 2020
Management of Critical Events
Alexander A. Hannenberg, *Editor*

March 2021
Neuroanesthesia
Jeffrey Kirsch and Cindy Lien, *Editors*

RECENT ISSUES

March 2020
Anesthesia at the Edge of Life
Ranjit Deshpande and Stanley H. Rosenbaum, *Editors*

December 2019
Cardiothoracic Anesthesia and Critical Care
Karsten Bartels and Stefan J.M. Dieleman, *Editors*

September 2019
Geriatric Anesthesia
Elizabeth L. Whitlock and Robert A. Whittington, *Editors*

Foreword

Gender, Racial, and Socioeconomic Issues in Perioperative Medicine

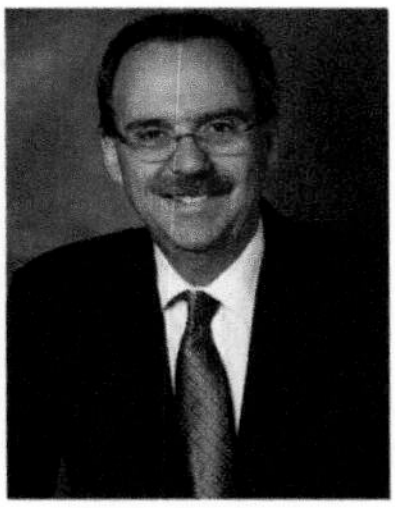

Lee A. Fleisher, MD, FACC, FAHA
Consulting Editor

Increasing attention has been focused on drivers of health with an emphasis on the impact of both social and environmental factors accounting for up to 40% of premature death. While race and gender were traditionally viewed as genetic factors, more recent evidence has demonstrated their impact on issues of access and other determinants of health disparities. Traditionally, the impact of these factors is considered outside of the domain of the anesthesiologist. The authors of this issue of *Anesthesiology Clinics* have written a series of important articles demonstrating the impact of these factors in perioperative care. In attempting to reduce the effect of disparities, we must diversify our workforce, which is also discussed in the final 2 articles.

In order to assemble a series of articles for Gender, Racial, and Socioeconomic Issues in Perioperative Medicine, I have enlisted a group of editors from the University of Virginia, Department of Anesthesiology. Katherine T. Forkin, MD is an Assistant Professor of Anesthesiology and focuses on caring for patients requiring general surgery and liver transplantation. Her research interests include medical education, gender and bias in medicine, and quality improvement. Lauren K. Dunn, MD, PhD is also Assistant Professor of Anesthesiology and focuses on caring for patients requiring neurosurgery. Her research interests include surgery-induced opioid dependence, sleep and fatigue. Edward C. Nemergut, MD, is the Frederic A. Berry Professor of Anesthesiology and vice-chair in the Department of Anesthesiology. Dr Nemergut has had a career-long interest in education and founded the University of Virginia Department of Anesthesiology's Medical Education Research Group to promote

Anesthesiology Clin 38 (2020) xiii–xiv
https://doi.org/10.1016/j.anclin.2020.03.002
1932-2275/20/© 2020 Published by Elsevier Inc.

more precise research in medical education. Together, they have assembled an all-star group of authors to educate in this area.

Lee A. Fleisher, MD, FACC, FAHA
Perelman School of Medicine
University of Pennsylvania
3400 Spruce Street, Dulles 680
Philadelphia, PA 19104, USA

E-mail address:
Lee.Fleisher@uphs.upenn.edu

Preface

Gender, Racial, and Socioeconomic Issues in Perioperative Medicine

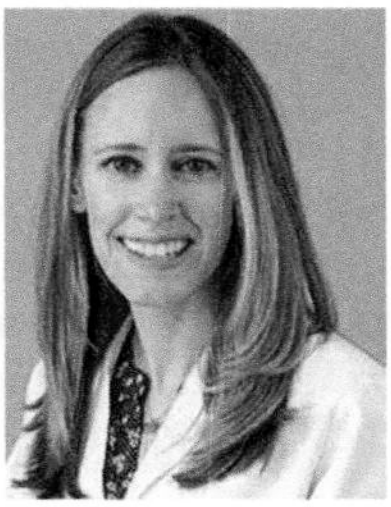
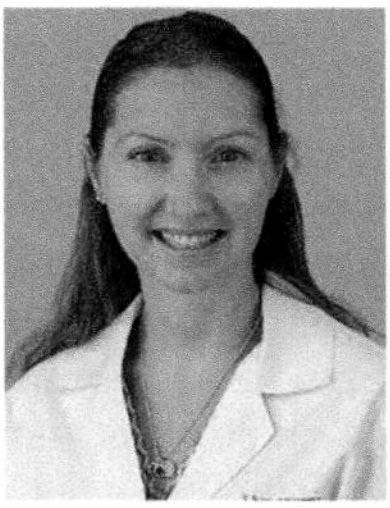
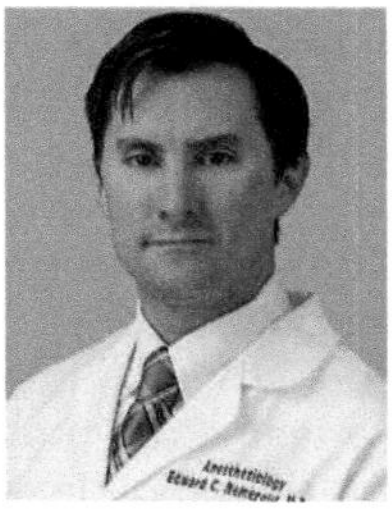

Katherine T. Forkin, MD Lauren K. Dunn, MD, PhD Edward C. Nemergut, MD
Editors

In diversity there is beauty and there is strength.

—*Maya Angelou*

Gender, race, and socioeconomic status influence both patients and health care providers. These factors should be recognized, appreciated, and given weight when approaching patient care and considering the physician workforce. Although the influences of these factors may seem subtle, the effects on health care delivery and patients' outcomes can be profound. In this issue of *Anesthesiology Clinics*, we explore how gender, race, and socioeconomic status shape patients' experiences throughout the perioperative period.

Gender and racial differences may come into play preoperatively and lead to biases in preoperative testing. Furthermore, socioeconomic status may impact patients' access to and timely referral for care and influence how early in the course of their condition they present for surgical intervention. Awareness of the impact of these factors may help us to better prepare patients for surgery and ensure they are better optimized.

Many articles within this issue explore how gender and racial differences influence patient care during the perioperative period. For instance, racial disparities in cesarean section and labor analgesia deserve special attention. In addition, sex of the organ donor and recipient impacts solid organ transplantation in a variety of ways, from listing to graft survival and even mortality. We then focus on other unique patient populations. The article on transgender patients highlights the unique considerations throughout the perioperative experience that anesthesiologists should familiarize themselves with to provide improved care for these patients (eg, barriers to care, issues arising from hormone therapy). Race and culture also contribute to differences

Anesthesiology Clin 38 (2020) xv–xvi
https://doi.org/10.1016/j.anclin.2020.03.001 anesthesiology.theclinics.com
1932-2275/20/© 2020 Published by Elsevier Inc.

and disparities in care of pediatric patients, such as in the use of premedication, administration of opioid analgesia, and adultification of minority patients. These differences may be addressed through increased diversity of health care providers, affordable health care to improve access for economically disadvantaged groups, and rigorous data collection and reporting standards to identify disparity in patient care and outcomes.

The effect of race and gender on care and outcomes of the critically ill is also presented. In addition, gender differences following cardiac surgery, such as coronary artery bypass graft, valve replacement, and left-ventricular assist device surgeries, are detailed. Women have increased risk of morbidity and mortality and present with different preoperative risk profile compared with men presenting for cardiac surgery.

In the final articles, we focus on the effect of differences in gender and race in the workforce. The workforce is slowly changing to reflect the diversity of our patient population in the United States. Diversity in perioperative teams likely improves patient care, but more research is needed. Strategies for improving communication within perioperative teams are provided. Many challenges remain in academic anesthesiology for women and underrepresented racial minorities.

It is our hope that this issue of *Anesthesiology Clinics* will help readers appreciate the impact of patients' gender, race, and socioeconomic status on their perioperative experience, from preoperative evaluation through hospital discharge. We also anticipate readers will be able to take away from this issue the importance of race and gender in teamwork, communication, and career advancement of anesthesiologists. Finally, we would like to sincerely thank our authors for donating their time and energy to writing these articles.

Katherine T. Forkin, MD
Department of Anesthesiology
University of Virginia Health System
PO Box 800710
Charlottesville, VA 22908-0710, USA

Lauren K. Dunn, MD, PhD
Department of Anesthesiology
University of Virginia Health System
PO Box 800710
Charlottesville, VA 22908-0710, USA

Edward C. Nemergut, MD
Department of Anesthesiology
University of Virginia Health System
PO Box 800710
Charlottesville, VA 22908-0710, USA

E-mail addresses:
ket2a@hscmail.mcc.virginia.edu (K.T. Forkin)
lak3r@hscmail.mcc.virginia.edu (L.K. Dunn)
en3x@hscmail.mcc.virginia.edu (E.C. Nemergut)

Special Considerations Related to Race, Sex, Gender, and Socioeconomic Status in the Preoperative Evaluation

Part 1: Race, History of Incarceration, and Health Literacy

Jeanna Blitz, MD[a], Jenna Swisher, MD[b], BobbieJean Sweitzer, MD[b,*]

KEYWORDS

• Low health literacy • Prisoners • Preoperative • Race • Ethnicity

KEY POINTS

- Vulnerable populations are at risk for increased adverse events with surgery and anesthesia.
- There are racial differences in health and treatment outcomes.
- Incarcerated patients have barriers to care.
- Studies support that matching the race of providers with patients has advantages.

INTRODUCTION

The Institute of Medicine framework of quality care includes 6 separate, equally important aims: safety, efficiency, patient-centeredness, efficacy, equity, and timeliness.[1] Provision of equitable care requires that the quality of care delivered must not vary by race, sex, gender, ethnicity, or other socioeconomic factors. Addressing health inequities can have a major impact, given that 80% to 90% of patients' health outcomes are ascribed to these factors.[2] Preparing for surgery is a pivotal time in a patient's life. The preoperative period may be marked by confusion and anxiety, because the patient has to coordinate care among multiple clinicians and preoperative appointments.

[a] Duke University School of Medicine, DUMC 3094, Durham, NC 27710, USA; [b] Northwestern University Feinberg School of Medicine, 251 East Huron, Feinberg 5-704, Chicago, IL 60611, USA
* Corresponding author.
E-mail address: bobbie.sweitzer@northwestern.edu
Twitter: @Jeanna_BlitzMD (J.S.); @BobbieJeanSwei1 (B.S.)

Anesthesiology Clin 38 (2020) 247–261
https://doi.org/10.1016/j.anclin.2020.01.005 anesthesiology.theclinics.com
1932-2275/20/

Even medically savvy patients may find it challenging to advocate for themselves or navigate the health care system. This challenge is amplified for patients from vulnerable or disenfranchised populations. Furthermore, underrepresented minorities and transgender patients may avoid or have limited access to health care before needing surgery, and these patients may thus enter the perioperative space with unidentified or poorly managed comorbid conditions. Homelessness, limited health literacy, and incarceration further hinder perioperative optimization initiatives and outcomes. All of these factors may result in avoidable postoperative complications, increases in length of hospitalization, and readmissions if they are not addressed.[3]

The so-called opportunity index within a value-based system describes the level of opportunity available to improve outcomes and decrease costs.[4] The preoperative evaluation clinic visit has a high opportunity index in vulnerable patients, because of the confluence of increased patient motivation to adhere to recommendations driven by desire for the best surgical outcome and access to a multidisciplinary team of providers focused on care coordination. Identifying patients who will benefit from additional resources is vital to reducing disparities in health and health care. One readily available piece of data that is predictive of life expectancy is a patient's zip code, which serves as a strong indicator of socioeconomic status and race.[5]

Causes of health disparities are not entirely elucidated but are likely multifactorial. Many marginalized patients avoid health care because of prior experiences with discrimination by health care workers or the perception that discrimination will occur. Provider-facing initiatives that result in a deeper understanding of racial, gender, sex, and socioeconomic differences related to how patients access health care may result in an improvement in health equity.[6] Initiatives include awareness of clinicians' own implicit biases as health care workers. Historically, women and vulnerable patient populations were not included in clinical research trials; therefore, it is often unclear how to interpret results for these patient populations.

A preoperative evaluation clinic visit may even improve a patient's long-term health trajectory by leveraging the visit as a teachable moment, improving health literacy, and providing individualized health interventions.

RACE AND ETHNICITY

Race-related and ethnicity-related health disparities exist in perioperative medicine and reflect the health disparities that are present in the broader health care delivery arena. They affect a wide spectrum of patient populations, from children and adolescents, to obstetric patients, to older patients presenting for orthopedic, cardiothoracic, and urologic surgery, whether planned or emergencies.[7–11] This burden is greatest for African American patients, but it affects Hispanic people, Asians, and other minorities.

African American women have a 3 times higher risk of maternal mortality, are more likely to receive general anesthesia for cesarean section, and experience neonatal mortality twice that of white obstetric patients.[8] White adolescents are more likely to undergo bariatric surgery than African American or Hispanic patients, despite no differences in efficacy of the procedure.[7] Black race has been associated with a higher rate of major complications following total joint arthroplasty, including infection, deep vein thrombosis (DVT), pulmonary embolism, and death. This significant difference in complication rates among patients of different races who present for major orthopedic surgery exists despite no difference in preexisting comorbidities.[11]

Although esophageal cancer is more prevalent in white people, African Americans experience a higher mortality from the disease. The reason for this disparity is not entirely understood but it may be partially caused by a difference in the disease. Squamous cell carcinoma is more prevalent in African Americans, whereas esophageal adenocarcinoma is most common in white people.[9] Furthermore, African American men are disproportionately affected by both cardiovascular disease and prostate cancer, and increased cholesterol level has been shown to be a risk factor for recurrence of prostate cancer.[10] By contrast, postoperative outcomes after abdominal surgery do not seem to differ by race.[12,13]

Predictors of difficult intubation also vary by race and ethnicity. One study reported that a modified Mallampati test, thyromental distance, and interincisor gap are the best predictors of difficult laryngoscopy in West Africans.[14] This finding is attributed to a longer sternomental distance compared with white people.

Although not fully understood, the causes of these racial and ethnic disparities are likely multifactorial. Disparities in perioperative outcomes may be related to differences in patient preferences. Hispanic people and African Americans are far less likely to undergo an elective endovascular repair of an aortic aneurysm.[15–17] Disparities in health may be caused by biological differences (such as a predilection toward diabetes or anatomic differences that predict difficulty with intubation), differences in the physician-patient interaction, and less access to high-quality care by nonwhite patients.[18] Language or cultural barriers may also contribute.

Far more population health research must be done in order to fully understand and mitigate the primary factors responsible for these disparities in perioperative outcomes. An immediately achievable goal is to consider race-related disparities when evaluating patients preoperatively. For example, an African American patient preparing for a total joint replacement may benefit from more aggressive prophylaxis against venous thromboembolism, given the increased risk of DVT and pulmonary embolism in this patient population. Heightened awareness of biological differences may be the most important consideration. Knowledge of racial differences in the incidence of diseases and responses to medications is required in order to provide a patient-centered, individualized perioperative plan. Evidence suggests that high-risk patients are often not identified preoperatively, and proven strategies to reduce risk are not implemented.[19] Risk assessment can lead to changes in preoperative medical management, the planned anesthetic and surgery, postoperative care, or recommendations to avoid surgery.

RACIAL DIFFERENCES IN COMORBIDITIES

Cardiovascular Disease

African American patients have the highest incidence of cardiovascular comorbidities, including hypertension, dyslipidemia, coronary artery disease, and peripheral arterial disease.[20] They are more likely than white patients to have multiple cardiac risk factors and to have associated metabolic conditions such as obesity and insulin resistance.[20] Furthermore, black patients are more likely to have poorly controlled hypertension, and may respond differently to certain first-line medications recommended in white patients.[20] Specifically, black patients may be less responsive to monotherapy with angiotensin-converting enzyme inhibitors, angiotensin receptor blockers, and β-blockers. Diuretics, calcium channel blockers, or combination therapy should be considered first.[21] As a group, black patients with a diagnosis of heart failure with preserved ejection fraction are younger and have more related comorbidities, including hypertension, diabetes, chronic kidney disease (CKD), and anemia.[22] African American patients with heart failure are less likely to benefit from enalapril than white patients.[23]

Racial differences in response to medications may reflect genetic differences, differences in the pathogenesis of diseases, or environmental factors, such as differences in diet and health-related behaviors.[22] For example, warfarin metabolism differs significantly among patients of different races: standard dosing may result in both an inappropriately high level in Asian patients as well as an underdosing in patients of African descent, compared with white patients.[24] Adherence to medications differs by race. On admission for a cardiac condition, nonwhite patients are more likely to report nonadherence to their prescribed home cardiac medications.[25]

Racial differences exist in the presentation of an acute myocardial infarction.[26] African American patients are more likely than white patients to have negative or nondiagnostic electrocardiograms at the time of presentation, complicating diagnosis.[27] Hispanic patients are less likely to undergo coronary revascularization, despite a higher incidence of diabetes.[26]

Chronic Kidney Disease

The incidence of CKD is highest in patients of African American, American Indian, Hispanic, or Pacific Islander descent.[28] Minority status increases the risk of dying from CKD.[29] CKD has long been recognized as a powerful independent predictor of major adverse cardiovascular events,[30] and is incorporated into many perioperative risk calculators.[30,31] Increased levels of inflammatory markers and a strong association with significant comorbidities such as hypertension, hyperlipidemia, diabetes mellitus, and cardiovascular disease may explain why CKD acts as a risk multiplier for morbidity, mortality, and cost in the perioperative period. Evidence suggests that CKD is under-recognized by patients and clinicians alike. Many patients who meet the criteria for CKD have not been formally diagnosed.[32] Awareness of CKD is particularly low among certain subsets of patients, including individuals who identify as black.[33] Although a formal diagnosis of CKD requires confirmation of a reduction in estimated glomerular filtration rate for 3 months or more, early stages of asymptomatic CKD may be uncovered by taking a careful medical history to screen for risk factors such as diabetes, hypertension, smoking, and exposure to nephrotoxic agents; measuring the patient's blood pressure; and obtaining laboratory studies.[28] Screening for CKD in high-risk patients should be a routine part of the preoperative assessment, given the well-documented impact of CKD on perioperative outcomes.

Pulmonary Diseases and Tobacco Use

Medication use, emergency department use, and patient-reported quality-of-life outcomes vary by race and ethnicity among adult patients with asthma.[34] Native Americans and Aleutians reported lower scores on the Mini Asthma Quality of Life Questionnaire than white people. African Americans are 5 times more likely to use emergency departments for asthma care, even after adjustment for socioeconomic factors, including income and education.[34] Biological differences exist among patients with chronic obstructive pulmonary disease (COPD) who are prescribed maintenance therapy. Tiotropium reduced the frequencies of antibiotic days and COPD-hospital days to a significantly greater extent in African Americans compared with white people.[35] Poor physical functioning and impairment in activities of daily life caused by pulmonary disease are greatest in smokers who identify as Hispanic.[36] However, Hispanic patients have the highest response to bronchodilators on pulmonary function testing. African American and Hispanic patients may benefit most from the initiation and optimization of preoperative bronchodilator therapy to prevent perioperative pulmonary complications.

No clear association between obstructive sleep apnea (OSA) and race or ethnicity has been established.[19] Nevertheless, diagnosis and treatment disparities exist for minority patients.[37] African Americans with OSA are at significantly greater risk of developing atrial fibrillation than those of other races.[38] The routine use of a screening tool such as the STOP-Bang (Snoring, tired, observed apnea, high blood pressure, BMI, age, neck circumference, gender) questionnaire is recommended as part of the preoperative evaluation. Patients who score 5 or higher are at high risk of moderate to severe OSA. They should be counseled about the risks related to sleep disordered breathing, and benefits of perioperative opioid-sparing analgesic regimens. Referral for polysomnography should be strongly considered in high-risk patients.

Exposure to tobacco increases perioperative complications, including surgical site infections, postoperative pulmonary complications, sepsis, and death.[39] Smokers require longer hospital stays and need postoperative intensive care more than nonsmokers. Studies have identified racial and ethnicity-related differences in smoking duration, as well as success with quitting. Black patients smoke for a longer period of time before a successful quit attempt compared with white patients. This finding may be explained in part by higher serum levels of the pharmacologically active nicotine metabolite compared with white or Hispanic patients.[40] Higher cotinine levels are attributed to a combination of slower cotinine clearance and greater nicotine intake per cigarette in black patients.[41] The difference in pharmacokinetics may indicate a higher exposure to carcinogenic compounds in cigarettes, and may explain the higher rates of lung cancer experienced in black smokers.[42] These findings support the need for individualized smoking cessation therapy plans in the preoperative evaluation clinic.

Diabetes Mellitus

Type 2 diabetes mellitus is more prevalent in African Americans, Hispanic people, Native Americans, and Native Hawaiians than in white people. Approximately half of all patients with diabetes remain undiagnosed in all races. Rates of medication adherence are lowest among African Americans, Latinos, Filipinos, Native Hawaiians, and other Pacific Islanders. This finding is attributed to high out-of-pocket medication costs relative to incomes.[43] Lack of adherence to medications, and resultant poor glycemic control, are reflected in racial differences in diabetes-associated complications. Rates of vision loss, amputations, and renal disease are 1.5 to 4 times higher in black people than in white people.[44] It is unclear whether or not dietary differences among groups contribute to the difference in complication rates.[45] White patients have approximately 40% more diabetes-related office visits annually compared with others. Despite the higher complication rates in minorities, and fewer office visits, diabetes-related mortality has declined significantly in the past decade, with the mortality in black patients less than in white patients.[44] Screening for diabetes in African Americans, Hispanic people, Native Americans, and Native Hawaiians should be a routine part of the preoperative assessment given the high rate of undiagnosed cases and the impact of poor glycemic control on postoperative outcomes.

RACIAL DIFFERENCES IN PREFERENCES FOR CARE AND THE PHYSICIAN-PATIENT RELATIONSHIP

Minority patients are less likely to pursue recommended elective surgical interventions, such as bariatric surgery[7] and endovascular repair of an aortic aneurysm.[15–17] This finding may in part be caused by negative experiences and mistrust from prior interactions with health care workers. Overt discrimination as well as more subtle, subjective mistreatment, such as low expectations for compliance with recommendations or less expressed empathy, are reported. Mistrust in health care providers may cause minority patients to disengage and defer necessary therapies.[19]

Therefore, it is critical that care providers are mindful of patients' preferences and how provider behavior influences patients' decisions. The impact is most powerful when there is racial discordance between the patient and physician. The average health maintenance visit is shortest between white physicians with African American patients.[19] Furthermore, African American patients characterized visits with nonblack physicians as having greater physician verbal dominance overall, and being least patient-centered.[19] Patient satisfaction is associated with compliance with recommendations and participation in treatment decisions, which is the foundation of high-quality care. Perioperative physicians must be aware of their own implicit biases that may affect their recommendations for patients of color.

PATIENTS WITH A HISTORY OF INCARCERATION

More than 12 million people cycle in and out of the prison system each year, and this number continues to grow.[46] Health disparities in individuals who have experienced incarceration are well documented. Rates of poorly controlled chronic diseases, mental health conditions, substance abuse disorders, and social isolation are higher compared with the general population.[46,47] These factors magnify baseline health disparities in already vulnerable populations, including incarcerated women and elderly individuals.[46,48]

Although no specific preoperative testing guidelines exist for this patient population, requirements should be guided by a thorough history and physical examination, combined with knowledge of conditions that commonly affect patients with a history of incarceration. Rates of common chronic diseases such as diabetes, COPD, and liver disease are reportedly twice as prevalent in those with a history of incarceration compared with the general population (**Box 1**).[46,47,49,50] By contrast, the incidence of obesity is lower.[50] The confluence of mental health disorders, sleep deprivation, poor nutrition, limited physical activity, and a low level of self-efficacy renders effective management of chronic medical conditions challenging in this vulnerable patient population.[46,50] Screening for common chronic health conditions and infectious diseases should be considered during the preoperative assessment. Incarcerated patients have significantly higher rates of communicable diseases such as hepatitis C, human immunodeficiency virus, and tuberculosis.[46,47] A chest radiograph is indicated in patients at high risk of active tuberculosis. Smoking, substance abuse, and poor nutrition, combined with low levels of education, predispose individuals to increased risks of postoperative complications such as surgical site infections, longer lengths of hospitalization, and high rates of readmission postoperatively.[51] Every encounter with this population may be the only window of opportunity to diagnose and initiate appropriate treatment.

Although more intensive screening in the prison patient population has its merits, it is fraught with challenges. Standardized screening tools, such as the Duke Activity Status Index and International Physical Activity Questionnaire, are not useful because of the unavailability of certain physical activities in a jail exercise area (shoveling snow, riding a bicycle, swimming). A prison-specific functional assessment known as the Prison Activities of Daily Living has been developed. To assess functional status in the currently incarcerated, providers can inquire about the patient's ability to perform yard duty, drop to the floor for alarms, stand for count, get to meals, hear orders, and climb onto the top bunk.[52] Similarly, questions regarding social interactions are problematic because of limited opportunities to interact with family and friends.[46]

Box 1
Common diseases in patients with a history of incarceration

Cardiovascular conditions
- Ischemic heart disease
- Heart failure
- Atrial fibrillation
- Cerebrovascular accident, transient ischemic attack

Pulmonary conditions
- Chronic obstructive pulmonary disease
- Asthma

Infectious diseases
- Hepatitis C
- Human immunodeficiency virus (HIV)/acquired immunodeficiency syndrome (AIDS)
- Tuberculosis
- Methicillin-resistant *Staphylococcus aureus* (MRSA)
- Gonorrhea, syphilis, chlamydia

Other chronic medical conditions
- Diabetes mellitus
- Cirrhosis
- Chronic kidney disease (CKD)
- Hypertension
- Hyperlipidemia
- Chronic pain conditions

Mental health disorders and behavioral health
- Depression
- Bipolar disorder
- Anxiety
- Alcohol and drug use disorders
- Tobacco use
- Schizophrenia
- Posttraumatic stress disorder (PTSD)
- Intellectual and learning disabilities

Adapted from Maruschak LM, et al. Medical Problems of Prisoners. Washington, DC: US Department of Justice, Bureau of Justice Statistics; 2008; with permission.

Individuals may face stigmatization associated with their incarceration, leading to a lack of stable housing and fragile social support system after release. These factors must be acknowledged when performing a global perioperative risk assessment and planning for postdischarge care. Furthermore, previously incarcerated patients often lack an established longitudinal relationship with a primary care physician. Although more than 75% of former prisoners rely on emergency department (ED) services as their primary source of health care,[46,52] use of EDs for routine health concerns often predates the patient's incarceration and is not a direct result of incarceration.[53] Achievement of optimal outcomes in this patient population requires an emphasis on thorough care coordination across the entire perioperative spectrum. This coordination includes identifying and resolving issues related to the patient's inability to access necessary preoperative medications or elements of the surgical preparation (eg, bowel preparation, preoperative carbohydrate drink, or decolonization soap), and confirming that the patient has an adequate level of health literacy to understand and implement the recommended treatment plan. Depression and social isolation are barriers to postoperative recovery.[54] Inquiring about the patient's current state of mental health and the stability of the social support network facilitates an understanding of the patient's psychological preparation for surgery. In addition to targeted preoperative intervention strategies, effective postoperative intervention checkpoints will be needed to disrupt the potential cycle of repeat readmissions and hospitalization. Coordination of robust postdischarge planning should begin during the preoperative evaluation visit whenever possible.

LOW HEALTH LITERACY

Comprehensive assessment of a patient's perioperative risk extends beyond an evaluation of the patient's medical conditions and physical status. Psychological preparedness and health literacy level are important factors to explore in order to anticipate a patient's postoperative course. Patients at highest risk of surgical complications often have a poor understanding of their health status, and overestimate their ability to manage their comorbidities.[3] Health literacy is defined as the skill set required for people to access, comprehend, and apply health information in order to participate in managing their health.[55,56] Furthermore, delivery of health information and services must align with the patient's capacity to understand and use them.[55]

The impact of health literacy is well documented in the perioperative period. Lower health literacy results in riskier behavior, less self-management, and increased hospitalization costs.[56] Furthermore, it is independently associated with patient dissatisfaction, longer hospitalization after major surgery, and increased mortality.[3,55,57–61] Inadequate health literacy affects one-third of surgical patients[3] and is most prevalent in vulnerable patient populations, including the elderly, those with low education levels, immigrants, and racial and ethnic minorities.[55,57,58] Surgical patients have to make complex decisions about their health, and adhere to multifaceted preoperative instructions. Misunderstandings can result in poor outcomes, reduce efficiency metrics (a surgical complication or cancellation related to noncompliance with medication instructions), and impair the informed consent process.[62] The ambulatory surgery setting may be particularly challenging for patients with low health literacy, given the increased need for support in the perioperative period. Therefore, preoperative interventions designed to increase health literacy and numeracy may be key components in prevention of postoperative complications in high-risk patients.[61]

Despite the importance and impact of health literacy, physicians are often unaware of their patients' literacy levels, or lack the ability to accurately identify low health literacy.[55] Furthermore, the assessment of health literacy is not always straightforward in a busy clinical environment. Multiple validated screening tools exist to assess different aspects of health literacy and numeracy, but it may not be readily apparent which tool is most appropriate for a particular patient population. In addition, routine health literacy screening is controversial, because vulnerable patients may be stigmatized or embarrassed by the results, leading them to avoid health care interactions in the future.[3,62]

The Test of Functional Health Literacy in Adults (TOFHLA) and Rapid Estimate of Adult Literacy in Medicine (REALM) are the most widely used measures of health literacy. Both tools predict knowledge, behaviors, and health outcomes.[61] Although the two tests are highly correlated, they measure different skills. TOFHLA is considered the most comprehensive assessment of health literacy and encompasses the domains of both comprehension and fluency. Because of its comprehensive nature, it requires at least 20 minutes to administer.[62] By contrast, REALM does not measure reading comprehension or numeracy. It measures word recognition and pronunciation. Despite its high degree of correlation with the longer TOFHLA assessment, it seems to be a more direct measure of basic literacy rather than true health literacy.

Box 2
Full 16-question version of health literacy screening tool

1. How often are appointment slips written in a way that is easy to read and understand?
   (1) Always (2) Often (3) Sometimes (4) Occasionally (5) Never
2. How often are medical forms written in a way that is easy to read and understand?
   (1) Always (2) Often (3) Sometimes (4) Occasionally (5) Never
3. How often are medication labels written in a way that is easy to read and understand?
   (1) Always (2) Often (3) Sometimes (4) Occasionally (5) Never
4. How often are patient educational materials written in a way that is easy to read and understand?
   (1) Always (2) Often (3) Sometimes (4) Occasionally (5) Never
5. How often are hospital or clinic signs difficult to understand?
   (1) Always (2) Often (3) Sometimes (4) Occasionally (5) Never
6. How often are appointment slips difficult to understand?
   (1) Always (2) Often (3) Sometimes (4) Occasionally (5) Never
7. How often are medical forms difficult to understand and fill out?
   (1) Always (2) Often (3) Sometimes (4) Occasionally (5) Never
8. How often are directions on medication bottles difficult to understand?
   (1) Always (2) Often (3) Sometimes (4) Occasionally (5) Never
9. How often do you have difficulty understanding written information your health care provider (eg, doctor, nurse, nurse practitioner) gives you?
   (1) Always (2) Often (3) Sometimes (4) Occasionally (5) Never
10. How often do you have problems getting to your clinic appointments at the right time because of difficulty understanding written instructions?
    (1) Always (2) Often (3) Sometimes (4) Occasionally (5) Never
11. How often do you have problems completing medical forms because of difficulty understanding the instructions?
    (1) Always (2) Often (3) Sometimes (4) Occasionally (5) Never
12. How often do you have problems learning about your medical condition because of difficulty understanding written information?
    (1) Always (2) Often (3) Sometimes (4) Occasionally (5) Never
13. How often are you unsure on how to take your medications correctly because of problems understanding written instructions on the bottle label?
    (1) Always (2) Often (3) Sometimes (4) Occasionally (5) Never
14. How confident are you filling out medical forms by yourself?
    (1) Extremely (2) Quite a bit (3) Somewhat (4) A little bit (5) Not at all
15. How confident do you feel that you are able to follow the instructions on the label of a medication bottle?
    (1) Extremely (2) Quite a bit (3) Somewhat (4) A little bit (5) Not at all
16. How often do you have someone (eg, family member, friend, hospital/clinic worker, or caregiver) help you read hospital materials?
    (1) Always (2) Often (3) Sometimes (4) Occasionally (5) Never

Modified from Chew LD, Bradley KA, Boyko EJ. Brief questions to identify patients with inadequate health literacy. Fam Med 2004;36(8):594; with permission.

The benefit of its use lies in its brevity: it requires only 3 minutes to administer.[61,62] The Medical Term Recognition Test (METER) is self-administered and assists in identifying how familiar a patient is with medical terminology. METER has been shown to correlate well with REALM, and the two may be used in conjunction.[62]

At present, no consensus exists regarding the best preoperative-specific screening tool.[3] However, The Brief Health Literacy Screen (BHLS) is commonly used. This questionnaire is available in various formats ranging from 1 to 16 questions in length and is administered via a patient interview (**Box 2**). Most commonly, a version with 3 or 4 questions is used, and includes the questions: "How often do you have someone (eg, family member, friend, or hospital worker) help you read hospital materials?" "How often do you have problems learning about your medical condition because of difficulty understanding written information?" "How confident are you in filling out forms by yourself?" (**Box 3**). Responses are scored on a Likert scale from 1 (always) to 5 (never) and correlated with basic health literacy (**Table 1**).[63,64] The question, "How confident are you in filling out medical forms?" has the greatest degree of reliability and can be used alone.[63]

Although low health literacy commonly occurs in conjunction with a low educational level, it may exist despite adequate basic literacy and numeracy skills. This distinction is important to acknowledge when designing a successful initiative to improve a patient's ability to access and understand preoperative information and instructions. Tests with high sensitivity, such as the BHLS, also identify persons who lack sufficient general literacy skills.[64] Recommendations for patients with low basic literacy emphasize face-to-face discussions, repeated oral instructions, and preoperative information that is presented via video or infographics.[63,65] By contrast, patients with adequate basic literacy may find value in printed materials when combined with an in-person discussion and use of the teach-back method.[66] The design of the health literacy intervention is also influenced by the practicality of implementation in the busy clinical setting of the preoperative evaluation clinic. A screening tool such as the BHLS may be administered during a brief phone call before the visit or administered in person on arrival. Patients with adequate basic literacy may be screened via a self-completed questionnaire. Universal preoperative health literacy screening should be the goal to ensure adequate communication, patient engagement, and equitable care delivery.

Perioperative medicine is evolving. As clinicians learn more about patient-specific risks, they are better able to adopt a tailored approach to preoperative assessment and optimization. Preparing patients for surgery often requires extensive evaluation and coordination of care. Knowledge and awareness of the impact of social

Box 3
Brief health literacy screening tool

1. How often do you have someone (eg, a family member, friend, hospital/clinic worker, or caregiver) help you read hospital materials?
   (1) Always. (2) Often. (3) Sometimes. (4) Occasionally. (5) Never.
2. How often do you have problems learning about your medical condition because of difficulty understanding written information?
   (1) Always. (2) Often. (3) Sometimes. (4) Occasionally. (5) Never.
3. How often do you have a problem understanding what is told to you about your medical condition?
   (1) Always. (2) Often. (3) Sometimes. (4) Occasionally. (5) Never.
4. How confident are you filling out medical forms by yourself?
   (1) Not at all. (2) A little bit. (3) Somewhat. (4) Quite a bit. (5) Extremely.

Adapted from Chew LD, Griffin JM, Partin MR, et al. Validation of screening questions for limited health literacy in a large VA outpatient population. J Gen Intern Med 2008;23(5):561-6.

Table 1
Scoring for 4-question version of brief health literacy screening tool

Health Literacy	Score	Skills and Abilities
Limited	4–12	Unable to read most low-literacy health materials. Need repeated oral instructions. Materials should be composed of illustrations or videotapes. Need low-literacy materials. May not be able to read a prescription label
Marginal	13–16	May need assistance. May struggle with patient education materials
Adequate	17–20	Able to read and comprehend most patient education materials

Data from Chew LD, Griffin JM, Partin MR, et al. Validation of screening questions for limited health literacy in a large VA outpatient population. J Gen Intern Med 2008;23(5):561-6.

determinants of health on perioperative outcomes is crucial. Racial minority patients and patients from marginalized or vulnerable groups of society have special concerns and needs that must be addressed during the preoperative evaluation visit. Identifying patients who will benefit from additional resource allocation and knowledge of their special challenges is vital to reducing disparities in health and health care.

DISCLOSURE

The authors have nothing to disclose.

REFERENCES

1. Crossing the Quality Chasm: A New Health System for the 21st Century Committee on Quality of Health Care in America, Institute of Medicine Washington, DC: National Academies Press; 2001.
2. Magnan S. Social determinants of health 101 for health care: five plus five. NAM Perspectives. Discussion Paper. Washington, DC: National Academy of Medicine; 2017. doi: 10.31478.
3. Roy M, Corkum JP, Urbach DR, et al. Health literacy among surgical patients: a systematic review and meta-analysis. World J Surg 2019;43:96–106.
4. Lee VS, Kawamoto K, Hess R. Implementation of a value-driven outcomes program to identify high variability in clinical costs and outcomes and association with reduced cost and improved quality. JAMA 2016;316(10):1061–72.
5. Available at: https://time.com/5608268/zip-code-health/. Accessed July 19, 2019.
6. Stone J, Moskowitz GB. Non-conscious bias in medical decision making: what can be done to reduce it? Med Educ 2011;45(8):768–76.
7. Nunez Lopez O, Jupiter DC, Bohanon FJ, et al. Health disparities in adolescent bariatric surgery: Nationwide outcomes and utilization. J Adolesc Health 2017;61:649–56.
8. Caughey AB. Racial and ethnic disparities in general anesthesia for cesarean: what are the implications? Anesth Analg 2016;122:297–8.
9. Sabra MJ, Crandall M, Smotherman C, et al. Does serum albumin explain observed racial disparities in mortality for cancer patients undergoing esophagectomy? Am J Surg 2018;216:778–81.
10. Allott EH, Howard LE, Aronson WJ, et al. Racial differences in the association between preoperative serum cholesterol and prostate cancer Recurrence: Results

from the SEARCH Database. Cancer Epidemiol Biomarkers Prev 2016;25(3):547–54.
11. Adelani MA, Archer KR, Song Y, et al. Immediate complications following hip and knee arthroplasty: does race matter? J Arthroplasty 2013;28:732–5.
12. Vohra RS, Evison F, Bejaj I, et al. The effect of ethnicity on in-hospital mortality following emergency abdominal surgery: a national cohort study using Hospital Episode Statistics. Public Health 2015;129:1496–502.
13. Uhr JH, Fields AC, Divino CM. Lack of a clinically significant impact of race on morbidity and mortality in abdominal surgery: an analysis of 186,466 patients from the American College of Surgeons National Surgical Quality Improvement Program database. Am J Surg 2015;210:236–42.
14. Merah N, Wong DT, Ffoulkes-Crabbe D, et al. Modified Mallampati test, thyromental distance and inter-incisor gap are the best predictors of difficult laryngoscopy in West Africans. Can J Anaesth 2005;52(3):291–6.
15. Williams TK, Schneider EB, Black JH 3rd, et al. Disparities in outcomes for Hispanic patients undergoing endovascular and open abdominal aortic aneurysm repair. Ann Vasc Surg 2013;27:29–37.
16. Yang Y, Lehman EB, Aziz F. African Americans are less likely to have elective endovascular repair of abdominal aortic aneurysms. J Vasc Surg 2019;70(2):462–70.
17. Osborne NH, Mathur AK, Upchurch GR Jr, et al. Understanding the racial disparity in the receipt of endovascular abdominal aortic aneurysm repair. Arch Surg 2010;145:1105–8.
18. Lucas FL, Stukel TA, Morris AM, et al. Race and surgical mortality in the United States. Ann Surg 2006;243:281–6.
19. Nelson AR. Unequal treatment: report of the Institute of Medicine on racial and ethnic disparities in healthcare. Ann Thorac Surg 2003;76:S1377–81.
20. Pool LR, Ning H, Lloyd-Jones DM, et al. Trends in racial/ethnic disparities in cardiovascular health among US adults from 1999-2012. J Am Heart Assoc 2017;6 [pii:e006027].
21. Ferdinand KC, Armani AM. The management of hypertension in African Americans. Crit Pathw Cardiol 2007;6:67–71.
22. Goyal P, Paul T, Almarzooq ZI, et al. Sex- and race-related differences in characteristics and outcomes of hospitalizations for heart failure with preserved ejection fraction. J Am Heart Assoc 2017;6 [pii:e003330].
23. Exner DV, Dries DL, Domanski MJ, et al. Lesser response to angiotensin-converting-enzyme inhibitor therapy in black as compared with white patients with left ventricular dysfunction. N Engl J Med 2001;344:1351–7.
24. Johnson JA. Ethnic differences in cardiovascular drug response: potential contribution of pharmacogenetics. Circulation 2008;118:1383–93.
25. Graham G. Racial and ethnic differences in acute coronary syndrome and myocardial infarction within the United States: From demographics to outcomes. Clin Cardiol 2016;39:299–306.
26. Bucholz EM, Ma S, Normand SL, et al. Race, socioeconomic status, and life expectancy after acute myocardial infarction. Circulation 2015;132:1338–46.
27. Nelson A. Unequal treatment: confronting racial and ethnic disparities in health care. J Natl Med Assoc 2002;94:666–8.
28. Blitz J. Chronic kidney disease. In: Sweitzer B, editor. Preoperative assessment and management. 3rd edition. Philadelphia: Wolters Kluwer; 2019. p. 269–75.
29. Assari S, Lankarani MM. Income gradient in renal disease mortality in the United States. Front Med (Lausanne) 2017;4:190.

30. Fleisher LA, Fleischmann KE, Auerbach AD, et al. 2014 ACC/AHA guideline on perioperative cardiovascular evaluation and management of patients undergoing noncardiac surgery: executive summary: a report of the American College of Cardiology/American Heart Association Task Force on practice guidelines. Circulation 2014;130:2215–45.
31. Gupta PK, Gupta H, Sundaram A, et al. Development and validation of a risk calculator for prediction of cardiac risk after surgery. Circulation 2011;124:381–7.
32. McClellan WM, Newsome BB, McClure LA, et al. Chronic kidney disease is often unrecognized among patients with coronary heart disease: the REGARDS Cohort Study. Am J Nephrol 2009;29:10–7.
33. Ackland GL, Laing CM. Chronic kidney disease: a gateway for perioperative medicine. Br J Anaesth 2014;113:902–5.
34. Mosen DM, Schatz M, Gold R, et al. Medication use, emergency hospital care utilization, and quality-of-life outcome disparities by race/ethnicity among adults with asthma. Am J Manag Care 2010;16:821–8.
35. Rice KL, Leimer I, Kesten S, et al. Responses to tiotropium in African-American and Caucasian patients with chronic obstructive pulmonary disease. Transl Res 2008;152:88–94.
36. Diaz AA, Petersen H, Meek P, et al. Differences in health-related quality of life between new Mexican Hispanic and non-Hispanic white smokers. Chest 2016;150:869–76.
37. Dudley KA, Patel SR. Disparities and genetic risk factors in obstructive sleep apnea. Sleep Med 2016;18:96–102.
38. Ghazi L, Bennett A, Petrov ME, et al. Race, sex, age, and regional differences in the association of obstructive sleep apnea with atrial fibrillation: Reasons for geographic and racial differences in stroke study. J Clin Sleep Med 2018;14:1485–93.
39. Wong J, Lam DP, Abrishami A, et al. Short-term preoperative smoking cessation and postoperative complications: a systematic review and meta-analysis. Can J Anaesth 2012;59:268–79.
40. Jones MR, Joshu CE, Navas-Acien A, et al. Racial/ethnic differences in duration of smoking among former smokers in the National Health and Nutrition Examination surveys. Nicotine Tob Res 2018;20:303–11.
41. Perez-Stable EJ, Herrera B, Jacob P 3rd, et al. Nicotine metabolism and intake in black and white smokers. JAMA 1998;280:152–6.
42. Caraballo RS, Giovino GA, Pechacek TF, et al. Racial and ethnic differences in serum cotinine levels of cigarette smokers: Third National Health and Nutrition Examination Survey, 1988-1991. JAMA 1998;280:135–9.
43. Harris MI. Noninsulin-dependent diabetes mellitus in black and white Americans. Diabetes Metab Rev 1990;6:71–90.
44. Sutton CX, Carpenter DA, Sumida W, et al. 2016 Writing contest undergraduate winner: The relationship between medication adherence and total healthcare expenditures by race/ethnicity in patients with diabetes in Hawai'i. Hawaii J Med Public Health 2017;76:183–9.
45. Nowlin SY, Cleland CM, Vadiveloo M, et al. Explaining racial/ethnic dietary patterns in relation to Type 2 diabetes: An analysis of NHANES 2007-2012. Ethn Dis 2016;26:529–36.
46. Trotter RT 2nd, Lininger MR, Camplain R, et al. A survey of health disparities, social determinants of health, and converging morbidities in a county jail: a cultural-ecological assessment of health conditions in jail populations. Int J Environ Res Public Health 2018;15 [pii:E2500].

47. Maruschak LM. Medical problems of prisoners, In: Bureau of Justice Statistics. Available at: https://www.bjs.gov/content/pub/html/mpp/mpp.cfm. Accessed February 15, 2020.
48. Sufrin C, Kolbi-Molinas A, Roth R. Reproductive Justice, Health Disparities And Incarcerated Women in the United States. Perspect Sex Reprod Health 2015; 47:213–9.
49. Bai JR, Befus M, Mukherjee DV, et al. Prevalence and predictors of chronic health conditions of inmates newly admitted to maximum security prisons. J Correct Health Care 2015;21:255–64.
50. Binswanger IA, Krueger PM, Steiner JF. Prevalence of chronic medical conditions among jail and prison inmates in the USA compared with the general population. J Epidemiol Community Health 2009;63:912–9.
51. Heng CK, Badner VM, Clemens DL, et al. The relationship of cigarette smoking to postoperative complications from dental extractions among female inmates. Oral Surg Oral Med Oral Pathol Oral Radiol Endod 2007;104:757–62.
52. Williams BA, Lindquist K, Sudore RL, et al. Being old and doing time: functional impairment and adverse experiences of geriatric female prisoners. J Am Geriatr Soc 2006;54:702–7.
53. Chodos AH, Ahalt C, Cenzer IS, et al. Older jail inmates and community acute care use. Am J Public Health 2014;104:1728–33.
54. Pan X, Wang J, Lin Z, et al. Depression and anxiety are risk factors for postoperative pain-related symptoms and complications in patients undergoing primary total knee arthroplasty in the United States. J Arthroplasty 2019;34(10): 2337–46.
55. Powers BJ, Trinh JV, Bosworth HB. Can this patient read and understand written health information? JAMA 2010;304:76–84.
56. Lytton M. Health literacy: an opinionated perspective. Am J Prev Med 2013;45: e35–40.
57. Williams MV, Parker RM, Baker DW, et al. Inadequate functional health literacy among patients at two public hospitals. JAMA 1995;274:1677–82.
58. Kobayashi LC, Wardle J, von Wagner C. Limited health literacy is a barrier to colorectal cancer screening in England: evidence from the English Longitudinal Study of Ageing. Prev Med 2014;61:100–5.
59. De Oliveira GS Jr, McCarthy RJ, Wolf MS, et al. The impact of health literacy in the care of surgical patients: a qualitative systematic review. BMC Surg 2015; 15:86.
60. Halleberg Nyman M, Nilsson U, Dahlberg K, et al. Association between functional health literacy and postoperative recovery, health care contacts, and health-related quality of life among patients undergoing day surgery: secondary analysis of a randomized clinical trial. JAMA Surg 2018;153:738–45.
61. Wright JP, Edwards GC, Goggins K, et al. Association of health literacy with postoperative outcomes in patients undergoing major abdominal surgery. JAMA Surg 2018;153:137–42.
62. Hovlid E, von Plessen C, Haug K, et al. Patient experiences with interventions to reduce surgery cancellations: a qualitative study. BMC Surg 2013;13:30.
63. Chew LD, Griffin JM, Partin MR, et al. Validation of screening questions for limited health literacy in a large VA outpatient population. J Gen Intern Med 2008;23: 561–6.
64. Duell P, Wright D, Renzaho AM, et al. Optimal health literacy measurement for the clinical setting: a systematic review. Patient Educ Couns 2015;98:1295–307.

65. Chew LD, Bradley KA, Boyko EJ. Brief questions to identify patients with inadequate health literacy. Fam Med 2004;36:588–94.
66. Ha Dinh TT, Bonner A, Clark R, et al. The effectiveness of the teach-back method on adherence and self-management in health education for people with chronic disease: a systematic review. JBI Database System Rev Implement Rep 2016;14: 210–47.

Special Considerations Related to Race, Sex, Gender, and Socioeconomic Status in the Preoperative Evaluation

Part 2: Sex Considerations and Homeless Patients

Jenna Swisher, MD[a], Jeanna Blitz, MD[b], BobbieJean Sweitzer, MD[a,*]

KEYWORDS

• Low health literacy • Undomiciled • Sex differences • Gender • Prisoners • Preoperative • Race • Ethnicity

KEY POINTS

- Vulnerable populations are at risk for increased adverse events with surgery and anesthesia.
- There are sex and racial differences in health and treatment outcomes.
- Undomiciled and incarcerated patients have barriers to care.
- Transgender individuals may be or feel discriminated against.
- Studies support that matching race of provider with patients has advantages.

INTRODUCTION

Part 2 explores the impacts of sex and homelessness on the preoperative evaluation. There are numerous sex differences in medical care related to symptoms, diagnosis, pathophysiology, medication management, and other treatment of diseases. This is compounded by the predominance of male patients in available research studies of outcomes and medication effects. This section focuses on sex differences in cardiovascular disease (CVD) diagnosis and treatment, atrial fibrillation, and perioperative hormonal medication considerations for male, female, and transgender patients.

[a] Northwestern University Feinberg School of Medicine, 251 East Huron, Feinberg 5-704, Chicago, IL 60611, USA; [b] Duke University School of Medicine, DUMC 3094, Durham, NC 27710, USA
* Corresponding author.
E-mail address: Bobbiejean.sweitzer@nn.org
Twitter: @Jeanna_BlitzMD (J.B.); @BobbieJeanSwei1 (B.S.)

https://doi.org/10.1016/j.anclin.2020.02.001

In addition, as previously highlighted in Part 1, the limited access to medical care for patients suffering from homelessness, low health literacy, and incarceration can hinder preoperative optimization and positive surgical outcomes. These factors may result in avoidable postoperative complications, increase in length of stay postoperatively, and readmissions if they are not adequately addressed in the preoperative setting.[1] The authors explore the consequences of homelessness on preoperative needs and postoperative discharge planning.

SEX CONSIDERATIONS

Cardiovascular Disease

The leading cause of death in women is CVD, which includes coronary artery disease (CAD), myocardial infarction (MI), heart failure (HF), cerebrovascular disease such as stroke and transient ischemic attack, peripheral artery disease, and aortic atherosclerosis including aneurysm. In women, the incidence of MI increases following menopause, and after the age of 65 years, one in three women will have symptoms of CVD.[2,3] The incidence of atrial fibrillation increases with age and the prevalence in women increases after age 75 years.[4] The risk factors for CVD in women, including sex-specific risks, are shown in **Table 1**.

Chest pain is the most common presentation of coronary ischemia for both sexes. However, women may experience chest pain with rest, sleep, and mental stress, as well as with exertion. This suggests that women who present for preoperative evaluation who state they have nonexertional chest pain may benefit from an evaluation for CAD. Women evaluated for acute coronary syndrome (ACS) are more likely to present with symptoms other than chest pain at higher rates than men (19% vs 13.7%). Another study shows that 42% of women versus 30.7% of men with MI lack symptoms of chest pain.[2] Noninvasive testing considerations for women should consider the following:

- Stress echocardiography is preferable to stress nuclear imaging or coronary cardiac computed angiography (CCTA) to minimize radiation exposure to breast tissue.[2]

Table 1
Risk factors for cardiovascular disease

Risk Factors in Common with Men	Risk Factors Unique to Women
• Age	• Early menarche ≤10 years old
• Family history	• Postmenopausal state
• Hypertension	• Hysterectomy
• Dyslipidemia: low HDL, high LDL	• Premenstrual syndrome
• Diabetes mellitus	• Oral contraceptive use
• Chronic kidney disease	• Polycystic ovarian syndrome with obesity, insulin resistance, diabetes mellitus, dyslipidemia
• Metabolic syndrome	• Gestational diabetes
• Smoking	• Preeclampsia
• Diet	• Spontaneous pregnancy loss
• Obesity	• Preterm birth (spontaneous delivery <37 wk estimated gestational age)
• Excess alcohol intake (>2 drinks/d)	
• Sedentary lifestyle	
• Depression	
• Inflammatory/rheumatic diseases	

Abbreviations: HDL, high-density lipoprotein; LDL, low-density lipoprotein.

Data from Poppas A. Overview of cardiovascular risk factors in women. In: UpToDate, Givens J, Downey BC (Eds), UpToDate, Waltham, MA, 2019; Accessed June 17 2019.

- Treadmill exercise testing has a higher false-positive rate in women.[2]
- The sensitivity and specificity of exercise echocardiography (86% and 79%) exceeds that of exercise electrocardiography (61% and 70%) and exercise thallium testing (78% and 64%).[2]
- CCTA may provide more prognostic information for women than men, because a positive result ($\geq$70% stenosis) is more strongly associated with subsequent events compared with a positive stress test.[2,5]
- Women are more likely to have elevated high-sensitivity C-reactive protein and brain natriuretic peptide than men and less likely to have troponin elevation during episodes of ischemia.[2]

The progression to invasive testing with coronary angiography and revascularization is different based on sex, even among patients hospitalized for ACS. Hansen and colleagues[6] found that between 2005 and 2011, women admitted for ACS were less likely to have diagnostic coronary angiography compared with men on day 1 (31% vs 42%, $P<.001$) and within 60 days (67% vs 80%, $P<.001$) and less likely to undergo percutaneous coronary intervention (58% vs 72%, $P<.001$) and coronary artery bypass grafting (6% vs 11%, $P<.001$) than men within 60 days. Studies have also shown prevalence of significant CAD on angiography to be lower in women than men during workup for presumed angina, with normal coronaries found in 41% women versus 8% men.[2] In these patients, a diagnosis of coronary microvascular disease (formerly known as syndrome X) may apply, which can be found in up to 20% to 50% of women with chest pain.[2]

Cardiac syndrome X was originally named as such due to uncertainty about its pathogenesis and is now more commonly referred to as microvascular angina (MVA) or coronary microvascular dysfunction (CMD). The broadest definition of this condition is angina with normal epicardial coronary arteries found on angiogram. In the period of 2014 to 2015, the Coronary Vasomotion Disorders International Study Group developed the following criteria for MVA:[7,8]

- Symptoms that suggest myocardial ischemia: angina with effort or rest or angina equivalent
- Objective documentation of myocardial ischemia: electrocardiogram, transient abnormal perfusion imaging, or wall motion abnormality
- Absence of obstructive CAD: defined as less than 50% stenosis on CCTA or coronary angiography
- Confirmation of a reduced coronary flow reserve (CFR) and/or inducible microvascular spasm

It is thought that CMD causes CFR limitations in the smaller coronary arteries and arterioles, possibly related to increased sensitivity to vasoconstrictor stimuli or lack of vasodilator capacity, even in the absence of obstructive epicardial disease. This leads to angina or ischemic-like symptoms.[7] CFR can be measured during angiography, with positron emission tomography or transthoracic echocardiogram.[8,9] Values less than 2.0 to 2.5 are consistent with CMD. Mygind and colleagues[9] examined 963 women with angina and less than 50% stenosis on coronary angiogram and found CFR less than 2.0 in 26% and CFR between 2.0 and 2.5 in 35%. Lower CFR were associated with older age, and after age-adjustment, impaired CFR was associated with hypertension (HTN), diabetes, current smoking, higher resting heart rate, and lower high-density lipoprotein cholesterol level. Another study that examined major adverse cardiac events in 1218 men and women referred for CAD evaluation found participants with CFR less than 2.0 had higher rates of cardiac mortality, overall mortality, MI, and HF within 2.3 years of the study follow-up.[10] These rates were not statistically significant between men and women. Management strategies for CMD proposed by Chaudhary[7] include the following:

- CVD risk factor modification
- As-needed sublingual nitroglycerin
- Aspirin and statin in patients with atherosclerotic CVD
- Physical training program to improve exercise capacity
- Second-line therapy with beta blockers or calcium channel blockers
- Third-line therapy with imipramine, particularly in patients with chronic pain syndromes

Women with CAD are more likely to develop symptomatic HF than men, possibly related to diastolic dysfunction. Risk factors for HF in women can be found in **Table 2**. Diabetes has the highest correlation with HF. There are sex-related differences in medication-prescribing patterns of providers. However, many of the benefits of goal-directed medical therapy apply to both sexes. It is well established that aspirin and statins are first-line therapies for patients with CVD. Beta blockers, angiotensin-converting enzyme inhibitors or angiotensin receptor blockers are included for those with MI or HF. However, women with CAD are more likely to receive nitrates, calcium channel blockers, diuretics, and sedatives than men and less likely to receive aspirin, statins, and beta blockers.[11] The results of several different studies that included women showed aspirin was beneficial, P2Y12 inhibitors were as safe and efficacious as in men, beta blockers are at least as beneficial in women compared with men after MI, and lipid-lowering drugs such as statins are beneficial in women with CAD.[11]

Atrial Fibrillation in Women

The incidence of atrial fibrillation in men and women increases with age, and in women older than 75 years the prevalence increases substantially; however, women comprise only one-third of patients included in studies of atrial fibrillation. Female patients with atrial fibrillation are more likely to be of advanced age and have higher rates of valvular disease, HTN, dysthyroidism, and diabetes.[4,12] Comparably, men have higher rates of CAD and HF.

At presentation, women typically have longer duration of disease. Their quality of life is more severely affected, possibly because of the higher atrioventricular penetrance and higher heart rates during paroxysms.[12] The sex-related differences in symptom burden are found in **Table 3**. Symptomatology leads to a 24% reduction in adjusted quality-of-life scores in women.[13]

Multiple studies have shown a higher prevalence of thromboembolic events in women (3.5%–25%) compared with men (1.8%–10%), even after correcting for other

Table 2
Risk factors for heart failure in women with coronary artery disease

Diabetes mellitus	Atrial fibrillation
Myocardial infarction	Hypertension (SBP >120 mmHg)
Current smoking	Body mass index >35
Left bundle branch block	Creatinine clearance <40 mL/min
Left ventricular hypertrophy on ECG	

Abbreviations: ECG, electrocardiogram; SBP, systolic blood pressure.
Data from Pagidipati N. Clinical features and diagnosis of coronary heart disease in women. In: UpToDate, Saperia GM (Eds), UpToDate, Waltham, MA, 2019; Accessed June 17 2019.

Table 3
Sex-associated differences in symptoms in patients with atrial fibrillation

	Female	Male	*P* Value
Asymptomatic	32.1%	42.5%	<.001
Palpitations	40%	27%	<.001
Dizziness/lightheadedness	23%	19%	<.001
Fatigue	28%	25%	<.001
Chest discomfort	11%	8%	<.001
Dyspnea at rest	11%	9%	.001
Dyspnea with exertion	29%	27%	.01

Data from Piccini JP, Simon DN, Steinberg BA, et al. Differences in clinical and functional outcomes of atrial fibrillation in women and men: Two-Year Results From the ORBIT-AF Registry. JAMA Cardiol 2016;1(3):282-91.

risk factors such as age, previous stroke, HF, CAD, diabetes mellitus (DM), and estrogen replacement therapy.[4,12,13] Despite this, women are prescribed oral anticoagulation therapy less frequently than men, at various reported rates of 25% to 76% versus 45% to 95% in men.[4] In addition, medication management in women more commonly involves rate control strategies using digoxin and calcium channel blockers rather than rhythm control.[4,13] Studies also indicate women have a higher rate of adverse events from antiarrhythmic drugs and are less likely to be referred for ablation procedures for rhythm control strategies, although there is no consensus that outcomes for ablation procedures are different based on sex.[4,12]

With these differences in mind, optimizing contributing factors such as HTN, DM, and dysthyroidism in women with atrial fibrillation is an important consideration in the preoperative setting, in addition to adequate rhythm or rate control. Because female sex is an independent risk factor for stroke, appropriate management and bridging of anticoagulant medications must be addressed preoperatively. Oral anticoagulation is recommended for a CHA_2DS_2-VASc score of 2 or higher, found in **Table 4**. Perioperative bridging guidelines can be found in the 2017 ACC Expert Consensus Decision Pathway for Periprocedural Management of Anticoagulation in Patients with Nonvalvular Atrial Fibrillation.[14]

Perioperative Hormonal Medication Considerations and Management

Venous thromboembolic (VTE) events in the perioperative period are affected by several factors such as hereditary risk factors, acquired risk factors, medications, and type of surgery. Estrogen therapy increases the risk of VTE. Many women are on estrogen-containing medications such as oral contraceptives (OC), postmenopausal hormone therapy, and selective estrogen receptor modulators for cancer treatment. Similarly, men may be taking testosterone supplementation, which carries a Federal Drug Administration (FDA) warning regarding cardiovascular (CV) risks. Patients' individual risk factors and type of surgery are considered when deciding a perioperative management plan for these drugs.

Oral Contraceptives

OC have restrictions that have been set by the Centers for Disease Control and Prevention and the World Health Organization (**Table 5**). The risk of VTE is highest in the first year after OC initiation. After the first year, the risk decreases but remains elevated until medication cessation and returns to premedication levels 1 to 3 months after

Table 4
CHA_2DS_2-VASc score

Congestive heart failure	1
Hypertension	1
Age ≥75 y	2
Diabetes mellitus	1
Stroke/TIA/thromboembolism	2
Vascular disease (prior MI, PAD, aortic plaque)	1
Age 65–74 y	1
Female sex	1
Maximum score	9

Abbreviations: MI, myocardial infarction; PAD, peripheral arterial disease; TIA, transient ischemic attack.

Adapted from January CT, Wann LS, Alpert JS, et al. 2014 AHA/ACC/HRS guideline for the management of patients with atrial fibrillation: a report of the American College of Cardiology/American Heart Association Task Force on Practice Guidelines and the Heart Rhythm Society. J Am Coll Cardiol 2014;64(21):e1-76; with permission.

cessation.[15–17] The estrogen dose and type of progestin included in the OC affects VTE risk. First-generation drugs with greater than or equal to 50mcg of ethinyl estradiol have higher risks.[17] A 2014 Cochran review including 26 studies, concluded OC use increases VTE risk 4-fold.[18] However, this review notes no increased risk for the levonorgestrel intrauterine device. The Practice Committee of the American Society for Reproductive Medicine (ASRM) concluded from 2 large studies that there was no difference in VTE risk among vaginal ring users compared with OC.[17] There is some controversy regarding VTE risk with the transdermal patch, but the evidence is insufficient to state the risk is different than OC.[15,17] Progestin-only contraceptives do not seem to increase risk of VTE.[16] The ASRM Practice Committee examined multiple studies to determine risk factors for VTE in OC users, summarized in **Table 6**.

Muluk and colleagues[19] suggest using the modified Caprini risk assessment model to guide perioperative estrogen management (**Table 7**)[20]. Several patient-, surgical-, and medication-related factors are tallied to classify patients as very low, low, moderate, or high risk for VTE. This risk stratification can then be used to recommend

Table 5
Contraindications for use of oral contraceptives

Age ≥35 y and smoking ≥15 cigarettes/d	Hypertension (systolic BP ≥160, Diastolic BP ≥100)
Venous thromboembolism	Known thrombogenic mutation
Ischemic heart disease	Complicated valvular heart disease
Major surgery with prolonged immobilization	Stroke
Cirrhosis	Solid organ transplant—complicated
Diabetes mellitus with nephropathy/neuropathy	Migraine with aura
Breast cancer	Antiphospholipid antibodies

Abbreviation: BP, blood pressure.

Modified from Centers for Disease Control and Prevention (CDC). Summary Chart of U.S. Medical Eligibility Criteria for Contraceptive Use, 2017. Available at: https://www.cdc.gov/reproductivehealth/contraception/pdf/summary-chart-us-medical-eligibility-criteria_508tagged.pdf. Accessed June 21 2019.

Table 6
Risk factors for venous thromboembolism in oral contraceptive users

Prolonged immobilization	Age >35 y	Obesity in patients older than 35 y
History of VTE	Family history of DVT	Active SLE
Smoking >15 cigarettes/d	Antiphospholipid syndrome	Current cancer diagnosis
Postpartum status (greatest for 6 wk; persists until 12 wk)	Inherited thrombophilia • Factor V Leiden • Prothrombin gene mutation	

Abbreviations: DVT, deep venous thrombosis; SLE, systemic lupus erythematosis; VTE, venous thromboembolism.

Data from Practice Committee of the American Society for Reproductive Medicine. Combined hormonal contraception and the risk of venous thromboembolism: a guideline. Fertil Steril 2017;107(1):43-51; and Martin K, Douglas P. Risks and side effects associated with combined estrogen-progestin oral contraceptives. In: UpToDate, Martin K, Eckler K (Eds), UpToDate, Waltham, MA, 2019; Accessed June 17 2019.

cessation of estrogen-containing drugs or continuation. For patients taking OC having surgery with low to moderate risk of VTE, the investigators recommend continuing the medication without interruption, assuming the patient receives appropriate perioperative VTE prophylaxis. For patients at high risk of VTE based on the risk assessment model, they recommend providers stop OC 4 weeks before surgery, discuss alternative forms of contraception, and obtain a serum pregnancy test immediately before surgery. The modified Caprini risk assessment model does not include the risk factor of smoking. It may be worth considering cessation of OC in patients who smoke and are found to be at moderate risk for VTE based on this model.

Postmenopausal Hormone Therapy and Selective Estrogen Receptor Modulators

The mean age of menopause is 51 years with a range of 45 to 55 years encompassing 95% of women.[21] Estrogen alone or estrogen combined with a progestin is used to control menopausal symptoms. As OC, the estimated risk of VTE due to postmenopausal estrogen is 2-fold and is highest in the first 1 to 2 years of therapy.[15,21,22] Additional risk factors include women who are older, obese and have Factor V Leiden or a history of VTE.[15,21,22] The use of aspirin or statin to decrease VTE in postmenopausal women is controversial, with some trials indicating a protective effect and others showing no difference.[21,22] In one study the odds ratio for VTE was 4.2 with oral versus 0.9 with transdermal estrogen compared with nonusers.[21] This was confirmed by another study in women with Factor V Leiden, showing transdermal estrogen did not increase risk for VTE in contrast to oral estrogen.[21] A large 3-year study of raloxifene showed a 3-fold increase in VTE.[22] Tamoxifen is frequently used in treatment of breast cancer and has been shown to increase VTE rates. The Breast Cancer Prevention Trial found a relative risk of pulmonary embolism of 3.01 in patients taking tamoxifen compared with placebo.[22]

Muluk recommends continuation of postmenopausal hormonal therapy for surgical patients at low to moderate risk of VTE (with appropriate VTE prophylaxis) but cessation at least 2 weeks before surgery for those at high risk of VTE, based on the modified Caprini risk assessment model.[20] The recommendations for selective estrogen receptor modulators (SERM) are slightly more complex, likely due to their use as treatment of breast cancer. Surgical patients at low to moderate risk of VTE can continue SERMs without interruption, with addition of appropriate

Table 7
Modified Caprini risk assessment model for venous thromboembolism in general surgical patients

Risk Score			
1 Point	**2 Points**	**3 Points**	**4 Points**
• Age 41–60 y • Minor surgery • BMI >25 • Swollen legs • Varicose veins • Pregnancy or postpartum • Prior unexplained or recurrent miscarriage • Oral contraceptives or hormone therapy • Sepsis (<1 mo) • Serious lung disease, including pneumonia (<1 mo) • Abnormal pulmonary function • Acute MI • CHF (<1 mo) • IBD • Medical patient at bed rest	• Age 61–74 y • Arthroscopic surgery • Major open surgery (>45 min) • Laparoscopic surgery (>45 min) • Malignancy • Confined to bed (>72 h) • Immobilizing plaster cast • Central venous access	• Age > or = 75 y • History of VTE • Family history of VTE • Factor V Leiden • Prothrombin gene mutation • Lupus anticoagulant • Anticardiolipin antibodies • Elevated serum homocysteine • HIT • Other congenital or acquired thrombophilia	• Stroke (<1 mo) • Elective arthroplasty • Hip, pelvis, or leg fracture • Acute spinal cord injury (<1 mo)

Interpretation		
Surgical Risk Category[a]	**Score**	**Estimated VTE Risk Without Prophylaxis (%)**
Very Low	0	<0.5
Low	1–2	1.5
Moderate	3–4	3.0
High	≥5	6.0

Abbreviations: BMI, body mass index; CHF, congestive heart failure; HIT, heparin-induced thrombocytopenia; IBD, inflammatory bowel disease; MI, myocardial infarction; VTE, venous thromboembolism.

[a] This table is applicable only to general, abdominal-pelvic, bariatric, vascular, plastic and reconstructive surgery.

Adapted from Gould MK, Garcia DA, Wren SM, et al. Prevention of VTE in nonorthopedic surgical patients: antithrombotic therapy and prevention of thrombosis, 9th ed: American College of Chest Physicians evidence-based clinical practice guidelines. Chest 2012;141(2 Suppl):e243S; with permission.

perioperative VTE prophylaxis. Those at high risk for VTE taking raloxifene for breast cancer prevention, or osteoporosis, should discontinue this drug 3 days before surgery. Patients at high risk of VTE should discontinue tamoxifen, if taken for breast cancer prevention, 2 weeks before surgery. If tamoxifen is used to treat breast cancer, it is recommended to continue perioperatively while also providing appropriate VTE prophylaxis.

Testosterone

Complications related to testosterone replacement in men have been controversial. Testosterone is generally prescribed to treat hypogonadism, defined as testosterone deficiency, and treatment can result in improvement in the following:

- Sexual dysfunction, including erectile dysfunction and decreased libido
- Mood, cognition, and energy
- Bone mineral density
- Increased lean muscle mass
- Decreased fat mass
- Improved insulin sensitivity, lower fasting plasma glucose, and lower glycosylated hemoglobin values (HbA_1c)
- Hematopoiesis, possibly leading to polycythemia

Interestingly, the FDA has never required new testosterone formulations to show efficacy, only suitable pharmacokinetic effects.[23] In 2014 the FDA issued a safety warning regarding possible increased risk of MI and strokes related to testosterone treatment. They further stated, "Health care professionals should prescribe testosterone therapy only for men with low testosterone levels caused by certain medical conditions and confirmed by laboratory tests,"which does not include hypogonadism related to normal aging."[24]

A review by Kloner and colleagues[23] in 2016 illustrated the continued controversy over CV risks associated with testosterone, including nonfatal MI, fatal MI, stroke, and CV mortality. The investigators concluded that patients with recent MI, revascularization, poorly controlled HF, or stroke within the last 6 months were poor candidates for testosterone therapy and that asymptomatic men without a history of heart disease should be counseled about the unknown CV risks. One effect of testosterone treatment that is less controversial is the resulting polycythemia. Limited studies have shown both an association of VTE related to testosterone use and no association.[23] Cessation of testosterone treatment perioperatively due to potential concerns of VTE, related to or independent from polycythemia, should be considered. Laboratory information, such as hemoglobin and hematocrit, and utilization of the modified Caprini assessment model previously mentioned, may aid in these discussions. With the unclear CV risks of testosterone, and the known increase in inflammatory markers related to surgery contributing to perioperative MI and stroke, the risk of continuation of the drug may outweigh the benefit in surgical patients.

Hormone Therapy and Perioperative Considerations for Transgender Patients

There is a paucity of research regarding adverse side effects of cross-sex hormone therapy (CSHT) in transgender patients. Streed and colleagues[25] conducted a review in 2017 that found some differences between transgender women and men. They concluded the following:

- CSHT improved psychological functioning of transgender persons

- In transgender men, CSHT with testosterone is associated with worse CV risk factors including elevated blood pressure, insulin resistance, and unfavorable lipid levels, but no increased CV morbidity and mortality
- In transgender women, CSHT with estrogen potentially increases VTE risk. Lower-dose transdermal or oral preparations are preferred over high-dose oral ethinyl estradiol formulations
- In all populations, reducing CV risk factors of HTN, DM, smoking, abnormal lipid levels, and body mass index greater than 25 is critical
- Older transgender women who have baseline CV risks may be at particular risk

Many of the studies are limited by small sample size, short duration of follow-up, or include only young patients with presumably low baseline CV risks. In addition, research on secondary prevention strategies for transgender persons taking CSHT who have had previous MI or stroke is limited.[25]

In 2018 Goodman and colleagues[26] performed a large cohort study of nearly 5000 transgender patients and nearly 100,000 cisgender individuals followed-up over several years, examining the incidence of VTE, MI, and stroke related to CSHT use. They concluded that transgender women had VTE risk increase by 4.1 and 16.7 at 2 and 8 years compared with cisgender men, and 3.4 and 13.7 compared with cisgender women. Stroke and MI rates in the 3 groups were similar. The evidence for risks in transgender men was inconclusive. The data, however, did not include statin use or various other comorbid conditions. They also hypothesized that the small number of MI events in the transgender men taking testosterone may have been related to the young age of the cohort.

The risks and benefits of continuation of CSHT in transgender patients perioperatively must be individually considered. Gender dysphoria is one disadvantage of discontinuation of CSHT. However, it seems the risk of perioperative VTE, especially in transgender women, can be substantial, especially in patients with other risk factors such as smoking and obesity. This highlights the importance of conversations and education about the perioperative risks of VTE and CV events and subsequent shared decision-making with patients.

For more information on the perioperative care of transgender patients, please review Luis E. Tollinche and colleagues' article, "Considerations for Transgender Patients Perioperatively," in this issue.

UNDOMICILED (HOMELESS) PATIENTS

The health care needs of homeless patients have long been known to be more challenging than their domiciled counterparts. Outpatient utilization of services is marginal compared with utilization of emergency departments (ED). Chronic medical conditions are poorly controlled or untreated, mental health and substance abuse are more prevalent, those who leave against medical advice and experience hospital readmission are more common, and overall mortality rates are substantially higher.[27]

Homeless, according to the US Department of Housing and Urban Development (HUD), is defined as someone who[28]

- Lacks a fixed, regular, and adequate nighttime residence
- Lives in a publicly or privately operated shelter designed to provide temporary living arrangements
- Has nighttime residence that is a public or private place not meant for human habitation
- Will imminently lose their primary nighttime residence
- Is fleeing their housing because of domestic violence

There are an estimated 553,000 homeless people in the United States.as of October 2018.[29] HUD estimates that more than 1.5 million people can be homeless at one point in any given year.[27,30]

Frequent health conditions encountered among the homeless population are found in **Table 8**.[27,31–33] Inadequate treatment leads to an age-adjusted mortality rate 2 to 11 times the general population.[27,34]

There have been very few studies examining surgical needs in the homeless population. Zuccaro and colleagues[34] found that the homeless patients referred from the ED for surgical treatment were predominantly men living in shelters who had traumatic injuries (**Box 1**). Urgent or emergency interventions were recommended in 78% who needed surgery.[34] Many also had poor postoperative care; 51% of patients failed to attend any outpatient follow-up appointments, and only 34% completed the full treatment course.

When caring for homeless patients, aspects of care shown in **Box 2** should be considered. Mistrust of the health care system is common among homeless individuals, and low-pressure techniques to engage patients, and allow them to dictate the pace of care, can be helpful.[27] The traumatic brain injury questionnaire, referenced in **Box 2**, includes a section that asks 12 questions about experiences commonly associated with head injury, such as motor vehicle accident, sports-related accidents, falls, domestic violence, assaults, or gunshots.[35] A second section assesses frequency and severity of 15 symptoms common after head injury, such as dizziness, headaches, trouble concentrating, and memory issues.[35] Further details are obtained if any experiences or symptoms are found to be positive.

It is useful to consider the fragmented care homeless patients receive and provide them with a wallet-sized list of medications.[36] Allowing for a drop-in system in outpatient settings will optimize opportunities for preoperative and follow-up care. Many patients have no convenient means of communication about testing results or further recommendations, so additional visits need to be coordinated ahead of time.[27] Steward and colleagues[37] examined patient-centered care for homeless persons by surveying 26 homeless individuals about their priorities in primary care. Both the homeless and the provider/expert groups agreed the highest priorities are

Table 8
Common medical conditions in homeless populations

Skin conditions • Cellulitis • Other skin & foot infections • Frostbite • Scabies, lice, and bed bug infestations	Cognitive impairments • Traumatic brain injury • Mental illness • Substance use disorders of alcohol or other illicit drugs
Respiratory infections • Tuberculosis • Viral or bacterial pneumonia	Blood-borne infections • HIV • Hepatitis C
Cardiac disease • Coronary artery disease • Hypertension	Sexually transmitted diseases
Smoking	Dental problems
Diabetes mellitus	Victims of violence

Abbreviation: HIV, human immunodeficiency virus.

Data from Baggett TP, Kertesz SG. Health care of homeless persons in the United States. In: UpToDate, Kunins L (Ed), UpToDate, Waltham, MA, 2019; Accessed June 6 2019.

Box 1
Type of surgical referrals

Traumatic injuries (64%)—80% for fractures referred to orthopedic surgery, plastic surgery, and otolaryngology

Genitourinary (9%)—urinary retention and obstruction

Infectious (9%)—peritonsillar abscess, frostbite, critical limb ischemia, and wound infection

Gastrointestinal (6%)—bowel perforation, small bowel obstruction, and acute cholecystitis

Data from Zuccaro L, Champion C, Bennett S, et al. Understanding the surgical care needs and use of outpatient surgical care services among homeless patients at the Ottawa Hospital. Can J Surg 2018;61(6):424–9.

accessibility of care, evidence-based decision-making, and cooperation and communication among all care providers. Homeless patients also ranked "shared knowledge and the free flow of information" fourth out of 16 constructs, whereas providers ranked this 14th. This is important to keep in mind when evaluating and optimizing homeless patients preoperatively. The investigators hypothesized access to information and understanding may play a role in alleviating distress, separate from the quality of treatment administered.

In the preoperative setting, it is important to note the high incidence of postoperative readmission rates for homeless individuals and ways to better optimize conditions to reduce this risk. Readmission rates of 21% to 51% have been reported among medical admissions in homeless populations. The likelihood of patients

Box 2
Routine outpatient care of homeless patients

Cognitive screening
- Mini-mental status examination
- Traumatic brain injury questionnaire

Single-item screens for alcohol and substance abuse
- "How many times in the past year have you used an illegal drug or used a prescription medication for nonmedical reasons?"
- "Do you sometimes drink beer, wine, or other alcoholic beverages?"

Universal HIV and HCV screening

Medication prescribing that is conducive to adherence
- Once-daily dosing
- Medications that can be stored at room temperature
- Accounting for street value of medications (ie, gabapentin, clonidine, inhalants, or opioids)

Considerations for medication/treatment
- Normal glycemic index targets may not be safe for homeless individuals
- Starting antihypertensive medications for low-risk outpatient surgery when patient has no means for follow-up blood pressure monitoring

Abbreviations: HCV, hepatitis C virus; HIV, human immunodeficiency virus.

Data from Baggett TP, Kertesz SG. Health care of homeless persons in the United States. In: UpToDate, Kunins L (Ed), UpToDate, Waltham, MA, 2019; Accessed June 6 2019; and Health Care for the Homeless Clinicians' Network. Adapting Your Practice: General recommendations for the care of homeless patients. National Health Care for the Homeless Council, Inc., 2010. Available at: https://nhchc.org/wp-content/uploads/2019/08/GenRecsHomeless2010.pdf. Accessed May 8 2019.

leaving against medical advice (AMA) is 9.3% to 14.3% in the homeless population compared with 1.3% in the general population.[30,33,38] Titan and colleagues[32] examined the 30-day readmission rates of homeless veterans after inpatient general, vascular, and orthopedic surgery. The strongest predictors of increased readmissions were the following:

- Discharge destination
- Alcohol abuse within the preceding 2 weeks
- Surgery in July through September
- Higher American Society of Anesthesiologists physical status classification

A common reason for readmission was wound infections, highlighting the challenge homeless patients' face with hygiene and self-care skills. Patients who abused alcohol, defined as greater than 2 drinks per day, within 2 weeks of surgery were 45% more likely to be readmitted ($P<.001$). This creates an opportunity for intervention in the preoperative setting, by referring these patients for prehabilitation preoperatively or on hospital discharge. In housed individuals, patients discharged to a nursing home are 15% more likely to experience readmission.[32] But, for homeless patients, discharge to a nursing or boarding home or other domiciliary was protective compared with discharge to the community.[30,32] Doran and colleagues[30] further specified that discharge to a motel with friends or family, rehabilitation facility, or skilled nursing facility lowered the 30-day readmission rate compared with discharge to streets or a shelter.

Medical respite programs were developed in 1985 by Boston Health Care for the Homeless Program and have since expanded to 78 programs nationwide.[31] These programs are designed to house homeless individuals who are too sick for the streets or a shelter but do not warrant an inpatient hospital stay. The services include[30,36]

- 24-hour shelter
- Meals
- Medical care by a physician, physician assistant, nurse practitioner, or nurse
- Health care coordination
- Social services
- Contact with a community health worker

The average length of stay is 42 days with a median length of stay of 30 days as of the 2016 report.[39] Kertesz has shown discharge of homeless patients to these facilities decreased odds of 90-day readmission by 50% compared with shelters or "own care."[38] Medical respite facilities listed by state can be found on the National Health Care for the Homeless Council's Website.[39] Many of these studies on readmission rates after hospital discharge were conducted on inpatients who received surgical or medical care. Discharge planning can be problematic in homeless patients having ambulatory surgery. These patients may not have an escort to leave with, a location to be discharged to, or a means of transport. It is imperative to contact social services early to start discharge planning for all surgical homeless persons.

In summary, the homeless population has more severe and poorly treated medical conditions, with age-adjusted mortality rates 10-fold that of housed individuals.[40] Surgical needs of the homeless most commonly include treatment of trauma, urologic, infectious, gastrointestinal, and vascular problems. Easy access to information and understanding are highly ranked priorities of homeless individuals and should be emphasized in the preoperative process. Homeless patients have higher rates of readmission and leaving AMA and are less likely to follow-up postdischarge. Availability of medical respite services is increasing and is associated with lower rates of readmissions for homeless individuals. Social services need to be involved early to meet the discharge needs of the homeless population anticipating both inpatient and ambulatory procedures.

SUMMARY

The perioperative period is a vulnerable time for many patients, especially those who experience health disparities related to race, sex, or as members of disenfranchised populations such as incarcerated or homeless, or those with low health literacy. The preoperative evaluation is an opportunity to change the trajectory of perioperative outcomes for these at-risk populations. Race, sex, and low socioeconomic status present unique considerations and goals for multidisciplinary care and preoperative optimization. Even postoperative discharge planning may be especially challenging. It is crucial to identify patients who will benefit from additional coordination of care and resource allocation to reduce health and health care disparities.

DISCLOSURE

The authors have nothing to disclose.

REFERENCES

1. Roy M, Corkum JP, Urbach DR, et al. Health literacy among surgical patients: a systematic review and meta-analysis. World J Surg 2019;43:96–106.
2. Douglas P, Pagidipati N. Clinical features and diagnosis of coronary heart disease in women. In: Saperia G, editor. UpToDate. 2018. Available at: https://www.uptodate.com/contents/clinical-features-and-diagnosis-of-coronary-heart-disease-in-women. Accessed June 17, 2019.
3. Douglas P, Poppas A. Overview of cardiovascular risk factors in women. In: Givens J, Downey B, editors. UpToDate. 2019. Available at: https://www.uptodate.com/contents/overview-of-cardiovascular-risk-factors-in-women. Accessed June 17, 2019.
4. Anselmino M, Battaglia A, Gallo C, et al. Atrial fibrillation and female sex. J Cardiovasc Med 2015;16(12):795–801.
5. Pagidipati NJ, Hemal K, Coles A, et al. Sex differences in functional and ct angiography testing in patients with suspected coronary artery disease. J Am Coll Cardiol 2016;67(22):2607–16.
6. Hansen KW, Soerensen R, Madsen M, et al. Developments in the invasive diagnostic-therapeutic cascade of women and men with acute coronary syndromes from 2005 to 2011: a nationwide cohort study. BMJ Open 2015;5(6):e007785.
7. Chaudhary I. Microvascular angina: Angina pectoris with normal coronary arteries. In: Saperia G, editor. UpToDate. 2018. Available at: https://www.uptodate.com/contents/microvascular-angina-angina-pectoris-with-normal-coronary-arteries. Accessed July 15, 2019.
8. Ong P, Camici PG, Beltrame JF, et al, Coronary Vasomotion Disorders International Study Group (COVADIS). International standardization of diagnostic criteria for microvascular angina. Int J Cardiol 2018;250:16–20.
9. Mygind ND, Michelsen MM, Pena A, et al. Coronary microvascular function and cardiovascular risk factors in women with angina pectoris and no obstructive

coronary artery disease: the iPOWERstudy. J Am Heart Assoc 2016;5(3): e003064.

10. Murthy VL, Naya M, Taqueti VR, et al. Effects of sex on coronary microvascular dysfunction and cardiac outcomes. Circulation 2014;129(24):2518–27.
11. Douglas P, Pagidipati N. Management of coronary heart disease in women. In: Saperia G, editor. UpToDate. 2019. Available at: https://www.uptodate.com/contents/management-of-coronary-heart-disease-in-women. Accessed June 24, 2019.
12. Andrade JG, Deyell MW, Lee AYK, et al. Sex differences in atrial fibrillation. Can J Cardiol 2018;34(4):429–36.
13. Piccini JP, Simon DN, Steinberg BA, et al, Outcomes Registry for Better Informed Treatment of Atrial Fibrillation (ORBIT-AF) Investigators and Patients. Differences in clinical and functional outcomes of atrial fibrillation in women and men: two-year results from the ORBIT-AF Registry. JAMACardiol 2016;1(3):282–91.
14. Doherty JU, Gluckman TJ, Hucker WJ, et al. 2017 ACCexpert consensus decision pathway for periprocedural management of anticoagulation in patients with nonvalvular atrial fibrillation: a report of the American College of Cardiology Clinical Expert Consensus Document Task Force. J Am CollCardiol 2017;69(7): 871–98.
15. Bauer K, Lip G. Overview of the causes of venous thrombosis. In: Finlay G, editor. UpToDate. 2019. Available at: https://www.uptodate.com/contents/overview-of-the-causes-of-venous-thrombosis. Accessed June 3, 2019.
16. Martin K, Douglas P. Risks and side effects associated with combined estrogen-progestin oral contraceptives. In: Martin K, Eckler K, editors. UpToDate. 2018. Available at: https://www.uptodate.com/contents/risks-and-side-effects-associated-with-combined-estrogen-progestin-oral-contraceptives. Accessed June 17, 2019.
17. Practice Committee of the American Society for Reproductive Medicine. Combined hormonal contraception and the risk of venous thromboembolism: a guideline. FertilSteril 2017;107(1):43–51.
18. de Bastos M, Stegeman BH, Rosendaal FR, et al. Combined oral contraceptives: venous thrombosis. CochraneDatabaseSyst Rev 2014;(3):CD010813.
19. Muluk V, Cohn S, Whinney C. Perioperative medication management. In: Kunins L, editor. UpToDate. 2019. Available at: https://www.uptodate.com/contents/perioperative-medication-management. Accessed June 17, 2019.
20. Gould MK, Garcia DA, Wren SM, et al. Prevention of VTE in nonorthopedic surgical patients: antithrombotic therapy and prevention of thrombosis, 9th ed: American College of Chest Physicians evidence-based clinical practice guidelines. Chest 2012;141(2 Suppl):e227S–77S.
21. Martin K, Rosenson R. Menopausal hormone therapy and cardiovascular risk. In: Mulder J, editor. UpToDate. 2017. Available at: https://www.uptodate.com/contents/menopausal-hormone-therapy-and-cardiovascular-risk. Accessed June 20, 2019.
22. Miller J, Chan BK, Nelson HD. Postmenopausal estrogen replacement and risk for venous thromboembolism: a systematic review and meta-analysis for the U.S. Preventive Services Task Force [Review]. Ann Intern Med 2002;136(9): 680–90 [Erratum in: Ann Intern Med. 2003;138(4):360].
23. Kloner RA, Carson C 3rd, Dobs A, et al. Testosterone and cardiovascular disease. J Am CollCardiol 2016;67(5):545–57.
24. U.S. Food and Drug Administration. FDA Drug Safety Communication: FDA cautions about using testosterone products for low testosterone due to aging; requires labeling change to inform of possible increased risk of heart attack and

stroke with use. 2015. Available at:https://www.fda.gov/drugs/drug-safety-and-availability/fda-drug-safety-communication-fda-cautions-about-using-testosterone-products-low-testosterone-due. Accessed June 21, 2019.
25. Streed CG Jr, Harfouch O, Marvel F, et al. Cardiovascular disease among transgender adults receiving hormone therapy: A narrative review. Ann Intern Med 2017;167(4):256–67.
26. Goodman M, Getahun D, Silverberg MJ, et al. Cross-sex hormones and acute cardiovascular events in transgender persons. Ann Intern Med 2019;170(2):143.
27. Baggett T, Kertesz S. Health care of homeless persons in the United States. In: Kunins L, editor. UpToDate. 2019. Available at: https://www.uptodate.com/contents/health-care-of-homeless-persons-in-the-united-states. Accessed June 6, 2019.
28. United States Interagency Council on Homelessness. Key federal terms and definitions of homelessness among youth. 2018. Available at:https://www.usich.gov/resources/uploads/asset_library/Federal-Definitions-of-Youth-Homelessness.pdf. . Accessed June 9, 2019.
29. HUD 2018 Continuum of Care Homeless Assistance Programs Homeless Populations and Subpopulations. 2018. Available at:https://files.hudexchange.info/reports/published/CoC_PopSub_NatlTerrDC_2018.pdf. . Accessed June 9, 2019.
30. Doran KM, Ragins KT, Iacomacci AL, et al. The revolving hospital door: hospital readmissions among patients who are homeless. Med Care 2013;51(9):767–73.
31. Koh HK, O'Connell JJ. Improving health care for homeless people. JAMA 2016; 316(24):2586–7.
32. Titan A, Graham L, Rosen A, et al. Homeless status, postdischarge health care utilization, and readmission after surgery. Med Care 2018;56(6):460–9.
33. Saab D, Nisenbaum R, Dhalla I, et al. Hospital readmissions in a community-based sample of homeless adults: a matched-cohort study. J Gen Intern Med 2016;31(9):1011–8.
34. Zuccaro L, Champion C, Bennett S, et al. Understanding the surgical care needs and use of outpatient surgical care services among homeless patients at the Ottawa Hospital. Can J Surg 2018;61(6):424–9.
35. Diamond PM, Harzke AJ, Magaletta PR, et al. Screening for traumatic brain injury in an offender sample: a first look at the reliability and validity of the Traumatic Brain Injury Questionnaire. J HeadTraumaRehabil 2007;22(6):330–8.
36. Health Care for the Homeless Clinicians' Network. General recommendations for the care of homeless patients: Summary of recommended practice adaptations. 2010. Available at:https://www.nhchc.org/wp-content/uploads/2011/09/General-Recommendations-for-Homeless-Patients.pdf. . Accessed May 8, 2019.
37. Steward J, Holt CL, Pollio DE, et al. Priorities in the primary care of persons experiencing homelessness: convergence and divergence in the views of patients and provider/experts. Patient Prefer Adherence 2016;10:153–8.
38. Kertesz SG, Posner MA, O'Connell JJ, et al. Post-hospital medical respite care and hospital readmission of homeless persons. J PrevIntervCommunity 2009; 37(2):129–42.
39. National Health Care for the Homeless Council. Inc. 2016 Medical respite program directory. 2016. Available at:https://www.nhchc.org/wp-content/uploads/2011/10/2016-MEDICAL-RESPITE-PROGRAM-DIRECTORY_FINAL2.pdf. Accessed June 15, 2019.
40. Roncarati JS, Baggett TP, O'Connell JJ, et al. Mortality among unsheltered homeless adults in Boston, Massachusetts,2000-2009. JAMA Intern Med 2018;178(9): 1242–8.

Racial Differences in Pregnancy-Related Morbidity and Mortality

Rebecca D. Minehart, MD, MSHPEd*, Jaleesa Jackson, MD,
Jaime Daly, MD

KEYWORDS

• Maternal mortality • Severe maternal morbidity • Racial disparities • Obstetrics
• Obstetric anesthesia

KEY POINTS

- Black women have experienced injustice and abuse in the United States since the 1600s.
- Institutionalized racism has led to black women's deep distrust of health care providers and medical research processes, leading to disparities in accessing care and dramatic underrepresentation in research.
- Black women die at a rate of 3 to 4 times greater compared with their white counterparts, regardless of socioeconomic factors.
- Hospital factors play a prominent role in black women experiencing greater morbidity and mortality, and anesthesiologists are uniquely positioned to help erase some of these disparities by focusing on these vulnerabilities.

INTRODUCTION

Over the last few years in the United States, there has been increasing scrutiny on maternal care as maternal morbidity rate and mortality soar.[1,2] As recently as May 2019, the Centers for Disease Control and Prevention (CDC) issued a Morbidity and Mortality Weekly Report that pregnant or postpartum women of color die at a staggering rate of 3 to 4 times greater than their white counterparts, regardless of socioeconomic factors.[3] This finding sent shockwaves through the country, as National Public Radio,[4] the Harvard Business Review,[5] the Associated Press,[6] and others called for accountability by the medical community. Although the American College of Obstetricians and Gynecologists (ACOG) had previously issued a Committee Opinion on racial and ethnic disparities in maternal care,[7] along with an ACOG

Department of Anesthesia, Critical Care and Pain Medicine, Massachusetts General Hospital, Harvard Medical School, 55 Fruit Street, GRJ 440, Boston, MA 02114, USA
* Corresponding author.
E-mail address: rminehart@mgh.harvard.edu
Twitter: @RDMinehart (R.D.M.)

Anesthesiology Clin 38 (2020) 279–296
https://doi.org/10.1016/j.anclin.2020.01.006
anesthesiology.theclinics.com

Postpartum Toolkit designed to provide resources to community health care providers and to patients,[8,9] clearly there remains an enormous need for understanding why these disparities exist, particularly between white and black mothers, where the disparities are the greatest.[3]

Anesthesiologists providing obstetric care are uniquely positioned to improve maternal care; recent ACOG Levels of Maternal Care Guidelines mandate that a board-certified anesthesiologist with special training or experience in obstetrics be available for care or consultation, particularly for those labor and delivery units who provide subspecialty obstetric care (level III) or regional perinatal health care centers (level IV), and even those centers providing specialty obstetric care (level II) are determined to require access to anesthesiology services at all times.[10] With maternal comorbidity burden increasing overall, this consolidation of maternal care is postulated to improve outcomes through the availability of these providers.[11] Through their integral role in labor and delivery processes, anesthesiologists aware of racial disparities may improve care for the diverse maternal population.

DISCREPANCIES IN MATERNAL HEALTH OUTCOMES

Before considering reasons why black mothers are becoming sicker and dying at higher rates than white mothers, this article first outlines the obstetric conditions leading to severe maternal morbidity (SMM) and mortality for which there are disparities. SMM, which has no formally accepted definition,[12] has alternately been described as "a life-threatening diagnosis or the need to undergo a life-saving procedure during a delivery hospitalization"[13,14] and as "unintended outcomes of the process of labor and delivery that result in significant short-term or long-term consequences to a woman's health."[15] ACOG and other investigators[15] recently proposed conditions and criteria for SMM, which may ultimately serve as an initiation point for building consensus among professional organizations (**Table 1**). Although the categorization and inclusion of these morbidities may need to be adjusted, this list fills an undeniable need for better classifying and understanding the extent of SMM through careful research.

Holdt Somer and colleagues[12] attempted to identify gaps in existing literature on disparities in SMM. Although their list of SMM definitions were not entirely congruent with the ACOG definitions, these investigators showed a large increase in SMM for multiple racial groups, predominantly African Americans. **Table 2** lists the disparities as well as gaps in the authors' literature search on a variety of morbid conditions. Specific conditions, such as inherited thrombophilias and sickle cell diseases, have a clear genetic basis. Almost all other conditions may be attributed to myriad factors involving the interplay between race and health, which are explored later.

THE LINKS BETWEEN RACE AND HEALTH

Race is a hotly debated topic, and many scholars advocate that it is in essence "an unscientific, societally constructed taxonomy that is based on an ideology that views some human populations as inherently superior to others on the basis of external physical characteristics or geographic origin,"[16] which nevertheless critically affects myriad outcomes, including health, longevity, and social status attainment.[16,17] In 2016, the National Health Interview Survey conducted by the CDC revealed that white men and women had consistently higher reports of health than black men and women.[18] To better visualize the relationship between race and health, Williams and colleagues[16] developed a framework (**Fig. 1**, **Table 3**) that is still useful to consider today. This article focuses on a subset of these factors, primarily racism, biological

Table 1
Examples of diagnoses and complications constituting severe maternal morbidity

SMM	Not Severe Morbidity (Insufficient Evidence If This Is the Only Criterion)
Hemorrhage	
Obstetric hemorrhage with ≥4 units of red blood cells transfused	—
Obstetric hemorrhage with 2 units of red blood cells and 2 units of fresh frozen plasma transfused (without other procedures or complications) if not judged to be overexuberant transfusion	Obstetric hemorrhage with 2 units of red blood cells and 2 units of fresh frozen plasma transfused and judged to be overexuberant
Obstetric hemorrhage with <4 units of blood products transfused and evidence of pulmonary congestion that requires >1 dose of furosemide	Obstetric hemorrhage with <4 units of blood products transfused and evidence of pulmonary edema requiring only 1 dose of furosemide
Obstetric hemorrhage with return to operating room for any major procedure (excludes dilation)	—
Any emergency/unplanned peripartum hysterectomy, regardless of number of units transfused (includes all placenta accrete spectrum conditions)	Planned peripartum hysterectomy for cancer/neoplasia
Obstetric hemorrhage with uterine artery embolization, regardless of number of units transfused	—
Obstetric hemorrhage with uterine balloon or uterine compression suture placed and 2–3 units of blood products transfused	Obstetric hemorrhage with uterine balloon or uterine compression suture placed and ≤1 units of blood products transfused
Obstetric hemorrhage admitted to ICU for invasive monitoring or treatment (either medication or procedure, not just observed overnight)	Any patient with obstetric hemorrhage who went to the ICU for observation only without further treatment
Hypertension/Neurologic	
Eclamptic seizures or epileptic seizures that were status	—
Continuous intravenous infusion of an antihypertensive medication	—
Nonresponsiveness or loss of vision, permanent or temporary (but not momentary), documented in physician's progress notes	—
Stroke, coma, intracranial hemorrhage	—
Preeclampsia with difficult-to-control severe hypertension (>160 mm Hg systolic blood pressure or >110 mm Hg diastolic blood pressure) that requires multiple intravenous doses, persistent ≥48 h after delivery, or both	Chronic hypertension that drifts up to severe range and needs postoperative medication dose alternation; preeclampsia blood pressure control with oral medication ≥48 h after delivery
Liver or subcapsular hematoma or severe liver injury admitted to the ICU (bilirubin >6 mg/dL or liver enzymes >600 U/L)	Abnormal liver function requiring prolonged postpartum length of stay but not in the ICU

(*continued on next page*)

Table 1
(*continued*)

SMM	Not Severe Morbidity (Insufficient Evidence If This Is the Only Criterion)
Multiple coagulation abnormalities or severe HELLP syndrome	Severe thrombocytopenia (<50,000/μL) alone that does not require a transfusion or ICU admission
Renal	
Diagnosis of acute tubular necrosis or treatment with renal dialysis	Oliguria treated with intravenous fluids (no ICU admission)
Oliguria treated with multiple doses of furosemide	Oliguria treated with 1 dose of furosemide (no ICU admission)
Creatinine level ≥2.0 mg/dL in women without preexisting renal disease	—
Sepsis	
Inflection with hypotension with multiple liters of intravenous fluid or pressors used (septic shock)	Fever >38.5° C with increased lactate level alone without hypotension
Inflection with pulmonary complications such as pulmonary edema or acute respiratory distress syndrome	Fever >38.5°C with presumed chorioamnionitis/endometritis with increased pulse but no other cardiovascular sign and normal lactate level Positive blood culture without other evidence of significant systemic
Pulmonary	
Diagnosis of acute respiratory distress syndrome, pulmonary edema, or postoperative pneumonia	Administration of oxygen without a pulmonary diagnosis
Use of a ventilator (with either intubation or noninvasive technique)	—
Deep vein thrombosis or pulmonary embolism	—
Cardiac	
Preexisting cardiac disease (congenital or acquired) with ICU admission for treatment	Preexisting cardiac disease (congenital or acquired) with ICU admission for observation only
Peripartum cardiomyopathy	Preexisting cardiac disease (congenital or acquired) without ICU admission for observation only
Arrhythmia requiring >1 does of intravenous medication but not ICU admission	Arrhythmia requiring 1 dose of intravenous medication but no ICU admission
ICU/Invasive Monitoring	
Any ICU admission that includes treatment or diagnostic or therapeutic procedure	ICU admission for observation of hypertension that does not require intravenous medication
Central line or pulmonary catheter used to monitor a complication	ICU admission for observation after general anesthesia
Surgical, Bladder, and Bowel complications	
Bowel or bladder injury during surgery beyond minor serosal tear	

(*continued on next page*)

Table 1
(*continued*)

SMM	Not Severe Morbidity (Insufficient Evidence If This Is the Only Criterion)
Small-bowel obstruction, with or without surgery during pregnancy/postpartum period	—
Prolonged ileus for ≥4 d	Postoperative ileus that resolved without surgery in ≤3 d
Anesthesia Complications	
Total spinal anesthesia	—
Aspiration pneumonia	Failed spinal anesthesia that requires general anesthesia
Epidural hematoma	Spinal headache treated with a blood patch

Abbreviations: HELLP, hemolysis, elevated liver enzymes, and low platelet count; ICU, intensive care unit.

Adapted from Main EK, Abreo A, McNulty J, et al. Measuring severe maternal morbidity: validation of potential measures. Am J Obstet Gynecol 2016;214(5):643.e1-643.e10; with permission.

factors, and risk factors and resources, as they relate to maternal health and well-being. As is explained later, there is considerable overlap and intertwining influence between these categories.

Racism

Although there are many historically relevant racial and ethnic narratives that are likely responsible for other disparities, each of which deserves equally thorough coverage, this discussion focusses on black women given the current enormous gap in maternal care. As late as 1972, the United States was still involved in the Tuskegee Syphilis study, in which black men were knowingly withheld treatment of syphilis.[19] This egregious display of governmentally endorsed, ethically corrupt, prolonged, and formalized racism is one of many that cultivated a deep distrust in many black Americans of the health care system. This distrust persists today and may be partially responsible for lower rates of participation in medical research by black patients, who have reported much higher rates of distrust in the medical research process.[20,21] This distrust leaves a knowledge vulnerability at the intersection of racial disparities in SMM with black women's potential unwillingness to participate in prospective research studies,[15,20,21] especially given that an overwhelming number of obstetric care providers (obstetricians, anesthesiologists, nurse midwives, certified registered nurse anesthetists, physician assistants, and nurses) are white.[22–26]

Disparities in maternal care in the United States must include a conversation of the historical treatment of black women, specifically African Americans. For these women, certain historical medical practices that shaped their interactions with health care have been collapsed by Prather and colleagues[27] into 4 distinct periods: during legalized slavery (AD 1619–1865), black codes/Jim Crow laws (AD 1865–1965), during the civil rights movement (AD 1955–1975), and the post–civil rights era (AD 1975 to present). They included institutional abuse, rape, and experimentation for perfecting surgical techniques, often without anesthesia (see **Table 4** for details). The horrors that these women endured as a result of their systematic and continued racism and disenfranchisement cannot be forgotten or discounted, because they affect current and future public health initiatives designed to reduce disparities.[27] An unsettling and

Table 2
Examples of racial/ethnic disparities in health outcomes classified by severe maternal morbidity indicator

Severe Maternal Morbidity Indicator	Disparities Identified in Current Literature Search
Acute MI	Increased cardiovascular risk factors among AA women; some literature finds increased MI risk among non-Hispanic white and AA women
ARF	Increased among AA and American Indian/Alaska native; AA and Hispanic women with lupus erythematosus at increased risk of ARF
Acute respiratory distress syndrome	Increased among AA and American Indian/Alaska native women
Amniotic fluid embolism	Conflicting reports in the literature; some suggest an increase among AA women
Aneurysm	No literature exists
Blood transfusion	Increased among AA women
Cardiac arrest or ventricular fibrillation	Increased among AA women
Cardiac monitoring	Increased among AA, Hispanic, Asian/Pacific Islander, and American Indian/Alaska native women
Conversion of cardiac rhythm	Increased among AA women
Disseminated intravascular coagulation	Increased among AA, Hispanic, Asian/Pacific Islander, and American Indian/Alaska native women
Eclampsia	Increased among AA and Hispanic women
Heart failure during procedure or surgery	Increased among AA, Hispanic, and Asian/Pacific Islander women
Hysterectomy	Increased among AA, Hispanic, and Asian/Pacific Islander women
Internal injuries of thorax, abdomen, and pelvis	Increased among AA women
Intracranial injuries	No literature exists
Operations on heart and pericardium	Increased among AA women
Puerperal cerebrovascular disorders	Subarachnoid hemorrhage increased among AA and Hispanic women, intracerebral hemorrhage and stroke increased among AA women
Pulmonary edema	Increased among AA and Asian/Pacific Islander women
Sepsis	Increased among AA and Hispanic women
Severe anesthesia complications	Increased among AA women; use of general anesthesia may also be increased among AA women
Shock	Increased among AA, Asian/Pacific Islander, and American Indian/Alaska native women
Sickle cell anemia with crisis	Increased among AA women
Temporary tracheostomy	Increased among AA women

(continued on next page)

Table 2
(*continued*)

Severe Maternal Morbidity Indicator	Disparities Identified in Current Literature Search
Thrombotic embolism	Increased among AA women; thrombotic risk factors differ among non-Hispanic white and AA women
Ventilation	Increased among AA, Hispanic, Asian/Pacific Islander, and American Indian/Alaska native women
Additional indicators of morbidity	—
Cardiomyopathy	Increased among AA women
Preeclampsia/HELLP	Increased among AA and American Indian/ Alaska native women
Hemorrhage	Increased among Hispanic and Asian/Pacific Islander women; conflicting data regarding AA women

Abbreviations: AA, African American; ARF, acute renal failure; MI, myocardial infarction.
Adapted from Holdt Somer SJ, Sinkey RG, Bryant AS. Epidemiology of racial/ethnic disparities in severe maternal morbidity and mortality. Semin Perinatol 2017;41(5):261; with permission.

enlightening *New York Times Magazine* edition, *The 1619 Project*, contains a collection of essays describing the previously untold sufferings of many black men and women in America, which augments understanding of the torture they endured, not just during slavery but for the subsequent centuries.[28]

As early as 2003, the Institute of Medicine highlighted racism, prejudice, and provider bias as drivers of health disparities in their sentinel report, *Unequal Treatment: Confronting Racial and Ethnic Disparities in Health Care*, which described that effects of socioeconomic differences could not explain the imbalance in care for conditions even with well-established, straightforward guidelines, such as cardiovascular catheterization, cancer diagnostic tests, and antiretroviral therapy for human immunodeficiency virus.[29] Even the hint of racism and prejudice precludes trusting provider-patient relationships; this dynamic apparently may be overcome by pairing black physicians with black patients, who are more likely to undergo recommended preventive tests, with a potential cardiovascular mortality benefit estimated near 20%.[30]

Overt racism may not be the sole reason behind widespread provider-driven disparities; much research into biases has shared that provider bias may be explicit (obvious, expressed openly) or implicit (hidden, subconscious). Although racism itself may be classified as an explicit bias, implicit biases act in a more insidious manner, often existing at the margins of awareness, directing behavior even while the person is not fully conscious of the negative bias.[31] Implicit biases are not unique to medicine and are found anywhere complex decisions are made and the need for cognitive shortcuts or heuristics is high, such as in the criminal justice system and law enforcement,[32] because biases are a primary pathway for the brain to recognize patterns, without the process of slower, analytical thinking.[33] It is well known that explicit biases can be spread easily through verbal messages.[34] However, what is striking is how pervasive these implicit biases can be, as seen through a social learning theory lens, which posits that nonverbal cues are influential in defining attitudes toward others. Thus, implicit biases can be created and perpetuated in everyday social

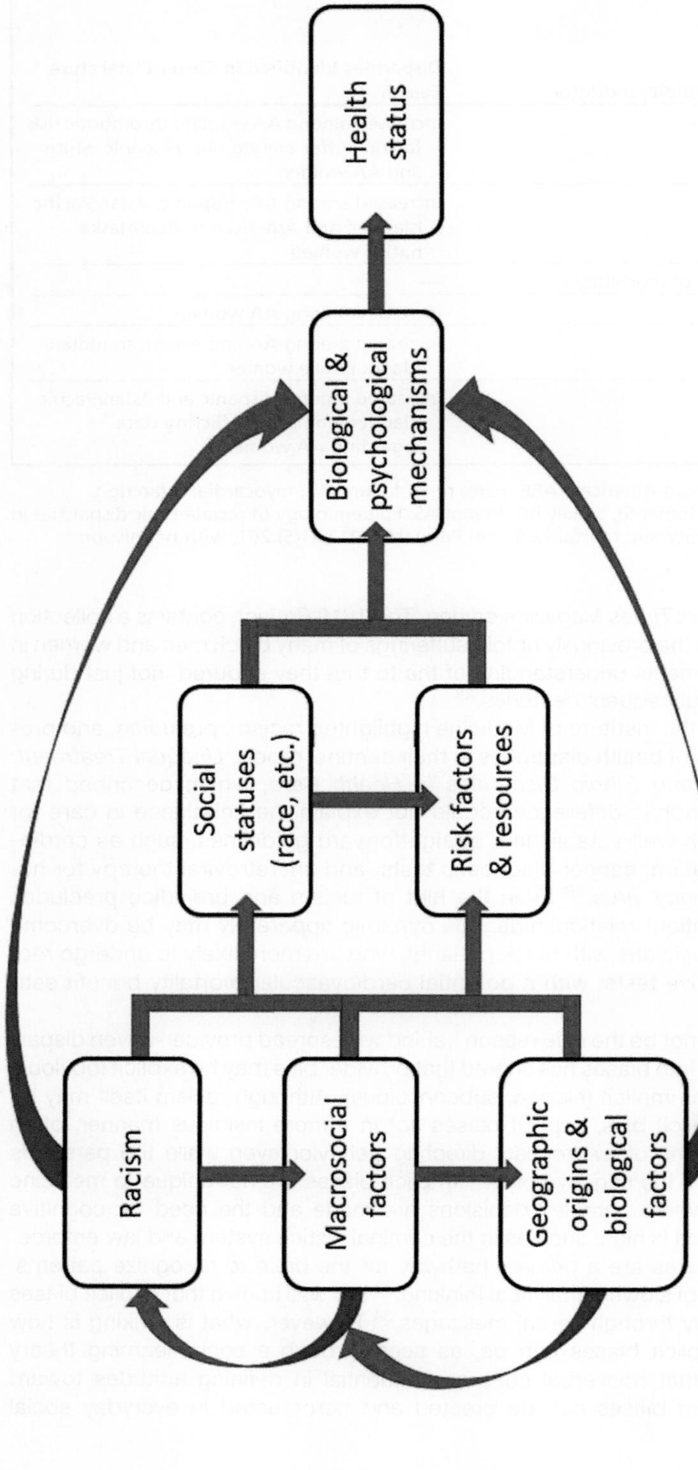

Fig. 1. A framework for understanding the relationship between race and health. (*Adapted from* Williams DR, Lavizzo-Mourey R, Warren RC. The concept of race and health status in America. Public Health Rep 1994;109(1):28; with permission.)

Table 3
Factors involved in the relationship between race and health

Factor	Definitions and Examples
Racism	Racial ideology (categorization or ranking), prejudice, or discrimination (individual or institutional) E.g., a black mother is not prescribed adequate opioid pain relief because her provider believes black women do not experience as much pain
Macrosocial factors	Historical conditions, economic structures, political order, legal codes, and social cultural institutions E.g., black people are generally underrepresented in medical research given their historical mistreatment and abuse, and therefore are more distrustful of medical researchers
Biological factors	Morphologic, physiologic, biochemical, or genetic factors E.g., chronic stress manifested physically results in higher rates of chronic hypertension, diabetes, and other cardiovascular comorbidities in black mothers than in white mothers
Social status	Race or ethnicity, socioeconomic status, sex, social roles, geographic location, or age E.g., black mothers are more likely to live in impoverished environments compared with white mothers, and are more likely to be uninsured
Risk factors and resources	Health behaviors; stress; medical care; social ties; or psychological, cultural, or religious factors E.g., black mothers are more likely to deliver in hospitals with much higher rates of severe maternal morbidity and mortality

Data from Williams DR, Lavizzo-Mourey R, Warren RC. The concept of race and health status in America. Public Health Rep 1994;109(1):26-41.

interactions in which people's nonverbal behaviors (body language, facial expressions) are shared.[34] Researchers have attempted to determine how much implicit bias shapes medical practice, but a recent systematic review revealed serious methodological limitations in published medical literature, much of which was lacking a strong theoretic basis.[31] A potential source of robust theory may come from the social psychology and organizational behavior literature on racial diversity, which has spent decades determining what processes are at play between individuals of different races and creating standardized tools to study those processes and interactions.[35–39]

Although provider bias training is advocated,[31] it has not been shown to change outcomes in bias when given in small "doses" related to raising awareness of bias.[40] Only intensive behavior-change techniques have been shown to be effective in altering implicit racial biases, which involve considerable time, financial resources, and personnel resources.[35,41] As investigators continue to explore the impacts of bias on disparities in care, through improving theoretic approaches and application of behavior-change principles, perhaps new frontiers will emerge as helpful in mitigating or modifying implicit biases (eg, more automated technology using risk stratification).

Biological Factors

The allure of a simple explanation for racial differences in health outcomes, especially those related to genetic factors, seems to be compelling, despite multitudinous evidence to the contrary.[16,17,30] As mentioned earlier, except for heritable diseases

Table 4
Historical and contemporary sexual-related and reproductive-related health and health care experiences of African American women

Period	Time Span	Number of Years	Personal Experiences of AA Women that Contribute to Disparities in Sexual and Reproductive Health	Health Care Experiences of AA Women that Contribute to Disparities
Slavery	1619–1865	246	Public, nude physical auction examinations to determine reproductive ability; raped for sexual pleasure and economic purpose; purposely aborting pregnancies where rape occurred; Jezebel stereotype emerged of black women being hypersexual; generational poverty	Nonconsensual gynecologic and reproductive surgeries performed at times repeatedly on female slaves without anesthesia, including cesarean sections and ovariotomy to perfect medical procedures
Black codes/ Jim Crow	1865–1965	100	Rape; lynching (genitalia/ reproductive mutilation); uncertain/unequal civil rights; stereotypes and negative media portrayals continued; generational poverty	Nonconsensual medical experiments continued; poor or no health care for impoverished blacks; compulsory sterilization; Jim Crow laws enforced lack of access to quality health care services and opportunities; effects of Tuskegee Untreated Syphilis Study on women (eg, some wives of untreated subjects acquired syphilis and their children incurred consequences of congenital syphilis)
Civil rights	1955–1975	20	Lynching, uncertain/ unequal civil rights and violence against women to show superiority and control; stereotypes and negative hypersexual medial portrayals continued; generational poverty	Nonconsensual medical experiments continued; compulsory sterilization for recipients of federal funding; effects of Tuskegee Untreated Syphilis Study on women; unequal health care services as a result of both overt and subtle racism
Post–civil rights	1975–2018	43	Black exploitation movies, media's hypersexual images continued; generational poverty	Unequal health care continued; targeted sterilizations, hysterectomies, abortions, and birth control

Adapted from Prather C, Fuller TR, Jeffries WL, et al. Racism, African American women, and their sexual and reproductive health: a review of historical and contemporary evidence and implications for health equity. Health Equity 2018;2(1):251; with permission.

such as certain thrombophilias and hemoglobinopathies, many of the biological changes are thought to be caused by chronic exposure to stress through experiences of prejudice and discrepancies in social standing, which manifests in tangible ways to produce "weathering," also known as the "physical consequence of social inequality."[42] Weathering is rarely found among white mothers but is overwhelmingly noted in African American women in poor neighborhoods; this manifests by low-birthweight neonates, preterm birth, and small-for-gestational-age births, and mitigates when African American mothers were situated in the upper half of neighborhoods for income and had also never resided in low-income neighborhoods.[43]

A possible biological explanation is that this is may be caused by leukocyte chromosomal telomere shortening from enhanced telomerase activity leading to accelerated aging; telomeres are otherwise known as protective "caps" at the end of chromosomes that consist of repeated nucleotides.[44] A link has been established between telomere shortening and both duration and amount of stress experienced by mothers caring for ill children,[45] and with shorter telomere length for African American women (but not men) living in poor and racially segregated neighborhoods.[46] More recently, the magnitude of distrust and anger expressed was associated with reduced telomere length in African American women involved in the Jackson Heart Study.[47] In addition, telomere length is heritable to some degree, as shown by black mothers having shorter telomeres than white mothers, and black male neonates having shorter telomeres than white male neonates.[48] It is unclear whether telomere length itself is the appropriate measure. Needham and colleagues[49] showed attenuation in racial and ethnic differences for telomere length when baseline telomere length was taken into consideration for 1169 participants in the Multi-Ethnic Study of Atherosclerosis (MESA), and most telomere shortening was eventually seen in older people and in men when adjusting for baseline length. Clearly, there is a great need to understand the links between psychological and physical stress and resulting mechanisms that lead to disease manifestation and worse health for black mothers.

Risk Factors and Resources

This category is broad and includes both patient-related factors as well as system-wide influences. This article mainly focuses on medical care delivered at a hospital level, because this is most pertinent to anesthesiologists intersecting with these women during their pregnancies; the factors influencing hospital care are represented in **Fig. 2**.[50] There is room for dramatic improvement to prevent SMM and mortality, because there exist enormous between-hospital differences in care, even within the same large metropolitan city (such as New York City), and these racial differences may account for nearly 48% of the racial disparity seen there.[50,51]

Black women may deliver in hospitals that primarily serve a black population, and these hospitals have been shown to have higher rates of SMM compared with hospitals primarily serving white women.[52] This trend may stem from a variety of factors, including organizational issues such as leadership influences, a culture of safety, active teamwork practices, and use of bundles to improve maternal care.[50] Safety practices such as bundle implementation are critical for maternal safety because they have been shown to empower all health care providers to initiate critical steps to mitigate delays in treatment.[53] Recently, the National Partnership for Maternal Safety developed a consensus statement introducing a maternal safety bundle designed to reduce peripartum racial and ethnic disparities in care.[54] A large proportion of the bundle is designed to improve safety culture, which is a known link to patient safety.[55,56]

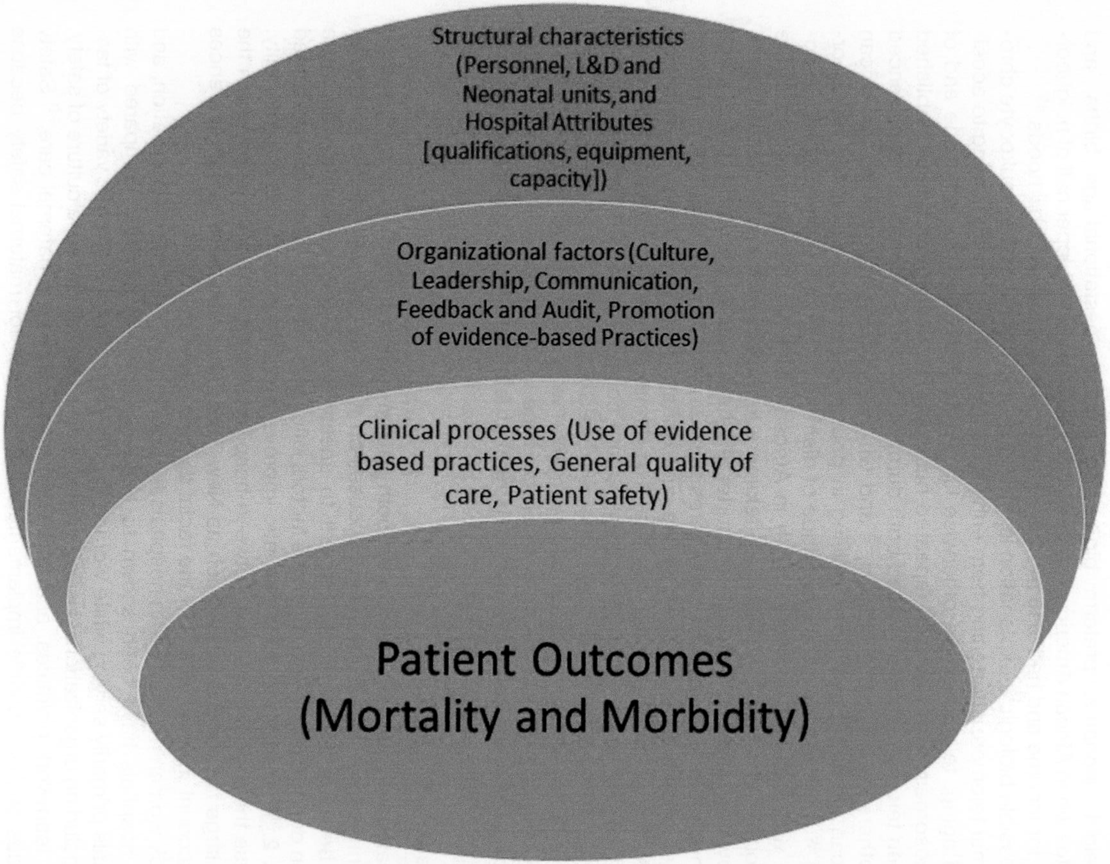

Fig. 2. Hospital quality and severe maternal morbidity: structural factors. L&D, labor and delivery. (*Adapted from* Howell EA, Zeitlin J. Improving hospital quality to reduce disparities in severe maternal morbidity and mortality. Semin Perinatol 2017;41(5):267; with permission.)

NATIONAL EFFORTS TO REDUCE RACIAL DISPARITIES IN OBSTETRICS

In the past, mothers were stratified to care centers based on their fetuses' well-being. Fetal deaths (>20 weeks' estimated gestational age) continue to be unacceptably high for black mothers. Black women's fetuses die at a rate of 10.8 per 1000 as of 2016, which is the highest of all racial and ethnic groups, and more than double that of white mothers (at 5 per 1000).[57] Historically, obstetric focus on fetal health and status has made providers systematically neglectful of mothers, especially black mothers. Since the ACOG Levels of Maternal Care initiative,[10] the Society for Obstetric Anesthesia and Perinatology (SOAP) has developed and implemented a designation of a SOAP Center of Excellence (COE)[58] in an effort to bring maternal health back to the forefront of obstetric care. To date, there have been 39 COEs designated, which represent a broad range of practice types (from academic centers to community hospitals) based in the United States as well as internationally.[59]

However, much of the care given in the labor and postpartum units is delivered by nurses, who may not be up to date on many of the maternal conditions, or on racial contributions to poorer maternal outcomes. A recent survey assessed postpartum nurses' reported knowledge and practices and found that only 54% of nurses knew of increasing maternal mortality, and 93% misattributed hemorrhage as the leading cause of death, rather than cardiovascular disease.[60] In addition, it has been reported that nurses may not always provide consistent, evidence-based discharge and postpartum education to patients, underscoring the need for sweeping, comprehensive educational efforts in this provider group as well.[61]

ANESTHESIOLOGISTS' ROLES IN IMPROVING MATERNAL CARE FOR BLACK MOTHERS

Anesthesiologists can make a substantial difference in maternal outcomes. After adjustment for many factors, including socioeconomic, demographic, prenatal care, and organizational features, severe obstetric hemorrhage was found to be associated with lack of an on-site, 24-hour anesthesiologist as well as with hospitals in which fewer than 500 deliveries per year occurred.[62] A recent article highlighted the role that anesthesiologists play in acting as the labor and delivery unit "peridelivery intensivist,"[63] submitting that anesthesiologists have cultivated a unique set of skills and knowledge to treat specific morbidities that other maternal care providers may not possess.

Outside of SMM and mortality, disparities exist in use of epidural analgesia for labor, specifically for black and Hispanic women who receive epidurals at lower rates.[64–66] The reasons for this are multifactorial,[65] and are postulated to be:

- Minority patients are less likely to have the same access to care as nonminority patients
- Physician bias toward nonminority patients may exist
- Minority patients mistrust the medical system, so compliance in following provider recommendations is poor
- Nonminority patients may demand more care than minority patients[65]

Lower use of labor epidural analgesia may be a precipitating factor for black women being more likely to receive general anesthesia for cesarean delivery.[66] Recent links have been shown between higher rates of morbidity in women who were deemed to be candidates to receive neuraxial anesthesia for cesarean delivery but received general anesthesia instead.[67] Guglielminotti and colleagues[67] found that racial or ethnic minority women were more likely to receive a potentially avoidable general anesthetic than white mothers, highlighting another area for anesthesiologists to improve care discrepancies through understanding and addressing problems present. Of note, it has been suggested that anesthesiologists who were obstetric fellowship-trained were less likely than non–fellowship-trained anesthesiologists to induce general anesthesia for cesarean delivery in the presence of an existing labor epidural catheter.[68] More research is needed to uncover and address the drivers of these differences.

In addition, obstetric anesthesiologists are leaders in patient safety and innovation[69] and have developed techniques to better understand teamwork and communication in obstetrics,[70] as well as proactively designed interventions to facilitate best teamwork practices, including encouraging speaking up.[71,72] Teamwork training in hospitals has been largely associated with better patient outcomes,[55,73] and large malpractice insurers, such as the Risk Management Foundation of the Harvard Teaching Institutions (also known as Controlled Risk Insurance Company [CRICO]), have incentivized a malpractice insurance premium reduction for anesthesiologists and obstetricians who undergo yearly team-based simulation training and drills in obstetric emergencies.[74,75]

SUMMARY

Racism in America has deep roots that affect maternal health, particularly through pervasive inequalities among black women compared with white. Anesthesiologists are optimally positioned to maintain vigilance for these disparities in maternal care, and to intervene with their unique acute critical care skills and knowledge. As leaders in patient safety, anesthesiologists should drive hospitals and practices to develop and implement national bundles for patient safety, as well as using team-based training practices designed to improve hospitals that care for racially diverse mothers.

DISCLOSURE

The authors have nothing to disclose.

REFERENCES

1. Kassebaum N. Global, regional, and national levels of maternal mortality, 1990-2015: a systematic analysis for the Global Burden of Disease Study 2015. Lancet 2016;388(10053):1775–812.
2. MacDorman MF, Declercq E, Cabral H, et al. Recent Increases in the U.S. maternal mortality rate: disentangling trends from measurement issues. Obstet Gynecol 2016;128(3):447–55.
3. Petersen EE, Davis NL, Goodman D, et al. Vital signs: pregnancy-related deaths, United States, 2011–2015, and strategies for prevention, 13 states, 2013–2017. MMWR Morb Mortal Wkly Rep 2019;68:423–9. https://doi.org/10.15585/mmwr.mm6818e1. Available at: https://doi.org/10.15585/mmwr.mm6818e1. Accessed August 14, 2019.
4. Neighmond P. Why racial gaps in maternal mortality persist. Washington, DC: National Public Radio; 2019. Available at: https://www.npr.org/sections/health-shots/2019/05/10/722143121/why-racial-gaps-in-maternal-mortality-persist. Accessed August 14, 2019.
5. Delbanco S, Lehan M, Montalvo T, et al. The rising U.S. maternal mortality rate demands action from employers. Harv Bus Rev 2019. Available at: https://hbr.org/2019/06/the-rising-u-s-maternal-mortality-rate-demands-action-from-employers. Accessed August 14, 2019.

6. Stobbe M, Marchione M. US pregnancy deaths are up, especially among minorities. New York: Associated Press; 2019. Available at: https://www.apnews.com/4907da5c58c84a708a548c4ea18fc5c7. Accessed August 14, 2019.
7. Racial and ethnic disparities in obstetrics and gynecology. Committee Opinion No. 649. American College of Obstetricians and Gynecologists. Obstet Gynecol 2015;126:e130–4.
8. ACOG Postpartum Toolkit. Racial disparities in maternal mortality in the United States: the postpartum period is a missed opportunity for action. 2018. Available at: https://www.acog.org/-/media/Departments/Toolkits-for-Health-Care-Providers/Postpartum-Toolkit/ppt-racial.pdf?dmc=1&ts=20190814T1957346976. Accessed August 14, 2019.
9. Black mamas matter alliance. 2019. Available at: http://blackmamasmatter.org/. Accessed March 1, 2018.
10. American College of Obstetricians and Gynecologists and Society for Maternal-Fetal Medicine, Menard MK, Kilpatrick S, Saade G, et al. Levels of maternal care. Am J Obstet Gynecol 2015;212(3):259–71.
11. Gelber K, Kahwajian H, Geller AW, et al. Obstetric anesthesiology in the United States: current and future demand for fellowship-trained subspecialists. Anesth Analg 2018;127(6):1445–7.
12. Holdt Somer SJ, Sinkey RG, Bryant AS. Epidemiology of racial/ethnic disparities in severe maternal morbidity and mortality. Semin Perinatol 2017;41:258–65.
13. Admon LK, Winkelman TNA, Zivin K, et al. Racial and ethnic disparities in the incidence of severe maternal morbidity in the United States, 2012-2015. Obstet Gynecol 2018;132:1158–66.
14. Callaghan WM, Creanga AA, Kuklina EV. Severe maternal morbidity among delivery and postpartum hospitalizations in the United States. Obstet Gynecol 2012;120:1029–36.
15. American College of Obstetricians and Gynecologists and Society for Maternal-Fetal Medicine, Kilpatrick SK, Ecker JL, Callaghan WM. Severe maternal morbidity: screening and review. Obstetric Care Consensus No. 5. Obstet Gynecol 2016;128:e54–60.
16. Williams DR, Lavizzo-Mourey R, Warren RC. The concept of race and health status in America. Public Health Rep 1994;109(1):26–41.
17. Dressler WW, Oths KS, Gravlee CC. Race and ethnicity in public health research: models to explain health disparities. Annu Rev Anthropol 2005;34:231–52.
18. U.S. Department of Health and Human Services, Centers for Disease Control and Prevention, National Center for Health Statistics. Summary health statistics: national health interview survey, 2016. Table A-11a, pages 1-9. Available at: https://ftp.cdc.gov/pub/Health_Statistics/NCHS/NHIS/SHS/2016_SHS_Table_A-11.pdf. Accessed August 15, 2019.
19. Kennedy BR, Mathis CC, Woods AK. African Americans and their distrust of the health care system: healthcare for diverse populations. J Cult Divers 2007;14(2):56–60.
20. Corbie-Smith G, Thomas SB, St. George DM. Distrust, race, and research. Arch Intern Med 2002;162(21):2458–63.
21. Shavers VL, Lynch CF, Burmeister LF. Racial differences in factors that influence the willingness to participate in medical research studies. Ann Epidemiol 2002;12:248–56.
22. Association of American Medical Colleges. Physician specialty data report. 1.3. Active physicians by sex and specialty, 2017. 2018. Available at: https://www.aamc.org/data/workforce/reports/492560/1-3-chart.html. Retrieved August 4, 2019.

23. Medscape lifestyle report 2017: race and ethnicity, bias and burnout. Available at: https://www.medscape.com/sites/public/lifestyle/2017. Accessed August 4, 2019.
24. Data USA: registered nurses. Available at: https://datausa.io/profile/soc/registered-nurses#demographics. Accessed August 5, 2019.
25. Data USA: nurse practitioners & nurse midwives. Available at: https://datausa.io/profile/soc/2911XX/#demographics. Accessed August 5, 2019.
26. National Commission on Certification of Physician Assistants. Statistical profile of certified physician assistants by specialty annual report. 2018. Available at: http://prodcmsstoragesa.blob.core.windows.net/uploads/files/2018StatisticalProfileofCertifiedPAsbySpecialty1.pdf. Accessed August 5, 2019.
27. Prather C, Fuller TR, Jeffries WL, et al. Racism, African American women, and their sexual and reproductive health: a review of historical and contemporary evidence and implications for health equity. Health Equity 2018;2(1):249–59.
28. The 1619 Project. The New York Times Magazine. 2019. Available at: https://www.nytimes.com/interactive/2019/08/14/magazine/1619-america-slavery.html. Accessed September 1, 2019.
29. Institute of Medicine. Unequal treatment: confronting racial and ethnic disparities in health care (with CD). Washington, DC: The National Academies Press; 2003. https://doi.org/10.17226/12875. Retrieved August 12, 2019.
30. Alsan M, Garrick O, Graziani GC. Does diversity matter for health? Experimental evidence from Oakland. Working Paper 24787, NBER Working Paper Series. 2019. Available at: https://www.nber.org/papers/w24787. Retrieved August 4, 2019.
31. Hall WJ, Chapman MV, Lee KM, et al. Implicit racial/ethnic bias among health care professionals and its influence on health care outcomes: a systematic review. Am J Public Health 2015;105(12):e60–76.
32. Pereda B, Montoya M. Addressing implicit bias to improve cross-cultural care. Clin Obstet Gynecol 2018;61(1):2–9.
33. Stiegler MP, Tung A. Cognitive processes in anesthesiology decision making. Anesthesiology 2014;120(1):204–17.
34. Skinner AL, Perry S. Are attitudes contagious? Exposure to biased nonverbal signals can create novel social attitudes. Pers Soc Psychol Bull 2019. 146167219862616. Retrieved September 1, 2019.
35. Hagiwara N, Elston Lafata J, Mezuk B, et al. Detecting implicit racial bias in provider communication behaviors to reduce disparities in healthcare: challenges, solutions, and future direction for provider communication training. Patient Educ Couns 2019;102:1738–43.
36. Boon H, Steward M. Patient-physician communication assessment instruments: 986 to 1996 in review. Patient Educ Couns 1998;35:161–76.
37. Schirmer JM, Mauksch L, Lang F, et al. Assessing communication competence: a review of current tools. Fam Med 2005;37:184–92.
38. Foldy EG, Rivard P, Buckley TR. Power, safety, and learning in racially diverse groups. Acad Manage Learn Educ 2009;8(1):25–41.
39. Avery DR, Richeson JA, Hebl MR, et al. It does not have to be uncomfortable: the role of behavioral scripts in black-white interracial interactions. J Appl Psychol 2009;94:1382–93.
40. Devine PG, Forscher PS, Austin AJ, et al. Long-term reduction in implicit race bias: a prejudice habit-breaking intervention. J Exp Soc Psychol 2012;48:1267–78.

41. Gawronski B, Bodenhausen GV. Associative and propositional processes in evaluation: an integrative review of implicit and explicit attitude change. Psychol Bull 2006;132:692–731.
42. Geronimus AT. Black/white differences in the relationship of maternal age to birthweight: a population-based test of the weathering hypothesis. Social Sci Med 1996;42(4):589–97.
43. Love C, David RJ, Rankin KM, et al. Exploring weathering: effects of lifelong economic environment and maternal age on low birth weight, small for gestational age, and preterm birth in African-American and White women. Am J Epidemiol 2010;172(2):127–34.
44. Aubert G, Landsorp PM. Telomeres and aging. Physiol Rev 2008;88(2):557–79.
45. Epel ES, Blackburn EH, Lin J, et al. Accelerated telomere shortening in response to life stress. Proc Natl Acad Sci U S A 2004;101(49):17312–5.
46. Gebreab SY, Riestra P, Gaye A, et al. Perceived neighborhood problems are associated with shorter telomere length in African American women. Psychoneuroendocrinology 2016;69:90–7.
47. Jordan CD, Glover LM, Gao Y, et al. Association of psychosocial factors with leukocyte telomere length among African Americans in the Jackson Heart Study. Stress Health 2019;35(2):138–45.
48. Weber KA, Heaphy CM, Joshu CE, et al. Racial differences in maternal and umbilical cord blood leukocyte telomere length and their correlations. Cancer Causes Control 2018;29(8):759–67.
49. Needham BL, Wang X, Carroll JE, et al. Sociodemographic correlates of change in leukocyte telomere length during mid- to late-life: the Multi-Ethnic Study of Atherosclerosis. Psychoneuroendocrinology 2019;102:182–8.
50. Howell EA, Zeitlin J. Improving hospital quality to reduce disparities in severe maternal morbidity and mortality. Semin Perinatol 2017;41(5):266–72.
51. New York City Department of Health and Mental Hygiene. Bureau of maternal and child health. Pregnancy-Associated Mortality New York City, 2006–2010. New York: NYC Health; 2015. Available at: https://www1.nyc.gov/assets/doh/downloads/pdf/ms/pregnancy-associated-mortality-report.pdf.
52. Howell EA, Egorova N, Balbierz A, et al. Black-white differences in severe maternal morbidity and site of care. Am J Obstet Gynecol 2016;214(1):122.e1-7.
53. U.S. Department of Health and Human Services Agency for Healthcare Research and Quality. Patient safety primer: maternal safety. 2019. Available at: https://psnet.ahrq.gov/primers/primer/50/Maternal-Safety. Accessed September 1, 2019.
54. Howell EA, Brown H, Brumley J, et al. Reduction of peripartum racial and ethnic disparities: a conceptual framework and maternal safety consensus bundle. Obstet Gynecol 2018;131:770–82.
55. Manser T. Teamwork and patient safety in dynamic domains of healthcare: a review of the literature. Acta Anaesthesiol Scand 2009;53:143–51.
56. Edmondson AC. Psychological safety and learning behavior in work teams. Administrative Sci Q 1999;44:350–83.
57. Healthy people 2020, fetal deaths (per 1,000 live births plus fetal deaths, 20+ weeks gestation) by race/ethnicity (of mother). Available at HealthyPeople.gov. Available at: https://www.healthypeople.gov/2020/data/Chart/4823?category=3&by=Race/Ethnicity%20(of%20mother)&fips=-1. Accessed August 14, 2019.
58. Society for Obstetric Anesthesia and Perinatology. Centers of excellence. Available at: https://soap.org/grants/center-of-excellence/. Accessed September 1, 2019.
59. Society for Obstetric Anesthesia and Perinatology. Society for Obstetric Anesthesia and Perinatology (SOAP) announces recipients of the 2018 SOAP Center

of Excellence (COE) designation. Available at: https://soap.org/wp-content/uploads/2019/06/2018-SOAP-Center-of-Excellence-Recipients-Press-Release.pdf. Accessed September 1, 2019.
60. Suplee PD, Bingham D, Kleppel L. Nurses' knowledge and teaching of possible postpartum complications. MCN Am J Matern Child Nurs 2017;42(6):338–44.
61. Suplee PD, Kleppel L, Santa-Donato A, et al. Improving postpartum education about warning signs of maternal morbidity and mortality. Nurs Womens Health 2017;20(6):552–67.
62. Bouvier-Colle M-H, Ould El Joud D, Varnoux N, et al. Evaluation of the quality of care for severe obstetrical haemorrhage in three French regions. BJOG 2001; 108(9):898–903.
63. McQuaid E, Leffert LR, Bateman BT. The role of the anesthesiologist in preventing severe maternal morbidity and mortality. Clin Obstet Gynecol 2018;61(2):372–86.
64. Glance LG, Wissler R, Glantz C, et al. Racial differences in the use of epidural analgesia for labor. Anesthesiology 2007;106:19–25.
65. Toledo P, Caballero JA. Racial and ethnic disparities in obstetrics and obstetric anesthesia in the United States. Curr Anesthesiol Rep 2013;3:292–9.
66. Lange EMS, Rao S, Toledo P. Racial and ethnic disparities in obstetric anesthesia. Semin Perinatol 2017;41:293–8.
67. Guglielminotti J, Landau R, Li G. Adverse events and factors associated with potentially avoidable use of general anesthesia in cesarean deliveries. Anesthesiology 2019;130(6):912–22.
68. Wagner JL, White RS, Mauer EA, et al. Impact of anesthesiologist's fellowship status on the risk of general anesthesia for unplanned cesarean delivery. Acta Anaesthesiol Scand 2019;63(6):769–74.
69. Birnbach DJ, Bateman BT. Obstetric anesthesia: leading the way in patient safety. Obstet Gynecol Clin North Am 2019;46:329–37.
70. Minehart RD, Pian-Smith MC, Walzer TB, et al. Speaking across the drapes: communication strategies of anesthesiologists and obstetricians during a simulated maternal crisis. Simul Healthc 2012;7(3):166–70.
71. Pian-Smith MC, Simon R, Minehart RD, et al. Teaching residents the two-challenge rule: a simulation-based approach to improve education and patient safety. Simul Healthc 2009;4(2):84–91.
72. Raemer DB, Kolbe M, Minehart RD, et al. Improving anesthesiologists' ability to speak up in the operating room: a randomized controlled experiment of a simulation-based intervention and a qualitative analysis of hurdles and enablers. Acad Med 2016;91(4):530–9.
73. Hughes AM, Gregory ME, Joseph DL, et al. Saving lives: a meta-analysis of team training in healthcare. J Appl Psychol 2016;101(9):1266–304.
74. Gardner R, Walzer TB, Simon R, et al. Obstetric simulation as a risk control strategy: course design and evaluation. Simul Healthc 2008;3(2):119–27.
75. CRICO. CRICO OB patient safety program. 2018. Available at: https://www.rmf.harvard.edu/Clinician-Resources/Article/2012/OB-Risk-Reduction-Program. Accessed September 1, 2019.

Perioperative Considerations Regarding Sex in Solid Organ Transplantation

Susan M. Walters, MD[a], Ellen W. Richter, MD[b], Tatiana Lutzker, MD[c], Suraj Patel, MD[c], Anita N. Vincent, MD[c], Amanda M. Kleiman, MD[a,*]

KEYWORDS

• Transplantation • Sex • Gender • Transplant listing • Mortality • Graft survival • Complications

KEY POINTS

- Sex and gender play a significant role in the preoperative and postoperative course of transplant surgeries.
- Differences are specific to the organ being transplanted.
- Pretransplant waiting list mortality and listing are affected by sex and gender.
- Sex affects graft survival, mortality, and complications following transplant.

Sex plays a pivotal role in all stages of the organ transplant process. In the preoperative phase, sex can affect being listed or considered for a transplant, and sex/size matching of organs is necessary for some organ transplants, thereby affecting organ availability. In the postoperative period, sex has a profound impact on complications as well as graft survival. Sex-related differences in organ transplantation are likely multifactorial related to biological and social characteristics. This article provides an overview of the impact of sex on various types of solid organ transplant, including kidney, pancreas, liver, lung, and heart transplants.

Funding: None.
[a] Department of Anesthesiology, University of Virginia Health System, PO Box 800710, Charlottesville, VA 22908, USA; [b] Department of Anesthesiology, Emory University School of Medicine, 1364 Clifton Road Northeast, Atlanta, GA 30322, USA; [c] Department of Anesthesiology and Critical Care Medicine, The George Washington University Medical Center, 900 23rd Street, Northwest, Washington, DC 20037, USA
* Corresponding author.
E-mail address: ak8zg@hscmail.mcc.virginia.edu

Anesthesiology Clin 38 (2020) 297–310
https://doi.org/10.1016/j.anclin.2020.01.008
1932-2275/20/Published by Elsevier Inc.

ORGAN DONATION

This article would be negligent without first briefly discussing overall sex-based differences in organ donation. Although deceased donors tend to be more men than women,[1] women show increased willingness to donate compared with men, which is further supported by the increased proportion of female living donors.[2] However, despite an increased willingness to donate, at their time of death, women tend to be older and more likely to die of cardiovascular causes, often preventing donation of organs.[2]

Table 1 summarizes the major preoperative and postoperative differences in the types of organ transplant discussed.

KIDNEY

Preoperative Care, Listing, and Donor Selection

According to the United Network for Organ Sharing (UNOS), the annual number of kidney transplants in 2018 was 21,167, with more than 450,000 in 30 years, making kidney the most common organ transplanted (59% of total organs transplanted).[3] There is a major gender discrepancy in kidney donation and

Table 1
Summary of sex and gender differences in solid organ transplantation

Organ	Preoperative	Postoperative
Kidney	• Higher rate of female donors & male recipients • Gender mismatch: female donor to male recipient worse outcomes for 5-y graft survival • Female recipients: higher risk of acute rejection; decreased risk of chronic rejection	• Male recipients: worst graft function, poorer long-term outcomes • Female recipients: increased psychosocial effects, poorer compliance, increased infection • Estrogen: positive effect on graft function. Testosterone: negative effect
Pancreas	• Female donors: higher rates of graft failure and shorter survival rates	• Female recipients: higher rates of acute rejection but better long-term outcomes
Liver	• Female recipients: higher waiting-list mortality caused by lower creatinine level and MELD for similar severity of illness; more likely to decline offer • Female donor to male recipient: worse graft function, outcomes	• Graft survival/mortality does not seem to differ by sex except in HCV • Female recipients: worse quality of life, higher rate of recidivism • Male recipients: higher rate of malignancy
Lung	• Female donors: worse outcomes, especially for male recipients	• Female recipients: improved graft function and long-term survival likely caused by estrogen effects; improved spirometry; lower quality of life • Male recipients: poorer outcomes; increased malignancy
Heart	• 75% of patients on waiting list are men • Women: improved waiting-list survival; paucity of appropriately sized organs for women • Gender mismatch = worse outcomes	• Comparable short-term survival • Female recipients: increased risk of antibody-mediated rejection; long-term survival advantage • Male recipients: higher rate of malignancy

Abbreviations: HCV, hepatitis C virus; MELD, Model for End-stage Liver Disease.

reception; specifically, more women are living kidney donors, whereas more men are kidney recipients even when accounting for the higher incidence of end-stage renal disease (ESRD) in men and slight predominance of women in the general population.[4] This phenomenon is present on a global level.[5] Notably, there is also a high rate of female-to-male spousal kidney donations, making up a large portion of the female-to-male donor-recipient discrepancy, because 80% of organ donations worldwide are blood related.[6] This finding may be representative of a pervasive cultural idea that women are more responsible for the health of their male partners or that men are generally unable to donate and be financially responsible for their families.[5] Some other reasons for this discrepancy have been postulated, including differences in incidence of renal disease, women being offered less aggressive care, and women being more risk averse to aggressive treatment options.[7] One study surveying US nephrologists showed they were less likely to recommend transplant to female patients.[8] This finding could partly be caused by the fact that female sex predicted better survival in patients with chronic kidney disease (CKD) managed conservatively, although the full explanation is unclear.[9] There is also less willingness for men to be kidney donors based on an American Society of Transplantation survey.[10] However, when considering open nephrectomy versus laparoscopic nephrectomy, the gender disparity between donors was significantly decreased in the laparoscopic nephrectomy group.[11]

The most common causes of ESRD in the United States are diabetic nephropathy and hypertensive nephrosclerosis, neither of which show a significant difference in incidence between the sexes.[12] Less common causes of ESRD include immunoglobulin A nephropathy, Fabry disease, and acquired immune deficiency syndrome nephropathy, which are more common in men, and lupus nephropathy, more common in women.[12] Overall, the incidence and prevalence of ESRD is greater in men, which is mainly attributable to the rate of renal function decline (slower in women with CKD),[13] likely caused by hormonal differences, with estrogen playing a protective role in renal pathophysiology.[14–16] The higher rate of kidney decline among men could contribute to women donating kidneys and men receiving kidneys at a higher rate.

The sex matching of donor and recipient also plays a significant role in outcomes. In 1 study, female-to-male donation resulted in worse 5-year graft survival compared with female-to-female, male-to-female, and male-to-male donation.[17] When breaking down survival into acute versus chronic rejection, female recipients have a higher risk of acute rejection but decreased risk of chronic rejection.[18] One study showed that the risk of early graft loss was increased if the donor was male.[19]

Postoperative Course and Outcomes

Recipient sex seems to more significantly affect renal allograft outcome compared with sex of the donor.[20] Male recipients had higher renal metabolic demands and worsened early graft function, represented by higher 24-hour urinary creatinine level and decreased estimated glomerular filtration rate (eGFR) after transplant.[21]

Hormonal influences also play a role in kidney function posttransplant. Ischemia-reperfusion injury occurs in 30% to 50% of renal allografts from deceased donors, contributing to delayed graft function or even primary nonfunction.[22] Estrogen seems to increase the tolerance of this process in renal allografts, helping reduce the incidence of delayed graft function.[23] In contrast, testosterone negatively affects renal graft function. One experimental rat model showed that removal of ovaries increases proteinuria and glomerulosclerosis after undergoing renal ablation.[24] However, ovariectomized rats treated with estradiol showed decreased proteinuria, glomerulosclerosis, and transforming growth factor (TGF)-β and platelet-derived growth factor levels after renal ablation.[24] Although tempting to assume that female hormonal factors are overwhelmingly protective, more recent studies have been inconsistent or even directly contrary to this finding, with no conclusive links between hormonal and genetic impacts on cellular apoptosis and antirejection drug metabolism, among other factors.[25]

Gender may play an important role in psychosocial issues surrounding renal transplants. A systematic review showed that female gender was associated with higher rates of noncompliance with medications posttransplant, along with patients who were unmarried, younger, or nonwhite.[26] Note that the review found that female gender, along with younger age, correlated with noncompliance. Although being married pretransplant is associated with better renal graft outcomes, this effect only remains present in male recipients when stratified by gender.[27] For women, psychosocial factors such as marital conflict are more often linked with worse physiologic and pathophysiologic outcomes, which could contribute to this discrepancy.[28] The negative association between female gender and psychosocial issues in renal transplantation may be caused by higher rates of psychiatric comorbidities, because female patients with ESRD have higher rates of depressed affect, anxiety, and personality disorder than male patients with ESRD.[29] With regard to health insurance coverage among kidney donors, male gender is associated with increased likelihood of being uninsured at the time of kidney donation, along with other factors, including minority status, unemployment, and less education.[30] For recipients, female gender and having public health insurance were independent factors associated with increased emergency department use in the first year after renal transplant.[31]

There are several adverse outcomes for renal allografts associated with male sex. Posttransplant glomerulonephritis can accelerate graft failure, and is more common in male transplant recipients.[32] Male sex is also an independent risk factor for posttransplant lymphoproliferative disorder, an abnormal proliferation of B cells in the setting of posttransplant immunosuppression.[33] Overall, long-term outcomes of renal allografts are less favorable for male recipients.[34] This finding may be attributable to women having lower renal metabolic demands than men, and estrogen possibly having a protective effect on long-term renal function supported by renal allograft protection from estradiol in rat studies.[35] In adults receiving a renal transplant because of focal segmental glomerulosclerosis, male sex was associated with a much higher rate of recurrence.[36] Another notable posttransplant gender difference is in the nutritional outcomes. Men tended to show signs of malnutrition for a longer period of time after renal transplant because they may require a larger protein and energy intake to return to normal body composition.[37] Also male donors are less likely to follow up with their primary care physicians, especially if unmarried.[38]

There are also several adverse outcomes for renal allografts associated with female sex. Posttransplant infection puts recipients at risk for graft failure, and female sex has been associated with increased incidence of posttransplant bacterial infection.[39] Specifically, women were shown to have higher rates of urinary tract infections posttransplant compared with male recipients, prompting discussions about considering antibiotic prophylaxis postoperatively.[40] Female renal transplant recipients also had higher rates of iron deficiency anemia posttransplant.[41] Overall, female recipients had a higher likelihood of delayed renal graft function and, thus, were at greater risk of acute transplant rejection.[42] With regard to medications after transplant, female sex had a positive association with alopecia from tacrolimus use, although the mechanism behind this relationship remains unclear.[43]

PANCREAS

Pancreas transplants are significantly less common and declining, with only 192 performed in the United States in 2018 and fewer than 500 worldwide. There are limited data on the effect of sex on pancreas transplants. Pancreas-only transplants are occasionally performed for patients without ESRD. In general, female recipient sex leads to higher rates of acute rejection but better long-term outcomes. As with kidney transplants, patients receiving organs donated by women have higher rates of graft failure and shorter survival rates.[44]

LIVER

Preoperative Care, Listing, and Donor Selection

There are significant differences in sex-based access to liver transplant. Women are 20% less likely to be transplanted than men and have higher 3-month mortality.[45,46] Differences in height and Model for End-stage Liver Disease (MELD) exception scores are thought to account for the decreased number of liver transplants in women. Because of differences in size and body composition, women derive fewer MELD points from creatinine than men with similar levels of renal dysfunction.[45] Therefore, women have higher bilirubin levels and International Normalized Ratio at a similar MELD score to men. However, modification of MELD to include eGFR did not improve mortality prediction.[46]

Another possible explanation for the variation is that women are less likely to receive exception points than men and thus are ranked lower on the waiting list.[47] Despite similar baseline illness severity, women on the liver transplant waiting list have more frequent hospitalizations and inpatient days pretransplant.[48] Likewise, waiting-list outcomes are worse in women, especially at higher MELD scores.[49] Smaller adults, most of whom are women, have greater mortality on the liver transplant waiting list because of a paucity of appropriately sized donor organs.[47] To this end, women receiving a first-offer pediatric donor liver have lower risk of waiting-list mortality compared with those receiving adult offers.[50]

Donor/recipient gender mismatch is a risk factor for graft failure. Female-to-male donation mismatch seems to be the most detrimental for graft survival and mortality,[51] possibly because of immunologic factors. Pediatric recipients of living-related donor liver transplants from female donors have higher levels of serum C5a, which may contribute to the immunologic response against their grafted livers.[52] Female donors and male recipients also showed more unfavorable characteristics (age, body mass index [BMI], renal function) that contribute to poorer long-term graft survival.[53] Female recipients with gender-matched livers also have better graft and overall survival.[52] There is lower graft survival among hepatitis C virus (HCV)–positive female recipients receiving a male donor liver, but not in female HCV-negative recipients.[54] There is significantly better graft survival in male donor–female recipient pairings than in female donor–male recipient and male-male/female-female pairings, but this may be related to differences in donor quality and recipient characteristics rather than the sex of the donor.

Postoperative Course and Outcomes

As in the preoperative period, there are significant sex-based differences in outcomes. Perhaps unexpectedly, posttransplant mortality and graft survival do not seem to differ by sex except in HCV.[49] As discussed previously, there is a clear difference in graft survival based on donor sex. Female donors tend to be older, shorter, and die more frequently of stroke, suggesting that gender differences in graft quality and gender mismatch between donor and recipient are more predictive of graft loss.[55] However, in female liver transplant recipients, lower Psychosocial Assessments of Candidates for Transplantation score and alcoholic cirrhosis were associated with greater risk of posttransplant mortality.[56] In contrast, women with alcoholic cirrhosis have greater pretransplant complications (eg, ascites and hepatic encephalopathy) but lower graft rejection than men with alcoholic cirrhosis.[57] Race may also play a role, with younger African American women having an increased risk of graft loss limited to the first 2 years posttransplant.[58]

There are additional sex-based differences in postoperative risks following liver transplant. Younger women with alcohol dependence before transplant are at a higher risk of alcohol recidivism despite a 6-month abstinence period pretransplant.[59] Women also have lower quality-of-life scores posttransplant.[49] Female sex is associated with increased incidence of postoperative respiratory failure.[60] However, men are more likely to develop posttransplant de novo malignancy.[61] Sex does not seem to predict risk of recurrent hepatocellular carcinoma posttransplant, suggesting that other sex-related differences are responsible for increased malignancy risk, including lifestyle differences.[49]

LUNG

Preoperative Care, Listing, and Donor Selection

Because of a lack of suitable organs for donation, only approximately 4000 lung transplants are performed worldwide each year. Men account for 55% of lung transplant recipients in the United States (Europe, 53%), whereas the US waiting list is composed of 40% men (Europe, 42%).[62]

In terms of organ allocation, gender-matching seems to have a role in terms of outcomes. Female sex is associated with worse long-term survival compared with men.[63] In a French study, men receiving lungs from female donors had the worst survival.[64] In addition, female-to-male donation was associated with an increased length of stay compared with gender-matched and male-to-female donation.[65] Gender mismatch also seems to be associated with an increased risk for primary graft dysfunction according to a study from the United Kingdom.[66] Likewise, 1 institution found the lowest 5-year survival rate (43%) when male recipients received lungs from female donors.[67]

Postoperative Course and Outcomes

Loor and colleagues[67] showed improved outcomes in female recipients at 1 institution with improved 5-year survival rates in women compared with men (71% vs 58%) and less long-term graft dysfunction in women (65% vs 75%). A retrospective analysis of the UNOS database found a statistically significant increase in 1-year mortality in men with interstitial pulmonary fibrosis older than 65 years of age. The same difference was not seen in patients less than 65 years of age.[68] In contrast, a study of patients with cystic fibrosis (CF) receiving a lung transplant found no difference in survival after lung transplant and time to the development of bronchiolitis obliterans syndrome. However, female patients with CF presented for transplant and died at an earlier age than male counterparts regardless of gender-mismatched donors.[69] Outside the United States, women have increased survival compared with men in Europe (7.6 vs 6.1 years) and internationally (6.2 vs 5.6 years).[62]

Several potential factors have been suggested to explain the gender differences in outcomes, including hormonal, immunologic, physiologic, and potentially psychosocial differences. Increased estrogen levels and improved tolerance of alloantigens likely play a role in improved survival and reduced rejection in women.[70] Some of the effect of gender on lung transplant outcomes may be explained by differences in ischemia-reperfusion injury. A recent animal study showed higher oxygen transfer ability and lower perfusion pressure (vascular compliance) in female rats compared with males.[71] In addition, women have a lower risk of cancer following lung transplant.[72] However, likely because of differences in estrogen, the postoperative risk of venous thromboembolism is increased in women.[73]

Men have better long-term exercise capacity with a significant difference in 6-minute walk distance, although this may be explained by differences in height and stride length.[74] Interestingly, men have lower stress levels posttransplant and decreased mood disturbance compared with female recipients.[75] In addition, women have lower health-related quality of life despite having better long-term improvements in spirometry, suggesting that differences in quality of life are unrelated to graft function.[76]

HEART

Preoperative Care, Listing, and Donor Selection

Although half of the overall heart failure (HF) population is female, 75% of the patients on the waiting list for an orthotopic heart transplant (OHT) in the United States are male.[77] Multiple factors may limit women's candidacy for heart transplant, including alloimmunization because of prior pregnancy and advanced age at diagnosis.[78,79] Social inequities may play a role as well; male physicians may be less likely to perform a comprehensive work-up and refer female patients with HF to a transplant center, and female patients may be less likely to have spousal support as they undertake the pretransplant evaluation.[80,81]

Compared with men, women on the waiting list tend to be younger, nonwhite, and have lower BMI. Women are less likely to have ischemic cardiomyopathy (ICM) or diabetes but more often have a higher percentage of panel-reactive antibodies.[77,82,83] Women are also less likely to be on antiarrhythmic therapy or have an implantable cardioverter-defibrillator or left ventricular assist device (LVAD).[77,83]

Sex-based differences in waiting-list mortality have been observed and have changed over time, likely in part because of the 2012 introduction of lower-profile LVADs suitable for use in smaller women.[83] Women seem to receive transplants more quickly than men after being listed, potentially because of increased severity of illness at the time of listing.[77,83] Among UNOS status 2 (nonurgent) patients, women have better hemodynamics and historically lower mortality.[77] At any given functional capacity (peak O_2 consumption), women seem to have better survival than men.[84]

Donors and recipients are usually matched by sex (preferable) and body size in order to ensure appropriate sizing of the donor heart for the recipient. Many centers use weight alone (with a goal of no more than 20%–30% difference between donor and recipient), but this method may not accurately estimate total heart mass, calculated using donor's age, height, weight, and sex. Women have lower cardiac mass by weight than men, complicating attempts to allocate sex-mismatched organs appropriately.[85] Female donors tend to be older than male donors and more likely to have died of stroke.[25,86] These demographic considerations have significant implications for recipients, because older donor age is a known risk factor for worse graft survival and higher posttransplant mortality.

Sex matching, particularly for male recipients, results in better long-term survival.[87] Several studies have shown higher mortality when men receive female-donor hearts.[88,89] By contrast, gender-matched men had the best long-term survival.[88] Sicker patients may be at increased risk of poor outcomes when they receive a sex-mismatched organ, with donor-to-recipient gender mismatch being an independent predictor of shorter graft survival in patients with mechanical circulatory support.[90] Similarly, female recipients of male allografts had lower 1-year survival compared with men who received male hearts.[91] Gender-matched organs are associated with improved survival.[88,92]

Postoperative Course and Outcomes

Female recipients are at a higher risk of rejection because of higher immunoreactivity and require greater immunosuppression (which may lead to infection, renal failure, and cancer).[93] Women seem to form anti–human leukocyte antigen antibodies earlier in the posttransplant period than men.[94] Several observational studies have found that women have an increased risk of antibody-mediated rejection (AMR) after OHT, their rejection episodes tend to be more severe and cause more hemodynamic compromise, and they more often require hospitalization in the first year after transplant.[82,95] There is evidence that AMR increases the risk of developing coronary allograft vasculopathy (CAV),[82] but women have been reported in other studies to have a lower risk of CAV.[95,96]

Sex hormone exposure of the cardiac allograft, both before and after transplant, seems to influence postoperative complications. Allografts from premenopausal women are more likely to show endothelial dysfunction and stenotic microvasculopathy after being transplanted into men than into premenopausal women.[97] Female recipients of male donor hearts have more acute rejection episodes, more inpatient days, higher incidence of CAV, and higher mortality than either sex-matched recipients or male recipients of female hearts.[98] There is some evidence that being postmenopausal may be beneficial for female recipient survival, presumably because of the decreased immunoreactivity that results from lower estrogen levels.[99]

Other complications also have sex-related differences. Heart transplant patients overall have been reported to have a 28.1% incidence of malignancy at 15 years posttransplant, and men seem to be at significantly higher risk than women of developing any type of cancer, including solid organ, hematologic, and skin cancers.[100] Immunosuppressant effects of androgens or differences in modifiable risk factors not captured on multivariate analysis may help explain this finding. Although women with HF have lower rates of cardiac arrhythmias than their male counterparts,[101] recipients of heart transplants are more likely to develop new-onset atrial fibrillation, a risk that is especially pronounced in women.[102]

Despite these apparent differences, men and women seem to have comparable short-term survival following OHT. On long-term follow-up, women have a survival advantage, with a median survival of 11.7 years versus 10.7 years for men.[96]

Quality of life after OHT may also be influenced by sex. Women and men report equal levels of stress and symptom distress after undergoing a heart transplant, but women seem to be more likely to report using negative coping strategies in response.[103] They also report worse functional ability 5 years after OHT.[104] On surveys, women simultaneously report more difficulty with posttransplant medication adherence and more adherence than do men, a finding that highlights some of the difficulties in assessing long-term quality-of-life outcomes.[103] Work status at 5 and 10 years posttransplant does not seem to differ between the sexes.[105]

SUMMARY

Sex has a significant impact on the preoperative and postoperative considerations for solid organ transplantation. More data are needed to elucidate whether these impacts are consistent when studied over larger groups, and whether they can lead to improve outcomes for future donors and recipients of solid organs. Future research should focus on whether female sex hormonal influences can be harnessed to improve graft outcome for recipients, whether male donation can specifically be encouraged to equal female donation rates, and whether gender socioeconomic factors can be improved for increased access and compliance rates.

DISCLOSURE

None.

CONFLICTS OF INTEREST

None.

REFERENCES

1. Ge F, Huang T, Yuan S, et al. Gender issues in solid organ donation and transplantation. Ann Transplant 2013;18:508–14.
2. Steinman JL. Gender disparity in organ donation. Gend Med 2006;3:246–52.
3. Hart A, Smith JM, Skeans MA, et al. OPTN/SRTR 2015 annual data report: kidney. Am J Transplant 2017;17(Suppl 1):21–116.
4. Kayler LK, Meier-Kriesche H-U, Punch JD, et al. Gender imbalance in living donor renal transplantation. Transplantation 2002;73(2):248–52.
5. Ghods AJ, Nasrollahzadeh D. Gender disparity in a live donor renal transplantation program: assessing from cultural perspectives. Transplant Proc 2003;35(7):2559–60.
6. Hermann HC, Klapp BF, Danzer G, et al. Gender-specific differences associated with living donor liver transplantation: a review study. Liver Transplant 2010;16(3):375–86.
7. Avula S, Sharma RK, Singh AK, et al. Age and gender discrepancies in living related renal transplant donors and recipients. Transplant Proc 1998;30(7):3674.
8. Thamer M, Hwang W, Fink NE, et al. U.S. nephrologists' attitudes towards renal transplantation: results from a national survey. Transplantation 2001;71(2):281–8.
9. Chandna SM, Da Silva-Gane M, Marshall C, et al. Survival of elderly patients with stage 5 CKD: comparison of conservative management and renal replacement therapy. Nephrol Dial Transplant 2011;26(5):1608–14.
10. Segev DL, Powe NR, Troll MU, et al. Willingness of the United States general public to participate in kidney paired donation. Clin Transplant 2012;26(5):714–21.
11. Tuohy KA, Johnson S, Khwaja K, et al. Gender disparities in the live kidney donor evaluation process. Transplantation 2006;82(11):1402–7.
12. Collins AJ, Foley RN, Chavers B, et al. United States Renal Data System 2011 annual data report: atlas of chronic kidney disease & end-stage renal disease in the United States. Am J Kidney Dis 2012;59(1 Suppl 1):A7, e1-420.
13. Berg UB. Differences in decline in GFR with age between males and females. Reference data on clearances of inulin and PAH in potential kidney donors. Nephrol Dial Transplant 2006;21(9):2577–82.
14. Neugarten J, Golestaneh L. Influence of sex on the progression of chronic kidney disease. Mayo Clin Proc 2019;94(7):1339–56.
15. Kwan G, Neugarten J, Sherman M, et al. Effects of sex hormones on mesangial cell proliferation and collagen synthesis. Kidney Int 1996;50(4):1173–9.

16. Pawluczyk IZA, Tan EKC, Harris KPG. Rat mesangial cells exhibit sex-specific profibrotic and proinflammatory phenotypes. Nephrol Dial Transplant 2009;24(6):1753–8.
17. Kwon OJ, Kwak JY. The impact of sex and age matching for long-term graft survival in living donor renal transplantation. Transplant Proc 2004;36(7):2040–2.
18. Zhou J-Y, Cheng J, Huang H-F, et al. The effect of donor-recipient gender mismatch on short- and long-term graft survival in kidney transplantation: A systematic review and meta-analysis. Clin Transplant 2013;27(5):764–71.
19. Zukowski M, Kotfis K, Biernawska J, et al. Donor-recipient gender mismatch affects early graft loss after kidney transplantation. Transplant Proc 2011;43(8):2914–6.
20. Valdes F, Pita S, Alonso A, et al. The effect of donor gender on renal allograft survival and influence of donor age on posttransplant graft outcome and patient survival. Transplant Proc 1997;29(8):3371–2.
21. Yoneda T, Iemura Y, Onishi K, et al. Effect of Gender Differences on Transplant Kidney Function. Transplant Proc 2017;49(1):61–4.
22. Noel S, Desai NM, Hamad AR, et al. Sex and the single transplanted kidney. J Clin Invest 2016;126(5):1643–5.
23. Aufhauser DD Jr, Wang Z, Murken DR, et al. Improved renal ischemia tolerance in females influences kidney transplantation outcomes. J Clin Invest 2016;126(5):1968–77.
24. Antus B, Yao Y, Song E, et al. Opposite effects of testosterone and estrogens on chronic allograft nephropathy. Transpl Int 2002;15(9–10):494–501.
25. Melk A, Babitsch B, Borchert-Mörlins B, et al. Equally Interchangeable? How sex and gender affect transplantation. Transplantation 2019;103(6):1094–110.
26. Jindal RM, Joseph JT, Morris MC, et al. Noncompliance after kidney transplantation: a systematic review. Transplant Proc 2003;35(8):2868–72.
27. Naiman N, Baird BC, Isaacs RB, et al. Role of pre-transplant marital status in renal transplant outcome. Clin Transplant 2007;21(1):38–46.
28. Kimmel PL, Patel SS. Psychosocial issues in women with renal disease. Adv Ren Replace Ther 2003;10(1):61–70.
29. Lew SQ, Patel SS. Psychosocial and quality of life issues in women with end-stage renal disease. Adv Chronic Kidney Dis 2007;14(4):358–63.
30. Rodrigue JR, Fleishman A. Health insurance trends in United States living kidney donors (2004 to 2015). Am J Transplant 2016;16(12):3504–11.
31. Lovasik BP, Zhang R, Hockenberry JM, et al. Emergency department use among kidney transplant recipients in the United States. Am J Transplant 2018;18(4):868–80. https://doi.org/10.1111/ajt.14578.
32. Chailimpamontree W, Dmitrienko S, Li G, et al. Probability, predictors, and prognosis of posttransplantation glomerulonephritis. J Am Soc Nephrol 2009;20(4):843–51.
33. Dharnidharka VR, Tejani AH, Ho P-L, et al. Post-transplant lymphoproliferative disorder in the United States: Young Caucasian males are at highest risk. Am J Transplant 2002;2(10):993–8.
34. Inoue S, Yamada Y, Kuzuhara K, et al. Are women privileged organ recipients? Transplant Proc 2002;34(7):2775–6.
35. Müller V, Szabó A, Viklicky O, et al. Sex hormones and gender-related differences: their influence on chronic renal allograft rejection. Kidney Int 1999;55(5):2011–20.

36. Moroni G, Gallelli B, Quaglini S, et al. Long-term outcome of renal transplantation in adults with focal segmental glomerulosclerosis. Transpl Int 2010;23(2): 208–16.
37. Coroas A, Oliveira JG, Sampaio S, et al. Nutritional status and body composition evolution in early post-renal transplantation: is there a female advantage? Transplant Proc 2005;37(6):2765–70.
38. Alejo JL, Luo X, Massie AB. Patterns of primary care utilization before and after living kidney donation. Clin Transplant 2017;31(7):1–7.
39. Dharnidharka VR, Agodoa LY, Abbott KC. Risk factors for hospitalization for bacterial or viral infection in renal transplant recipients–an analysis of USRDS data. Am J Transplant 2007;7(3):653–61.
40. Sorto R, Irizar SS, Delgadillo G, et al. Risk factors for urinary tract infections during the first year after kidney transplantation. Transplant Proc 2010;42(1):280–1.
41. Kahng K, Kang C, Kwak J. Changes in hemoglobin levels after renal transplantation. Transplant Proc 1998;30(7):3023–4.
42. Jushinskis J, Trushkov S, Bicans J, et al. Risk factors for the development of delayed graft function in deceased donor renal transplants. Transplant Proc 2009; 41(2):746–8.
43. Tricot L, Lebbe C, Pillebout E, et al. Tacrolimus-induced alopecia in female kidney-pancreas transplant recipients. Transplantation 2005;80(11):1546–9.
44. Li Z, Mei S, Xiang J, et al. Influence of donor-recipient sex mismatch on long-term survival of pancreatic grafts. Sci Rep 2016;6:29298.
45. Allen A, Heimbach J, Larson J, et al. Reduced access to liver transplantation in women: role of height, MELD exception scores, and renal function underestimation. Transplantation 2018;102(10):1710–6.
46. Myers R, Shaheen A, Aspinall A, et al. Gender, renal function, and outcomes on the liver transplant waiting list: assessment of revised MELD including estimated glomerular filtration rate. J Hepatol 2011;54:462–70.
47. Nephew L, Goldberg D, Lewis J, et al. Exception points and body size contribute to gender disparity in liver transplantation. Clin Gastroenterol Hepatol 2017;15:1286–93.
48. Rubin J, Sinclair M, Rahimi R, et al. Women on the liver transplantation waitlist are at increased risk of hospitalization compared to men. World J Gastroenterol 2019;25(8):980–8.
49. Sarkar M, Watt K, Terrault N, et al. Outcomes in liver transplantation: does sex matter? J Hepatol 2015;62:946–55.
50. Ge J, Gilroy R, Lai J. Receipt of a pediatric liver offer as the first offer reduces waitlist mortality for adult women. Hepatology 2018;68(3):1101–10.
51. Lai Q, Giovanardi F, Melandro F, et al. Donor-to-recipient gender match in liver transplantation: a systematic review and meta-analysis. World J Gastroenterol 2018;24(20):2203–10.
52. Hussein MH, Hashimoto T, Suzuki T, et al. Liver transplantation from female donors provokes higher complement component C5a activity. Ann Transplant 2017;22:694–700.
53. Schoening W, Helbig M, Buescher N, et al. Gender matches in liver transplant allocation: matched and mismatched male-female donor-recipient combinations; long-term follow-up of more than 2000 patients at a single center. Exp Clin Transplant 2016;2:184–90.
54. Zhang Y. Impact of donor recipient gender and race mismatch on graft outcomes in patients with end-stage liver disease undergoing liver transplantation. Prog Transplant 2017;27(1):39–47.

55. Lai J, Feng S, Roberts J, et al. Gender differences in liver donor quality are predictive of graft loss. Am J Transplant 2011;11:296–302.
56. Schneekloth T, Hitschfeld M, Patterson T, et al. Psychosocial risk impacts mortality in women after liver transplantation. Psychosomatics 2019;60:56–65.
57. Legaz I, Noguera E, Bolarin J, et al. Patient sex in the setting of liver transplant in alcoholic liver disease. Exp Clin Transplant 2019;17(3):355–62.
58. Dave S, Dodge J, Terrault N, et al. Racial and ethnic differences in graft loss among female liver transplant recipients. Transplant Proc 2018;20:1413–23.
59. Zeair S, Cyprys S, Wisniewska H, et al. Alcohol relapse after liver transplantation: younger women are at greatest risk. Ann Transplant 2017;22:725–9.
60. Avolio A, Gaspari R, Teofili L, et al. Postoperative respiratory failure in liver transplantation: risk factors and effect on prognosis. PLoS One 2019;14(2): e0211678.
61. Bhat M, Mara K, Dierkhising R, et al. Gender, race and disease etiology predict de novo malignancy risk after liver transplantation: insights for future individualized cancer screening guidance. Transplantation 2019;103(1):91–100.
62. Chambers DC, Yusen RD, Cherikh WS, et al. The registry of the International Society for Heart and Lung Transplantation: thirty-fourth adult lung and heart-lung transplantation report-2017; focus theme: allograft ischemic time. J Heart Lung Transplant 2017;36(10):1047–59.
63. Thabut G, Mal H, Cerrina J, et al. Influence of donor characteristics on outcome after lung transplantation: a multicenter study. J Heart Lung Transplant 2005;24: 1347–53.
64. Sato M, Gutierrez C, Waddell TK, et al. Donor-recipient gender mismatch in lung transplantation: impact on obliterative bronchiolitis and survival. J Heart Lung Transplant 2005;24(11):2000–1.
65. Banga A, Mohanka M, Mullins J, et al. Hospital length of stay after lung transplantation: independent predictors and association with early and late survival. J Heart Lung Transplant 2017;36(3):289–96.
66. Singh SSA, Banner NR, Rushton S, et al. ISHLT primary graft dysfunction incidence, risk factors, and outcome: a UK national study. Transplantation 2019; 103:336–43.
67. Loor G, Brown R, Kelly RF, et al. Gender differences in long-term survival post-transplant: a single-institution analysis in the lung allocation score era. Clin Transplant 2017;31(3).
68. Sheikh SI, Hayes D Jr, Kirkby SE, et al. Age-dependent gender disparities in post lung transplant survival among patients with idiopathic pulmonary fibrosis. Ann Thorac Surg 2017;103(2):441–6.
69. Raghavan D, Gao A, Ahn C, et al. Lung transplantation and gender effects on survival of recipients with cystic fibrosis. J Heart Lung Transplant 2016;35: 1487–96.
70. Zou Y, Steurer W, Klima G, et al. Estradiol enhances murine cardiac allograft rejection under cyclosporin and can be antagonized by the antiestrogen tamoxifen. Transplantation 2002;74(3):354–7.
71. Mrazkova H, Lischke R, Herget J. Influence of gender on ischemia-reperfusion injury in lungs in an animal model. Physiol Res 2016;65:953–8.
72. Berastegui C, LaPorta R, López-Meseguer M, et al. Epidemiology and risk factors for cancer after lung transplantation. Transplant Proc 2017;49(10):2285–91.
73. Aboagye JK, Hayanga JW, Lau BD, et al. Venous thromboembolism in patients hospitalized for lung transplantation. Ann Thorac Surg 2018;105:1071–6.

74. Mejia-Downs A, DiPerna C, Shank C, et al. Predictors of long-term exercise capacity in patients who have had lung transplantation. Prog Transplant 2018;28: 198–205.
75. Lanuza DM, McCabe M, Norton-Rosko M, et al. Symptom experiences of lung transplant recipients: comparisons across gender, pretransplantation diagnosis, and type of transplantation. Heart Lung 1999;28(6):429–37.
76. Rodrigue JR, Baz MA. Are there sex differences in health-related quality of life after lung transplantation for chronic obstructive pulmonary disease? J Heart Lung Transplant 2006;25(1):120–5.
77. Hsich EM, Blackstone EH, Thuita L, et al. Sex differences in mortality based on United Network for Organ Sharing status while awaiting heart transplantation. Circ Heart Fail 2017;10(6).
78. Alba AC, Tinckam K, Faroutan F, et al. Factors associated with anti-human leukocyte antigen antibodies in patients supported with continuous-flow devices and effect on probability of transplant and post-transplant outcomes. J Heart Lung Transplant 2015;34(5):685–92.
79. Hsich EM, Grau-Sepulveda MV, Hernandez AF, et al. Relationship between sex, ejection fraction, and B-type natriuretic peptide levels in patients hospitalized with heart failure and associations with inhospital outcomes: findings from the get with the guideline-heart failure registry. Am Heart J 2013;166(6):1063–71.
80. Cleland JG, Swedbreg K, Follath F, et al. The EuroHeart Failure survey programme—a survey on the quality of care among patients with heart failure in Europe. Part 1: patient characteristics and diagnosis. Eur Heart J 2003;24(5): 442–62.
81. Regitz-Zagrosek V, Petrov G, Lehmkuhl E, et al. Heart transplantation in women with dilated cardiomyopathy. Transplantation 2010;89(2):236–44.
82. Grupper A, Nestorovic EM, Daly RC, et al. Sex related differences in the risk of antibody-mediated rejection and subsequent allograft vasculopathy post-heart transplantation: a single-center experience. Transplant Direct 2016;2(10):e106.
83. Morris AA, Cole RT, Laskar SR, et al. Improved outcomes for women on the heart transplant wait list in the modern era. J Card Fail 2015;21(7):555–60.
84. Hsich E, Chadalavada S, Krishnaswamy G, et al. Long-term prognostic value of peak oxygen consumption in women versus men with heart failure and severely impaired left ventricular systolic function. Am J Cardiol 2007;100(2):291–5.
85. Hsich EM. Sex differences in advanced heart failure therapies. Circulation 2019; 139:1080–93.
86. Eifert S, Kofler S, Nickel T, et al. Gender-based analysis of outcome after heart transplant. Exp Clin Transplant 2012;10(4):368–74.
87. Kittleson MM, Shemin R, Patel JK, et al. Donor-recipient sex mismatch portends poor 10-year outcomes in a single-center experience. J Heart Lung Transplant 2011;30(9):1018–22.
88. Al-Khaldi A, Oyer PE, Robbins RC. Outcome analysis of donor gender in heart transplantation. J Heart Lung Transplant 2006;25(4):461–8.
89. Weiss ES, Allen JG, Patel ND, et al. The impact of donor-recipient sex matching on survival after orthotopic heart transplantation: analysis of 18 000 transplants in the modern era. Circ Heart Fail 2009;2(5):401–8.
90. Maltais S, Jaik NP, Feurer ID, et al. Mechanical circulatory support and heart transplantation: donor and recipient factors influencing graft survival. Ann Thorac Surg 2013;96(4):1252–8.

91. Kaczmarek I, Meiser B, Beiras-Fernandez A, et al. Gender does matter: gender-specific outcome analysis of 67,855 heart transplants. Thorac Cardiovasc Surg 2013;61(1):29–36.
92. Khush KK, Kubo JT, Desai M. Influence of donor and recipient sex mismatch on heart transplant outcomes: analysis of the International Society for Heart and Lung Transplantation Registry. J Heart Lung Transplant 2012;31(5):459–66.
93. Lietz K, John R, Kocher A, et al. Increased prevalence of autoimmune phenomena and greater risk for alloreactivity in female heart transplant recipients. Circulation 2001;104(12 Suppl 1):I177–83.
94. Mifsud NA, Purcell AW, Chen W, et al. Immunodominance hierarchies and gender bias in direct T(CD8)-cell alloreactivity. Am J Transplant 2008;8(8):1749–54.
95. Hickey KT, Doering LV, Chen B, et al. Clinical and gender differences in heart transplant recipients in the NEW HEART study. Eur J Cardiovasc Nurs 2017;16(3):222–9.
96. The International Society for Heart and Lung Transplantation. International Thoracic Organ Transplant Registry 2018 data slides: Adult Heart Transplantation Statistics. Available at: https://ishltregistries.org/registries/slides.asp. Accessed August 15, 2019.
97. Hiemann NE1, Knosalla C, Wellnhofer E, et al. Beneficial effect of female gender on long-term survival after heart transplantation. Transplantation 2008;86(2):348–56.
98. Jalowiec A, Grady KL, White-Williams C. Mortality, rehospitalization, and post-transplant complications in gender-mismatched heart transplant recipients. Heart Lung 2017;46(4):265–72.
99. Morgan AE, Dewey E, Mudd JO, et al. The role of estrogen, immune function and aging in heart transplant outcomes. Am J Surg 2019;218(4):737–43.
100. Bhat M, Mara K, Dierkhising R, et al. Immunosuppression, race, and donor-related risk factors affect de novo cancer incidence across solid organ transplant recipients. Mayo Clin Proc 2018;93(9):1236–46.
101. Seegers J, Conen D, Jung K, et al. Sex difference in appropriate shocks but not mortality during long-term follow-up in patients with implantable cardioverter-defibrillators. Europace 2016;18(8):1194–202.
102. Hu WS, Lin CL. Risk of new-onset atrial fibrillation among heart, kidney and liver transplant recipients: insights from a national cohort study. Intern Emerg Med 2019;14(1):71–6.
103. Grady KL, Andrei AC, Li Z, et al. Gender differences in appraisal of stress and coping 5 years after heart transplantation. Heart Lung 2016;45(1):41–7.
104. Grady KL, Naftel DC, Young JB, et al. Patterns and predictors of physical functional disability at 5 to 10 years after heart transplantation. J Heart Lung Transplant 2007;26(11):1182–91.
105. White-Williams C, Wang E, Rybarczyk B, et al. Factors associated with work status at 5 and 10 years after heart transplantation. Clin Transplant 2011;25(6):E599–605.

Considerations for Transgender Patients Perioperatively

Luis E. Tollinche, MD*, Christian Van Rooyen, MD, Anoushka Afonso, MD, Gregory W. Fischer, MD, Cindy B. Yeoh, MD

KEYWORDS

• Transgender • Anesthesia • Perioperative • Hormone therapy • Surgery

KEY POINTS

- Barriers to health care: The transgender community is arguably the most marginalized and underserved population in medicine. Personal, structural, and financial barriers restrict access to health services for this patient population.
- Preoperative assessment: Health care facilities should be safe and welcoming places with progressive and inclusive hospital policies. Clinicians should use a gender-affirming approach when interviewing or examining a transgender patient and must be aware of the effect cross-hormone therapy can have on laboratory results.
- Risk assessment: All patients scheduled to undergo surgery should be assessed for the risk of a perioperative cardiovascular event. Transgender patients are at an increased risk of myocardial infarction, diabetes, venous thromboembolism, and pulmonary complications.
- Intraoperative management: Clinicians should be aware of altered anatomy that could affect intraoperative airway management, possible drug interactions, and the increased risk of venous thromboembolism.
- Postoperative management: The postoperative period is a vulnerable time for the transgender patient. A multidisciplinary approach must be taken when managing pain, respecting privacy and ensuring mental well-being.

INTRODUCTION

Recent studies estimate that 25 million people (0.5%–1.3%) identify as transgender worldwide, approximately 1.4 million of whom reside in the United States.[1–3] These

Department of Anesthesiology and Critical Care Medicine, Memorial Sloan Kettering Cancer Center, 1275 York Avenue, C330F, New York, NY 10065, USA
* Corresponding author.
E-mail address: tollincl@mskcc.org

https://doi.org/10.1016/j.anclin.2020.01.009

estimates are likely conservative because of the limited amount of studies that have attempted to measure the transgender population.

A recent survey by the French global market and research company Ipsos interviewed American panelists and showed that most (60%) of the 19,747 respondents aged 16 to 64 believe that their country is becoming more tolerant and want their government to do more to protect and support transgender people.[4] Health governing bodies, such as the American Psychiatric Association and the World Health Organization, are following suit by reclassifying "gender identity disorder" to "gender dysphoria" and moving "gender incongruence" from the panels' mental health disorders chapter to the sexual health chapter, respectively.

With this increase in visibility and acceptance, it is likely that more transgender people will present to a general surgical setting. Thus, there is a need for anesthesia providers to develop cultural competence and acquire the knowledge and skills necessary for safely managing transgender patients during the perioperative period.

Terminology

Critical to the understanding of what it means to be transgender is recognizing that although they are often used interchangeably, gender and sex are distinct. "Sex" refers to the sex assigned at birth, based on assessment of internal and external sex organs, chromosomes, and hormonal activities within the body. "Gender," however, is socially, culturally, and personally defined. It includes how individuals see themselves, how others perceive them and expect them to behave, and the interactions that they have with others.

The conceptualization of gender as binary has dominated Western societies and continues to be enforced by the media, religion, mainstream education, and political, cultural, and social systems. However, the binary paradigm is not embraced by many cultures worldwide. Some examples include the Muxes in Juchitan de Zagroza[5]; the two spirit native North American Navajo culture; the Fa'afines in Samoa[6]; and the Hijras in South Asia, who have recently been legally recognized as a third gender in several South Asian countries.[7]

Some people have a gender that is neither male nor female and may identify as both at the same time, as different genders at different times, as no gender at all, or dispute the very idea of only two genders. Definitions of these categories vary and continue to evolve over time with an array of terms describing one's gender or genders (**Table 1**).[8]

It is also important to note that there is a difference between gender nonconformity and gender dysphoria. Gender nonconformity refers to the extent to which a person's gender identity, role, or expression differs from the cultural norms prescribed for people of a particular sex. Gender dysphoria based on the Diagnostic and Statistical Manual of Mental Disorders–5th edition criteria refers to the clinically significant impairment in social, occupational, or other important areas of functioning caused by a discrepancy between a person's gender identity and that person's sex assigned at birth.[9,10]

Barriers to Health Care

The transgender community is arguably the most marginalized and underserved population in medicine. Although being transgender does not determine a person's health, the appalling effects of social and economic marginalization are associated with various adverse health outcomes. These include increased rates of human immunodeficiency virus (HIV) infection, smoking, some cancers, drug and alcohol use, and suicide attempts compared with the general population.[11–14]

Table 1
Gender classification definition

Terminology	Definition
Cisgender	People whose gender identity matches their sex assigned at birth
Transgender male (female to male)	A person who was assigned female at birth, but identifies as a man or on the masculine spectrum
Transgender female (male to female)	A person who was assigned male at birth, but identifies as a woman or on the feminine spectrum
Gender nonconforming, genderqueer	A person whose gender identity differs from that assigned at birth, but may be more complex, fluid, multifaceted, or less clearly defined than a transgender person
Nonbinary	Transgender or gender nonconforming person who identifies as neither male nor female
Transitioning	A person's process of developing and assuming a gender expression to match their gender identity
Transsexual	A clinical term previously used to describe those transgender people who sought medical intervention

From Kuper LE, Nussbaum R, Mustanski B. Exploring the diversity of gender and sexual orientation identities in an online sample of transgender individuals. J Sex Res 2012;49(2-3):244-254; with permission.

Access to health care as defined by the Institute of Medicine is "timely use of personal health services to achieve the best possible outcome." To understand a transgender patient's presurgical needs, one first needs to address the unique barriers to accessing health care they face. These barriers are divided into three groups: (1) personal, (2) structural, and (3) financial barriers.

Personal barriers are largely driven by transgender stigma, the inferior status and relative powerlessness that society collectively assigns to this group of people. These widespread stigmas can prevent a transgender patient from attempting to access quality care.[15]

Structural barriers are faced at an institutional level including health care systems and insurance policies. Protransgender laws (eg, the nondiscrimination provision of the Affordable Care Act) make health care discrimination against transgender and gender nonconforming people illegal under existing federal law.

Despite these nondiscrimination provisions, transgender patients are still less likely to have health insurance coverage compared with their cisgender counterparts.[16] Not only are they more likely to be uninsured than the general population, they are also less insured than lesbian, gay, and bisexual persons.[17] In a 2015 US Transgender Survey, 55% of patients who sought surgery and 25% of those on hormones reported difficulty obtaining insurance coverage.[18]

Even with these laws in place, having access to health care does not equate to having adequate high-quality care. Transgender patients report that lack of providers with expertise in transgender medicine represents the single largest component inhibiting access.[19] They often encounter ignorance about basic aspects of transgender health. In one widely disseminated study, 50% of respondents reported having to teach providers some aspect of their health needs.[13] Poor patient–provider communication is strongly associated with adverse health behaviors, such as decreased levels of adherence to physician advice and decreased rates of satisfaction.[20] Transgender populations experience health inequities in part because of the exclusion of transgender-specific health needs from medical school and residency curricula. Of all LGBTQ topics, transgender health is the least well understood. Seventy-four percent of medical students report receiving less than 2 hours of curricular time devoted to transgender clinical competency.[21]

The rising cost of health care is another hurdle transgender patients must overcome to access quality care. A survey reported that transgender people are experiencing an unemployment rate of 14%, double the national average at the time, and 15% reported a household income less than $10,000 a year.[13] The paucity of insurance coverage for hormone therapy and gender-affirming surgery, even among those who are able to secure health insurance, contributes to a high financial burden.[22]

GENDER-AFFIRMING THERAPIES

The World Professional Association for Transgender Health has established internationally accepted standards of care for the treatment of gender dysphoria. There are a wide range of therapeutic options that are divided into four broad categories, discussed next.[9]

Behavioral Modification

Transgender people may use techniques, such as genital tucking (pushing the testes into the inguinal canal and securing the penis back between the legs with an undergarment), packing (placing of a penile prosthesis in one's underwear), or chest binding (methods of flattening breast tissue) to reduce the symptoms of gender dysphoria.[23]

Psychotherapy

The aim of psychotherapy is to treat the dysphoria and associated symptoms, not the person's gender identity. Its goal is alleviating internalized transphobia, symptoms of depression, anxiety, fear, guilt, low self-esteem, shame, and self-hatred.[9]

Medical Management

Medical management consists of cross-sex hormone therapy (CSHT) as the primary intervention. CSHT is divided into feminizing and masculinizing therapy.

The goal of feminizing hormone therapy is the development of female secondary sex characteristics and suppression of male secondary sex characteristics. Therapy consists mainly of estrogen, progestogens, and antiandrogens. Estrogen (17-β estradiol) is most commonly delivered via a transdermal patch, oral or sublingual tablet, or injection of a conjugated ester. Antiandrogens include spironolactone and 5α-reductase inhibitors, such as finasteride and dutasteride.[24] Most physical changes occur over the course of 2 years depending on the dose, route of administration, and medications used.

The goal of masculinizing hormone therapy is the development of male secondary sex characteristics, and suppression of female secondary sex characteristics. Therapy consists of several forms of parenteral or oral testosterone.[25]

Health care providers need to be cognizant of the risks when subjecting patients to CSHT. According to the American Congress of Obstetricians and Gynecologists, transgender youth who receive inadequate treatment are at an increased risk for engaging in self-harm or obtaining injected hormones through illegal means.[26]

Surgical Management

The number of patients presenting for gender-related medical and surgical care is increasing dramatically. This is thought to be, in large part, a result of the Affordable Care Act, which states that it is unlawful for an insurance carrier to "have or implement a categorical coverage exclusion or limitation for all health services related to gender transition."

Female to male surgeries include:

- Bilateral mastectomy (top surgery)
- Removal of female genitalia and creating male genitalia through phalloplasty, scrotoplasty
- Implantation of testicular prostheses (bottom surgery)
- Nongenital nonbreast surgeries (voice surgery and liposuction)[9,27]

Many transgender men choose to retain their uterus and ovaries, which impacts future fertility options.

Male to female surgeries include:

- Augmentation mammoplasty (top surgery)
- Removal of male genitalia and constructing female genitalia through vaginoplasty, clitoroplasty, and vulvoplasty (bottom surgery)
- Nongenital nonbreast surgeries (thyroid cartilage reduction, voice surgery)

PREOPERATIVE

A health care facility might be a traumatizing place for a transgender patient with a large portion of patients reporting harassment in a medical setting or violence at a doctor's office.[13] A culturally appropriate environment in which the patient feels safe and welcomed needs to be provided. It is imperative that all staff including nursing, front desk, and allied health personal be aware of transgender terminology and health issues. Waiting areas should include transgender-themed posters, legal rights, and pamphlets to emphasize the importance of this marginalized community. Bathroom policies should be clearly defined as either being gender-neutral or allowing the patient to choose bathrooms based on their own preference.

Transgender patients may have a chosen name and gender identity that differs from their current legally designated name and sex. It is important to record each patient's preferred name and pronoun (**Table 2**) so that they are used throughout the health

Table 2
Gender pronouns

Terminology	Pronoun
Cismale	He/him/himself
Cisfemale	She/her/herself
Transgender male	He/him/himself
Transgender female	She/her/herself
Gender nonconforming	They/them/themself
Gender neutral	Zhe/zhim/zher/zhers/zhimself

Adapted from Deutsch MB, Buchholz D. Electronic health records and transgender patients–practical recommendations for the collection of gender identity data. J Gen Intern Med 2015;30(6):846; with permission.

care facility.[28] Incorrect use or disregard of patients' preferences reinforces stigmas and may lead the patient to not return for further care.

The best practice for collecting gender identity data (sex assigned at birth, gender identity, preferred name and preferred pronoun) is through a two-step questionnaire using gender identity followed by sex assigned at birth (**Box 1**).[29] This process has been made easier through The Joint Commission, which now requires that all electronic health record systems certified under the Meaningful Use incentive program have the capacity to collect sexual orientation and gender identity information.[30]

This, however, does not negate that transgender patients may still present to the preanesthetic clinic with legal documents incongruent with their preferred name and/or gender identity. To ensure proper documentation for legal and insurance purposes the patients' legal photograph identification and insurance card should be noted.

Interview

Careful consideration should be taken when interviewing a transgender patient. Specific details regarding transgender status and transition history, including an inventory of organs and information on hormone use should be recorded.[28] Clinicians should inquire about silicone or other filler use because many are injected by unlicensed medical providers. Improper use can lead to devastating effects, such as acute respiratory distress syndrome, sepsis, embolization, hypersensitivity pneumonitis, or hypercalcemia.[31,32]

A detailed smoking history should be recorded, especially in transgender females, because hormone therapy (estrogen) and smoking are independent factors for venous thromboembolism (VTE).[33,34]

Physical Examination

As part of the preoperative assessment a focused physical examination must be performed. The examination should be relevant to the anatomy that is present, regardless of gender presentation, and without assumptions as to the anatomy or identity of the patient. During the examination the provider should be aware of the patient's preferred pronoun and use a gender-affirming approach. Gender affirmation refers to a process whereby a person receives social recognition and support for their gender identity and expression through social interactions.[35]

Box 1
Collection of gender identity on a patient intake form

1. What is your current gender identity? (check and/or circle all that apply)
   - ☐ Female
   - ☐ Male
   - ☐ Transgender male/transman/FTM
   - ☐ Transgender female/transwoman/MTF
   - ☐ Genderqueer
   - ☐ Additional category (please specify):__________
   - ☐ Decline to answer
2. What sex were you assigned at birth? (check one)
   - ☐ Male
   - ☐ Female
   - ☐ Decline to answer

Adapted from Tate CC, Ledbetter JN, Youssef CP. A two-question method for assessing gender categories in the social and medical sciences. J Sex Res 2013;50(8):767-776; with permission.

A chaperone should be present during physical examinations, with the appropriate gender of the chaperone decided by the patient. Transgender and gender-nonconforming patients should have the option to be examined by medical students or residents to help further the education and cultural sensitivity of future providers, but have the right to refuse if it makes them uncomfortable.

While examining the patient, be aware that secondary sex characteristics may present along a spectrum of development in patients undergoing hormone therapy.

Routine Tests

Appropriate laboratory testing is an important process in the preprocedural preparation of the patient. These investigations are helpful to stratify risk, direct anesthetic choices, and guide postoperative management. The use of these tests is generally guided by the patient's clinical history, comorbidities, and findings on physical examination. When interpreting preoperative laboratory results of a transgender patient it is important to understand how hormone therapy can affect these parameters.

The effects of testosterone and estrogen on a patient's blood chemistry can vary depending on the drug and duration of therapy. CSHT decreases hemoglobin, hematocrit, and creatinine levels in transgender women and increases these levels in transgender men. Additionally, a decrease in calcium, albumin, and alkaline phosphatase levels is expected in transgender woman with increased triglycerides and decreased high-density lipoprotein levels in transgender men (**Table 3**).[36–39]

Preliminary research suggests that transgender patients on CSHT for longer than 6 months should have their laboratory values compared with that of their ciscounterparts rather than with those of their sex assigned at birth.[40] Clearly new reference intervals need to be established for transgender patients. In the interim the Guidelines for the Primary and Gender-Affirming Care of Transgender and Gender Nonbinary People has created tables as tools for health care providers to interpret chemistry levels (**Tables 4** and **5**).[41]

Health care providers also need to be aware that transgender females are often prescribed spironolactone to suppress testosterone production. It is particularly important to monitor serum potassium and creatinine levels in these patients.[37]

Table 3
Changes in laboratory values for transgender people on hormone therapy

	Transgender Woman on Hormone Therapy	Transgender Man on Hormone Therapy
Increased	Red blood cell count Hemoglobin concentration Hematocrit Creatinine Triglycerides	Red blood cell count Hemoglobin concentration Hematocrit Creatinine Alkaline phosphate Aspartate aminotransferase Alanine aminotransferase Triglycerides
Decreased	Calcium Albumin Alkaline phosphate	High-density lipoprotein

Modified from SoRelle JA, Jiao R, Gao E, et al. Impact of Hormone Therapy on Laboratory Values in Transgender Patients. Clin Chem 2019;65(1):174.

Table 4
Interpreting selected laboratory tests in transgender women using feminizing hormone therapy

Laboratory Measure	Lower Limit of Normal	Upper Limit of Normal
Creatinine	Not defined	Male value
Hemoglobin/hematocrit	Female value	Male value

Adapted from UCSF Transgender Care, Department of Family and Community Medicine, University of California San Francisco. Guidelines for the Primary and Gender-Affirming Care of Transgender and Gender Nonbinary People; 2nd edition. Overview of feminizing hormone therapy. Deutsch MB, ed. June 2016. Available at transcare.ucsf.edu/guidelines; with permission.

Pregnancy Testing

The American Society of Anesthesiologists Practice Advisory for Preanesthesia Evaluation recommends that pregnancy testing be offered to (biologic) female patients of childbearing age for whom the result would alter the patient's medical management. This rule extends to transgender men with intact female reproductive organs.[42]

In a recent study, 54% of transgender men reported that they desired to have children.[43] Despite uncertainty about predictable fertility effects, transgender men with intact female reproductive organs have successfully conceived and carried a pregnancy after using testosterone. Transgender men may also have unintended pregnancies while taking or still amenorrheic from testosterone, which was previously thought to preclude pregnancy.[44]

Preoperative Risk Assessment

All patients scheduled to undergo surgery should be assessed for the risk of perioperative cardiovascular events. Risk models have been designed to estimate patients' perioperative risk based on information obtained from the history, physical examination, electrocardiogram, and type of surgery. Special attention should be paid to transgender patients because they face a unique set of risks of which anesthesiologists may be unaware (**Fig. 1**). Currently there is no guidance on whether to use risk calculators based on natal sex or affirmed gender.

Cardiovascular risk factors

Sex is an independent predictor of cardiovascular health outcomes. Few studies have investigated cardiovascular disease (CVD) risk and burden among transgender people on hormone therapy thereby limiting appropriate primary and specialty care.

Table 5
Interpreting selected laboratory tests in transgender men using masculinizing hormone therapy

Laboratory Measure	Lower Limit of Normal	Upper Limit of Normal
Creatinine	Not defined	Male value
Hemoglobin/hematocrit	Male value[a]	Male value

[a] If menstruating regularly, consider using female lower limit of normal.

Adapted from UCSF Transgender Care, Department of Family and Community Medicine, University of California San Francisco. Guidelines for the Primary and Gender-Affirming Care of Transgender and Gender Nonbinary People; 2nd edition. Overview of masculinizing hormone therapy. Deutsch MB, ed. June 2016. Available at transcare.ucsf.edu/guidelines; with permission.

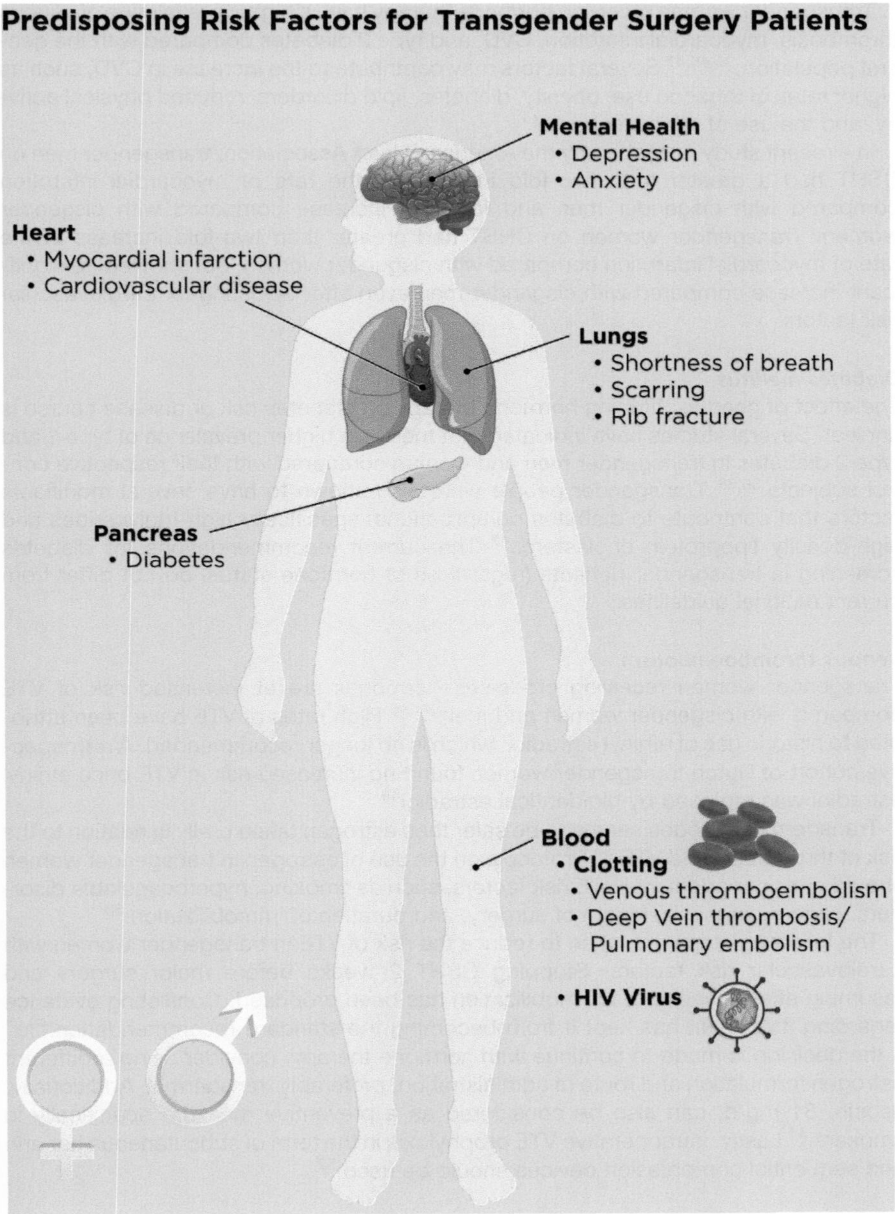

Fig. 1. Consideration for transgender patients perioperatively. (©2019, Memorial Sloan Kettering Cancer Center.)

For transgender adults on hormone therapy, an association with increased CVD risk factors, such as blood pressure elevation, insulin resistance, and lipid derangements, has been appreciated. Up to recently, these changes have not been associated with an increase in morbidity or mortality in transgender men.[45,46]

Transgender women receiving hormone therapy have a higher prevalence of venous thrombosis, myocardial infarction, CVD, and type 2 diabetes compared with the general population.[36,46,47] Several factors may contribute to the increase in CVD, such as higher rates of tobacco use, obesity, diabetes, lipid disorders, reduced physical activity, and the use of ethinyl estradiol.

In a recent study published by the American Heart Association, transgender men on CSHT had a greater than two-fold increase in the rate of myocardial infarction compared with cisgender men and four-fold increase compared with cisgender women. Transgender women on CHST had greater than two-fold increase in the rate of myocardial infarction compared with cisgender women, but showed no significant increase compared with cisgender men even after adjusting for cardiovascular risk factors.

Diabetes mellitus

The effect of gender-affirming hormone therapy on diabetes risk or disease course is unclear. Several studies have indicated that there is a higher prevalence of type 1 and type 2 diabetes in transgender men and women compared with their respective control subjects.[36,38] Transgender people were also shown to have several modifiable factors that contribute to diabetes complications, specifically high triglycerides and high-density lipoprotein cholesterol.[48] The current recommendations for diabetes screening in transgender patients (regardless of hormone status) do not differ from current national guidelines.

Venous thromboembolism

Transgender women receiving cross-sex hormones are at increased risk of VTE compared with cisgender women and men.[34,46] High rates of VTE have been attributed to historic use of ethinyl estradiol, which is no longer recommended. A retrospective cohort of Dutch transgender women found no increased risk in VTE once ethinyl estradiol was replaced by bioidentical estradiol[49]

Transdermal estrogen seems to be safer than estrogen taken orally in relation to the risk of thrombosis and VTE.[34] Protocols on the use of estrogen in transgender women should consider additional VTE risk factors, such as smoking, hypercoagulable disorders, cancer diagnosis, length of surgery, and duration of immobilization.[50]

The following steps are taken to reduce the risk of VTE in transgender women with cardiovascular risk factors. Stopping CSHT 2 weeks before major surgery and resuming after 3 weeks of full mobilization has been proposed. Conflicting evidence regarding its benefit has kept it from becoming the standard recommendation.[49,51] If the decision is made to continue with hormone therapy, consider using a different estrogen formulation and route of administration, preferably transdermal. Additionally, aspirin, 81 mg/d, can also be considered as a preventive measure specifically in smokers.[41] Lastly, intraoperative VTE prophylaxis in the form of subcutaneous heparin and sequential compression devices should be used.[52]

Pulmonary

Chest binding, or compressing the chest tissue, is a common practice among transgender males. There is a lack of research that directly assesses the long-term health impacts of chest binding, but negative physical symptoms have been reported. Symptoms range from chest pain and shortness of breath to scarring and rib fractures.[53] Providers must clearly explain to patients that these devices should not be present during the intraoperative and immediate postoperative period to mitigate the associated cardiopulmonary derangements of binders.

Human immunodeficiency virus

HIV has a high prevalence in the transgender community with an estimated 14% of transgender women infected with the virus.[54] Perioperative risks linked to HIV infection include hepatic and renal dysfunction, coronary artery disease, pulmonary arterial hypertension and cardiac abnormalities, respiratory complications, drug allergies, and hematologic abnormalities.[55]

Patient's perspective

The anesthesiologist's preoperative consultation is central to the enhancement of trust and the creation of a safe environment where the patient feels comfortable. All staff should address the patient with the name, pronouns, and gender identity that the patient prefers.[56] Discussion between the anesthesiologist and the patient should include room assignment, where they will wait during the preoperative period, how they will get to the operating room, and where they will go postoperatively.

INTRAOPERATIVE

Drug Interactions

No drug interactions between estrogen, the various androgen blockers, and testosterone with anesthesia medications have been reported.

Because of the high prevalence of HIV in the transgender community there is a chance that patients may be on antiretroviral therapy. Some antiretroviral therapy medications, specifically the protease inhibitors and nonnucleoside reverse-transcriptase inhibitors, are primarily metabolized by cytochrome P-450 enzymes. The clinician needs to be aware that these drugs may have significant interactions with sedatives, hypnotics, anxiolytics, and antibiotics.[57]

Anatomic Considerations

Transgender patients, especially transgender females, may alter aspects of their voice through surgical procedures, such as laryngoplasty and/or chondroplasty, to alleviate the symptoms of gender dysphoria. Risks of these procedures include vocal cord damage, reduction of tracheal lumen or stenosis, dysphagia, or tracheal perforation, all of which can affect intraoperative airway management.[23,58]

Gender-confirming surgery involving the urethra (vaginoplasty, phalloplasty, or metoidioplasty with urethral lengthening) may require using a smaller urinary catheter. If there is uncertainty, consult a urologist or practitioner experienced with transgender anatomy.[23]

POSTOPERATIVE

The postoperative period is a challenging and vulnerable time for the transgender patient as they deal with postoperative pain, withdrawal, anxiety, and depression. It is important that there are detailed reports and hand-offs between care providers at different stages in the postoperative period. This is a vulnerable period for the patient because the effects of residual anesthesia can impact and the patient's ability to accurately confirm medical history and preferred names and pronouns.

Pain

Pain management is of great importance during the postoperative period, even more so for the transgender patient. Contributing elements to postoperative and chronic pain include psychological factors, such as depression, fear, and anxiety, and medical factors, such as hormone-induced osteoporosis, previous surgeries, and an impaired immune system. A multimodal approach, including nonpharmacologic psychological pain therapies, should be used while being cognizant of the high drug addiction rate among transgender patients. Community and social work support is an important component of the long-term management of these patients and regular follow-up might be required.[59]

Psychosocial

The transgender community is at higher risk of psychiatric morbidity because of depression and anxiety disorder. Budge and colleagues[60] estimated the rates of depression in transgender men and women at 48.3% and 51.4%, respectively. This is relevant to surgery because patients with a history of these disorders are at higher risk for poorer outcomes, including increased opioid use and mortality.[61,62] Furthermore, surgery and prolonged inpatient hospital stays may worsen these conditions.[63] It is important to have a holistic approach when managing a transgender patient during the postoperative period. Incorporate all team members in the decision-making process and consult mental health care, social work, and spiritual care to address the patient's specific needs.

Room Assignment

Postanesthesia care unit room assignment should ideally be discussed during the preoperative assessment. Where room assignments are gender-based, transgender patients should be assigned to rooms based on their self-identified gender.[64] Consider a private room if there is availability, because the increased privacy may provide additional comfort to the patient. Clear communication with postanesthesia care unit staff is needed to avoid unnecessary confrontations and potentially embarrassing situations for the patient.

SUMMARY

Transgender and gender nonconforming people face rampant discrimination in every area of life. Access to quality health care should not be denied to this large, underrepresented population. Anesthesiologists need to acquire an in-depth understanding of the transgender patient's medical and psychosocial needs. A thoughtful approach throughout the entirety of the perioperative period is key to the successful management of the transgender patient.

DISCLOSURE

The authors' work was supported and funded in part by NIH/NCI Cancer Center Support Grant P30 CA008748. L.E. Tollinche serves a paid consultancy and advisory role for Merck & Company Inc. L.E. Tollinche is a grant recipient through Merck Investigators Studies Program to fund clinical trial at MSKCC (NCT03808077).

REFERENCES

1. Flores AR, Herman JL, Gates GJ, et al. How many adults identify as transgender in the United States? Los Angeles (CA): The Williams Institute; 2016.
2. Reisner SL, Poteat T, Keatley J, et al. Global health burden and needs of transgender populations: a review. Lancet 2016;388(10042):412–36.
3. Zucker KJ. Epidemiology of gender dysphoria and transgender identity. Sex Health 2017;14(5):404–11.

4. Clark J, Boyon N, Jackson C. Global attitudes toward transgender people. Paris (France): Ipsos; 2018.
5. Gomez FR, Semenyna SW, Court L, et al. Familial patterning and prevalence of male androphilia among Istmo Zapotec men and muxes. PLoS One 2018; 13(2):e0192683.
6. Semenyna SW, Vasey PL. Striving for prestige in Samoa: a comparison of men, women, and Fa'afafine. J Homosex 2019;66(11):1535–45.
7. Hossain A. The paradox of recognition: hijra, third gender and sexual rights in Bangladesh. Cult Health Sex 2017;19(12):1418–31.
8. Kuper LE, Nussbaum R, Mustanski B. Exploring the diversity of gender and sexual orientation identities in an online sample of transgender individuals. J Sex Res 2012;49(2–3):244–54.
9. World Professional Association for Transgender Health. Standards of care for the health of transsexual, transgender, and gender nonconforming people. World Professional Association for Transgender Health; 2011.
10. Davy Z, Toze M. What is gender dysphoria? A critical systematic narrative review. Transgend Health 2018;3(1):159–69.
11. Dean L, Meyer IH, Robinson K, et al. Lesbian, gay, bisexual, and transgender health: findings and concerns. J Gay Lesbian Med Assoc 2000;4(3):102–51.
12. Herbst JH, Jacobs ED, Finlayson TJ, et al. Estimating HIV prevalence and risk behaviors of transgender persons in the United States: a systematic review. AIDS Behav 2008;12(1):1–17.
13. Grant JM, Motter LA, Tanis J, et al. Injustice at every turn: A report of the national transgender discrimination survey. Washington, DC: National Center for Transgender Equality (NCTE) and National LGBTQ Task Force; 2011.
14. Barboza GE, Dominguez S, Chance E. Physical victimization, gender identity and suicide risk among transgender men and women. Prev Med Rep 2016;4: 385–90.
15. Safer JD, Pearce EN. A simple curriculum content change increased medical student comfort with transgender medicine. Endocr Pract 2013;19(4):633–7.
16. Roberts TK, Fantz CR. Barriers to quality health care for the transgender population. Clin Biochem 2014;47(10–11):983–7.
17. Daniel H, Butkus R, Health and Public Policy Committee of American College of Physicians. Lesbian, gay, bisexual, and transgender health disparities: executive summary of a policy position paper from the American College of Physicians. Ann Intern Med 2015;163(2):135–7.
18. James S, Herman J, Rankin S, et al. US Transgender survey report on health and healthcare. Washington, DC: National Center for Transgender Equality; 2016.
19. Sanchez NF, Sanchez JP, Danoff A. Health care utilization, barriers to care, and hormone usage among male-to-female transgender persons in New York City. Am J Public Health 2009;99(4):713–9.
20. Brown J, Noble LM, Papageorgiou A, et al. Clinical communication in medicine. John Wiley & Sons; 2016.
21. Dubin SN, Nolan IT, Streed CG Jr, et al. Transgender health care: improving medical students' and residents' training and awareness. Adv Med Educ Pract 2018; 9:377–91.
22. Lane M, Ives GC, Sluiter EC, et al. Trends in gender-affirming surgery in insured patients in the United States. Plast Reconstr Surg Glob Open 2018; 6(4):e1738.
23. Tollinche LE, Walters CB, Radix A, et al. The perioperative care of the transgender patient. Anesth Analg 2018;127(2):359–66.

24. Hembree WC, Cohen-Kettenis P, Delemarre-van de Waal HA, et al. Endocrine treatment of transsexual persons: an endocrine society clinical practice guideline. J Clin Endocrinol Metab 2009;94(9):3132–54.
25. Gardner IH, Safer JD. Progress on the road to better medical care for transgender patients. Curr Opin Endocrinol Diabetes Obes 2013;20(6):553–8.
26. Committee on Health Care for Underserved Women. Committee Opinion no. 512: health care for transgender individuals. Obstet Gynecol 2011;118(6):1454–8.
27. Berli JU, Knudson G, Fraser L, et al. What surgeons need to know about gender confirmation surgery when providing care for transgender individuals: a review: what surgeons need to know about gender confirmation surgery. JAMA Surg 2017;152(4):394–400.
28. Deutsch MB, Buchholz D. Electronic health records and transgender patients: practical recommendations for the collection of gender identity data. J Gen Intern Med 2015;30(6):843–7.
29. Tate CC, Ledbetter JN, Youssef CP. A two-question method for assessing gender categories in the social and medical sciences. J Sex Res 2013;50(8):767–76.
30. Cahill SR, Baker K, Deutsch MB, et al. Inclusion of sexual orientation and gender identity in stage 3 meaningful use guidelines: a huge step forward for LGBT health. LGBT Health 2016;3(2):100–2.
31. Hage JJ, Kanhai RC, Oen AL, et al. The devastating outcome of massive subcutaneous injection of highly viscous fluids in male-to-female transsexuals. Plast Reconstr Surg 2001;107(3):734–41.
32. Visnyei K, Samuel M, Heacock L, et al. Hypercalcemia in a male-to-female transgender patient after body contouring injections: a case report. J Med Case Rep 2014;8:71.
33. Cheng Y-J, Liu Z-H, Yao F-J, et al. Current and former smoking and risk for venous thromboembolism: a systematic review and meta-analysis. PLoS Med 2013;10(9):e1001515.
34. Chan W, Drummond A, Kelly M. Deep vein thrombosis in a transgender woman. CMAJ 2017;189(13):E502–4.
35. Sevelius JM. Gender affirmation: a framework for conceptualizing risk behavior among transgender women of color. Sex Roles 2013;68(11–12):675–89.
36. Wierckx K, Elaut E, Declercq E, et al. Prevalence of cardiovascular disease and cancer during cross-sex hormone therapy in a large cohort of trans persons: a case-control study. Eur J Endocrinol 2013;169(4):471–8.
37. Roberts TK, Kraft CS, French D, et al. Interpreting laboratory results in transgender patients on hormone therapy. Am J Med 2014;127(2):159–62.
38. Defreyne J, Vantomme B, Van Caenegem E, et al. Prospective evaluation of hematocrit in gender-affirming hormone treatment: results from European Network for the Investigation of Gender Incongruence. Andrology 2018;6(3):446–54.
39. SoRelle JA, Jiao R, Gao E, et al. Impact of hormone therapy on laboratory values in transgender patients. Clin Chem 2019;65(1):170–9.
40. Goldstein Z, Corneil TA, Greene DN. When gender identity doesn't equal sex recorded at birth: the role of the laboratory in providing effective healthcare to the transgender community. Clin Chem 2017;63(8):1342.
41. Deutsch MB. Guidelines for the primary and gender-affirming care of transgender and gender nonbinary people. University of California, San Francisco; 2016. Available at: www.transhealth.ucsf.edu/guidelines.
42. Committee on Standards and Practice Parameters, Apfelbaum JL, Connis RT, Nickinovich DG, et al. Practice advisory for preanesthesia evaluation: an updated

report by the American Society of Anesthesiologists Task Force on Preanesthesia Evaluation. Anesthesiology 2012;116(3):522–38.
43. Wierckx K, Van Caenegem E, Pennings G, et al. Reproductive wish in transsexual men. Hum Reprod 2011;27(2):483–7.
44. Light AD, Obedin-Maliver J, Sevelius JM, et al. Transgender men who experienced pregnancy after female-to-male gender transitioning. Obstet Gynecol 2014;124(6):1120–7.
45. Smith FD. Perioperative care of the transgender patient. AORN J 2016;103(2):151–63.
46. Alzahrani T, Nguyen T, Ryan A, et al. Cardiovascular disease risk factors and myocardial infarction in the transgender population. Circ Cardiovasc Qual Outcomes 2019;12(4):e005597.
47. Irwig MS. Cardiovascular health in transgender people. Rev Endocr Metab Disord 2018;19(3):243–51.
48. Elbers JM, Giltay EJ, Teerlink T, et al. Effects of sex steroids on components of the insulin resistance syndrome in transsexual subjects. Clin Endocrinol 2003;58(5):562–71.
49. Asscheman H, Giltay EJ, Megens JA, et al. A long-term follow-up study of mortality in transsexuals receiving treatment with cross-sex hormones. Eur J Endocrinol 2011;164(4):635–42.
50. Tangpricha V, den Heijer M. Oestrogen and anti-androgen therapy for transgender women. Lancet Diabetes Endocrinol 2017;5(4):291–300.
51. Boskey ER, Taghinia AH, Ganor O. Association of surgical risk with exogenous hormone use in transgender patients: a systematic review. JAMA Surg 2019;154(2):159–69.
52. Kozek-Langenecker S, Fenger-Eriksen C, Thienpont E, et al. European guidelines on perioperative venous thromboembolism prophylaxis: surgery in the elderly. Eur J Anaesthesiol 2018;35(2):116–22.
53. Jarrett BA, Corbet AL, Gardner IH, et al. Chest binding and care seeking among transmasculine adults: a cross-sectional study. Transgend Health 2018;3(1):170–8.
54. Becasen JS, Denard CL, Mullins MM, et al. Estimating the prevalence of HIV and sexual behaviors among the US transgender population: a systematic review and meta-analysis, 2006–2017. Am J Public Health 2019;109(1):e1–8.
55. Committee MCC. Perioperative management. 2012. Available at: https://www.hivguidelines.org/hiv-care/perioperative-management/#tab_1. Accessed May 20, 2019.
56. Rosa DF, Carvalho MVdF, Pereira NR, et al. Nursing care for the transgender population: genders from the perspective of professional practice. Rev Bras Enferm 2019;72:299–306.
57. Oluwabukola A, Adesina O. Anaesthetic considerations for the HIV positive parturient. Ann Ib Postgrad Med 2009;7(1):31–5.
58. Nolan IT, Morrison SD, Arowojolu O, et al. The role of voice therapy and phonosurgery in transgender vocal feminization. J Craniofac Surg 2019;30(5):1368–75.
59. Pisklakov S, Carullo V. Care of the transgender patient: postoperative pain management. Topics in Pain Management 2016;31(11):1–8.
60. Budge SL, Adelson JL, Howard KAS. Anxiety and depression in transgender individuals: the roles of transition status, loss, social support, and coping. J Consult Clin Psychol 2013;81(3):545–57.

61. Armaghani SJ, Lee DS, Bible JE, et al. Preoperative opioid use and its association with perioperative opioid demand and postoperative opioid independence in patients undergoing spine surgery. Spine (Phila Pa 1976) 2014;39(25):E1524–30.
62. Connerney I, Sloan RP, Shapiro PA, et al. Depression is associated with increased mortality 10 years after coronary artery bypass surgery. Psychosom Med 2010; 72(9):874–81.
63. Nickinson RSJ, Board TN, Kay PR. Post-operative anxiety and depression levels in orthopaedic surgery: a study of 56 patients undergoing hip or knee arthroplasty. J Eval Clin Pract 2009;15(2):307–10.
64. Lambda Legal. Creating equal access to quality health care for transgender patients: transgender-affirming hospital policies. Lambda Legal; 2016.

Racial Disparities in Pediatric Anesthesia

Anne Elizabeth Baetzel, MD[a,*], Ashlee Holman, MD[a], Nicole Dobija, MD[a], Paul Irvin Reynolds, MD[a], Olubukola Olugbenga Nafiu, MD, FRCA, MS[b]

KEYWORDS

• Health care disparities • Inequity • Minority health • Pediatric anesthesia • Implicit bias

KEY POINTS

- Health care disparities exist in pediatric anesthesia. By 2020, more than 50% of children born in the United States will be considered part of a minority group.
- Measures must be instituted to protect this vulnerable population during the especially stressful time of surgery. Potential solutions to correct health care disparities should include changes at the provider, patient, and health care system levels.
- Anesthesia providers are providers uniquely positioned to lead the way because of increasing usage of protocol-driven health care.

I've learned that people will forget what you said, people will forget what you did, but people will never forget how you made them feel.

—Maya Angelou

INTRODUCTION

More than 2 decades ago, Gornick and colleagues[1] described disparities in health care of Medicare patients based on race and income level. Despite increased recognition and countermeasures to correct these differences, disparities in health outcomes owing to race, ethnicity, gender, and social status persist. Data on health care disparities have largely been from adult patients. A 2003 systematic review on health care disparities published by the Institute of Medicine included only 5 pediatric-specific studies.[2] That same year, the first National Healthcare Disparities Report was published with the intent of describing differences in the quality of and access to health care, with particular emphasis on modifiable health outcomes.[3] Racial disparities in the adult population have been demonstrated on a variety of health care fronts, including examination of rates of mammography,[3] recommendation for

[a] University of Michigan, CS Mott Children's Hospital, 4-911, 1540 East Medical Center Drive, Ann Arbor, MI 48109, USA; [b] Nationwide Children's Hospital, 700 Children's Drive, Columbus, OH 43205, USA

* Corresponding author.

E-mail address: abaetzel@med.umich.edu

Anesthesiology Clin 38 (2020) 327–339
https://doi.org/10.1016/j.anclin.2020.01.010
anesthesiology.theclinics.com

angiography,[4] and treatment of cancer.[5,6] Outcomes related to racial disparities in the pediatric population are less frequently studied, and those specific to pediatric anesthesia are even more infrequent. In this review, the authors summarize the literature regarding health care disparities in pediatric anesthesia at the health care provider, patient, and system level (**Fig. 1**). Racial differences in health care outcomes may be nonmodifiable (because of genetic susceptibility); however, disparities in health care delivery (such as failing to treat a child with adequate analgesia despite documented high pain scores or preferential administration of expensive medications to a particular race or ethnicity) are modifiable. Therefore, this review focuses on modifiable health care disparities in the pediatric perianesthesia setting.

HEALTH CARE PROVIDER FACTORS

The Institute of Medicine identified health care provider bias and stereotyping as possible contributors to health care disparities.[2] Although attitudes provide a framework to subjectively organize the environment and orient ourselves to those people and things within it, attitudes also have the potential to bias us in ways that may unduly influence us. Explicit attitudes are measured by self-report. Implicit attitudes automatically function without a person's full awareness or control and are not necessarily congruent with self-reported attitudes.[7] Implicit attitudes are more likely to influence responses when the chance to assess consequences of various actions does not exist, for example, when time pressure or the motivation to do so is absent.[8,9]

Although there are no studies specifically looking at bias among pediatric anesthesiologists, discrepancies in physician-patient communication have been examined in other specialties. One such retrospective study examined primary care physicians and

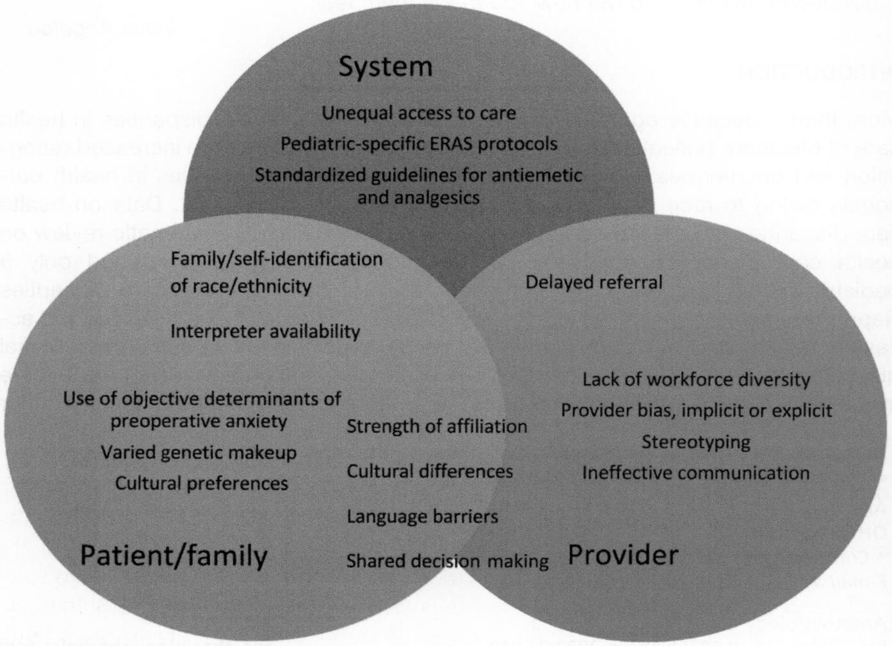

Fig. 1. Factors influencing health care disparities in pediatric anesthesia.

adult patients who identified their race/ethnicity as white or African American with the purpose of surveying the quality of their interactions with patients of different races during their office visits.[10] Patient-physician communication during these visits was the primary study outcome, focusing on duration of visit and speech speed, physician verbal dominance (reported as the ratio of physician's talk time divided by the patient's talk time), physician patient-centeredness score, and patient and physician positive-affect scores.[10] This study found that physicians were 23% more verbally dominant and 33% less patient centered with African American patients compared with their interactions with white patients. In addition, for both physicians and African American patients, positive affect was lower than when compared with visits with white patients. Physician specialty was not associated with outcomes in this specific study; however, Paasche-Orlow and Roter[10] found that family medicine physicians, in comparison with internal medicine physicians, were more patient centered with minority patients but more verbally dominant with female patients.

Sabin and colleagues[11] examined data from test takers who voluntarily completed the Race Implicit Attitude Test (IAT). Test results examining implicit attitudes among physicians aligned with the same pattern seen in the overall population. When measuring implicit attitudes by physician race and ethnicity, they found that white physicians showed the strongest preference for whites. In addition, white, male, physician bias applied to other social characteristics, including sexuality, weight, ability, age, and religion.[12] African American physicians did not show an implicit preference for either white Americans or black Americans. When considering physician gender, Sabin and colleagues[11] observed a strong preference for white Americans among male physicians and a weaker but still appreciable preference for white Americans among female physicians. A different study found that female physicians, in comparison to their male colleagues, were more likely to spend more time with their patients regardless of race, were more likely to be more collaborative with treatment plans, and were more likely to address social and emotional patient concerns.[13] Patient satisfaction was also higher for patients of female physicians, which the research team speculated could be a result of differences in implicit attitudes and effect on nonverbal behavior.[14]

Sabin and colleagues[15] conducted a similar study of implicit and explicit attitudes among pediatricians (including attendings, fellows, and residents) at 1 institution. They observed that pediatricians displayed less overall implicit preference for whites compared with most IAT test takers; however, a moderate implicit association was found describing European Americans as more likely to be a "compliant patient." No difference was observed in treatment recommendations as associated with patient race and implicit measures, as was previously demonstrated in studies performed by Bogart and colleagues.[16] This study did, however, show a significant positive correlation between physician age and presence of implicit bias toward European Americans. Of note, a female gender response bias was described in this study, but the investigators did not speculate on the reason for this bias nor its effect on the responses.[13]

A study of pediatric patients within Managed Care Organizations found that the pediatric patient-physician interpersonal relationship was often shorter in duration and weaker in quality for minorities (including black, Hispanic, and Asian patients) compared with white patients, regardless of insurance status.[17] Reasons for this included language barriers, difficulty in finding a primary care physician of the same race, and cultural differences in seeking care related to limitations instituted by managed care policies.[18] Interestingly, pediatricians were reported to have better interpersonal relationships with patients than other generalists in this study.

In 2010, the American Academy of Pediatrics published a technical report summarizing literature on racial and ethnic disparities in the pediatric population.[19] In this review, African American children experienced higher risk of unmet health care needs, lower rates of access to primary care physicians, lower rates of referral to a specialist for evaluation, and higher risk of not receiving adequate time and information from physicians compared with white children.[19] In addition, African American children were found to have lower scores for primary care provider interpersonal relationships, comprehensiveness, and strength of affiliation. African American families also displayed lower physician-visit rates with higher odds of going more than 1 year between physician visits and placing fewer calls to physician offices. Similar findings have been reported for Asians/Pacific Islander, Latino, American Indian, and Alaska Native children.[19] Although there are no studies to date specifically examining provider bias among pediatric anesthesia caregivers, the preceding findings are important given that a strong patient-physician relationship is crucial for providing high-quality care and making long-term treatment decisions as well as promoting adherence to treatment plans, coordinating care, increasing patient and family satisfaction, and working toward better health outcomes.

PATIENT LEVEL FACTORS

Several studies have examined patient-specific factors contributing to health care disparities in pediatric anesthesia (**Table 1**). In 2010, Jimenez and colleagues[20] evaluated the effect of race/ethnicity on the perioperative pain treatment of children who underwent adenotonsillectomy. The investigators demonstrated Latino children were administered 30% fewer postoperative opioids compared with their white peers. This difference was in the setting of Latino children being more likely to have received shorter-acting intraoperative opioids than their white peers and no significant difference in the documented median pain scores between the groups. The cause for this difference was not determined; however, the investigators postulated that this may be related to language barriers and cultural preferences. For example, either parental presence for induction or use of oral premedication was offered to all children participating in this study to mitigate peri-induction anxiety. Most Latino families (73%) chose parental presence at induction, whereas white families more often chose oral premedication (42%). Investigators hypothesized that Latino families may have relied more on nonpharmacologic comfort measures, whereas white families more often chose pharmacologic interventions. The investigators also theorized that biological factors may contribute to differences in opioid administration, because previous pharmacokinetic and pharmacodynamic studies have demonstrated differences in mu-opioid receptors and effect of morphine metabolites on ventilatory response to hypercapnia between Latino and white patients.[21,22]

In a prospective, observational study, Sadhasivam and colleagues[23] examined the early postoperative pain treatment of children aged 6 to 15 years old who underwent adenotonsillectomy. All study subjects received standardized preoperative care, uniform surgical technique, and a standard intraoperative dose of morphine, which was decreased by half in the presence of demonstrated obstructive sleep apnea. Postoperative care included assessment of pain score with either the Faces, Legs, Activity, Cry, Consolability (FLACC) scale or the Numerical Rating Scale, and scores of $\geq$4/10 received morphine 0.05 mg/kg intravenously (IV). Adverse opioid events were recorded, with emphasis on clinical respiratory depression. In addition, all children received intraoperative ondansetron and dexamethasone for antiemetic prophylaxis. Overall, black children had higher FLACC scores in the recovery room, higher odds of needing

Table 1
Summary of literature on racial disparities in pediatric anesthesia

Study	Design	Purpose	Sample Size	Findings	Limitations
Jimenez et al,[20] 2010	Retrospective review	Primary outcome: administration of opioids following tonsillectomy Secondary outcomes: nonopioid analgesics, opioid side effects, pain scores	Latino: 47 children White: 47 children	30% less opioids given to Latino children; no difference in nonopioid analgesics; no difference in peak pain score; no difference in side effects	Retrospective, missing data, assumption of language barriers, single institution
Sadhasivam et al,[23] 2012	Prospective observational	Outcomes: maximum postoperative pain score, postoperative opioid requirement, analgesic interventions, opioid-related adverse effects	African American: 34 children White: 160 children	Higher FLACC scores, more interventions needed, great postoperative morphine requirement in African American children; higher rate of opioid-related adverse effects in white children	Unknown variables (eg, socioeconomic status, pain coping skills), only 2 races represented, variations among clinical care providers (observational study)
Nafiu et al,[25] 2017	Prospective observational	Primary outcome: PACU analgesic administration Secondary outcome: PACU LOS	White: 619 children Minorities: 152 children	No difference between racial groups; minority children received IV opioid more often; minority children had longer PACU LOS	Aggregation of all minority groups, variety of surgical procedures, no data on pain coping skills, socioeconomic status, or genetic makeup; single institution
Rosenbloom et al,[26] 2017	Retrospective cohort study	Perioperative medication administration for emergency appendectomy, first and highest recorded pain scores	White: 1329 children Black: 351 children	No difference in perioperative or intraoperative medication administration; no difference in pain scores	Small sample size, limited data on preoperative and postoperative periods; no data on anesthesiologist characteristics; single institution
Baetzel et al,[28] 2019	Retrospective review	Primary outcome: inhalation vs IV induction Secondary outcomes: presence of family member at induction, use of preoperative anxiolytic, use of child life therapy	White: 33,717 children Black: 3901 children	Black children <15 yo less likely to have family present at induction; black children <5 yo less likely to have preoperative midazolam	Potential errors in data entry, unmeasured variables, insufficient provider information; single institution

intervention, and increased postoperative morphine consumption. White children had more instances of opioid-related side effects and prolonged postanesthesia care unit (PACU) length of stay (LOS) as a result of the adverse side effects of administered opioids. Even when morphine dosing was equivalent, black children tended to have higher pain scores than white children. Of note, the investigators found no significant evidence of racial difference in the odds of treatment of documented moderate to severe pain. Indeed, ethnic minority children were more likely than their white peers to receive IV opioids for the management of mild recovery room pain. Follow-up studies have demonstrated that black children have a higher morphine clearance, which may be associated with a variant of the OCT1 gene.[24] The investigators also speculated that individual clinical providers, including nurses in the recovery room, may have exhibited bias toward subjective pain scores leading to differential treatment.

Another prospective study examined differences in analgesic administration in the recovery room among white children compared with minority children, including African American, Latino, Asian, Pacific Islander, and American Indian/Alaska Native children.[25] Unlike previous studies that examined only 1 surgical procedure, Nafiu and colleagues[25] looked at all procedures considered to be painful, defined by intraoperative use of IV opioid, local anesthetic infiltration, and/or nerve block. The primary outcome of the study was administration of any analgesic medication in the PACU. Secondary outcomes included PACU LOS. The investigators showed no difference in the rate of any analgesic medication administration in the recovery room when comparing white and minority children. However, minority children were twice as likely to receive IV opioids to treat minor pain when compared with their white peers. Not surprisingly, children who received opioid analgesics had a longer stay in the recovery room, although this result was not significantly associated with race or ethnicity. Unlike findings in other studies whereby black children had higher pain scores and required intervention with opioid analgesics more frequently,[23] this study showed no difference between pain scores for white and minority children.[25] One reason for this may be that minority children were examined as a group compared with their white peers, as opposed to comparing individual races or ethnicities. Grouping several races and ethnicities together may underrepresent outcomes for different racial identities and therefore obscure results for all minority patients.

Rosenbloom and colleagues[26] performed a retrospective study of differences in the administration of anesthetic drugs perioperatively in children undergoing emergency laparoscopic appendectomy. Self-reported race was the primary exposure variable. A total of 1680 children were included, 351 of whom were black. The investigators compared medication administration, including preoperative midazolam, intraoperative morphine and fentanyl, intraoperative lidocaine for prevention of propofol-related pain and endotracheal intubation, intraoperative ondansetron and ketorolac, as well as initial and highest recorded postoperative pain scores. The study found no significant difference in the administration of anesthetic or analgesic medications and no difference between first or highest pain scores when comparing black and white children. There was a difference in the rate of preoperative administration of midazolam, similar to the results described in the Jimenez study,[20] with only 49% of black children receiving preoperative midazolam compared with 56% of white children; however, this difference was not significant after controlling for covariates such as age, gender, and attending anesthesiologist. Limitations of this study include a small study size and lack of data on attending anesthesiologist characteristics, objective determinants of preoperative anxiety, and parental preferences for premedication. Despite adjusting for numerous variables, the investigators noted that their analysis was limited by practice variation at their institution. Another study examining racial disparities in emergency department pain management of children with appendicitis found that black patients reporting moderate or severe pain were less likely to receive opioids compared with white patients.[27]

In a recent retrospective study, Baetzel and colleagues[28] described "adultification" of black children in the perioperative setting. "Adultification" is a term used in the fields of justice and education and is a process that serves to "remove or reduce the consideration of childhood as a mediating factor in youth's behavior."[29] In their study of more than 37,000 children who underwent elective surgery, the investigators examined differences in the use of strategies for mitigating peri-induction anxiety between black and white children. They compared administration of oral midazolam premedication, presence of family for induction of anesthesia, and use of child life therapy, as well as use of inhalation induction versus IV induction across racial groups.[29] Children with preexisting IV access and those in whom a rapid sequence induction was planned were excluded. Overall, black children were more likely than their white peers to have undergone inhalational induction and were less likely to have received preoperative midazolam or have a family member present for induction. Race was a significant predictor of the use inhalational induction and appeared to influence whether a family member was present for induction. The latter is a critical finding given that parental presence at induction is one of the most common nonpharmacologic methods of comfort and a decision largely made at the discretion of the attending anesthesiologist. Causality can only be inferred because of the retrospective, cross-sectional study design. Nevertheless, the investigators postulated that this finding may be a result of weaker interpersonal relationships between care providers and parents of minority children as well as less shared decision making with parents of minority children, which is consistent with studies in the pediatric primary care setting.[19] Using comfort measures, such as family member presence for induction or pharmacologic premedication with midazolam, may also reflect racial bias in the form of "adultification," perceiving that black children need less nurturing and protection and have a greater fund of knowledge about adult topics when compared with their white peers.

SYSTEM-LEVEL FACTORS

In 1999, the US Congress tasked the Institute of Medicine with evaluating health care disparities between minorities and nonminorities, resulting in the report "Unequal Treatment: Confronting Racial and Ethnic Disparities in Health Care."[2] This report identified system level factors influencing care, including access to medical and surgical services, method of payment for services, and ability of the patient to understand what procedures or services are available for treatment.[2]

Access to pediatric anesthesia services is determined by the primary surgeon or proceduralist and is thus an initial systems issue. Within pediatric surgery and emergency medicine, acute appendicitis and progression to appendiceal perforation (AP) have been used as a surrogate for evaluation of access to care.[30,31] A delay in diagnosis and treatment of acute appendicitis may lead to perforation, with resultant increase in morbidity and LOS. A disparity in the numbers of AP between the minority and white population exists.[32–34] A study at Kaiser Permanente in California[31] demonstrated no difference in perforation rates for patients treated for acute appendicitis only after access to care was reliably available for all patients, regardless of race or socioeconomic status. Equal access for all patients remains a significant obstacle in health care delivery. Data provided by Hayes and colleagues[35] from 2013 to 2015 showed that the disparity in access to care between white, black, and Hispanic patients had decreased. One confounding factor is a patient's or family's willingness to undergo surgery once surgery is determined to be required, a preference that is influenced by culture and race. In the adult population, Lathan and colleagues[36] showed that black patients were more likely than white patients to decline surgery in the early stages of treatment of non–small cell lung cancer. Pediatric literature also shows an association between religious and cultural beliefs for healing and health care and parent's refusal of medical care.[37]

The practice of anesthesia is increasingly protocol driven, with implementation of enhanced recovery after surgery (ERAS) protocols, the perioperative surgical home, checklists, and care bundles intended to minimize physiologic stress and promote early recovery. One adult study found that institution of ERAS protocols eliminated racial differences in LOS after colorectal surgery when comparing black and white patients.[38] The investigators noted that before usage of ERAS protocols, the ACS-NSQIP Risk Calculator would have predicted no difference in LOS when comparing black and white patients; yet black patients stayed an average of 3 days longer compared with white patients in the pre-ERAS period.[38] No differences for LOS or any of the secondary outcomes, including readmission, mortality, and 30-day complication rates, were found when comparing black and white patients in the post-ERAS time period.[38] Few studies look specifically at ERAS protocols in the pediatric population, and of these, none looked at racial differences.[39,40] Whether implementation of ERAS protocols has the potential to decrease racial disparities in outcomes following common pediatric procedures remains an important area for future investigation.

Administration of antiemetic medication is considered a standard of care with clear guidelines for adult patients,[41] has been associated with improvement in patient outcomes, and is the responsibility of the anesthesia provider.[42] Andreae and colleagues[43] postulated that antiemetic prophylaxis could serve as a marker of anesthesia quality and examined its use in both pediatric and adult surgery. They collected demographic data, including age, gender, race, and insurance status, from approximately 92,000 electronic anesthesia records from the National Anesthesia Clinical Outcomes Registry and found a large difference in the use of antiemetic medications with only 40% of patients with Medicaid receiving antiemetic therapy, compared with 60% of patients with commercial insurance.[43] Proving bias among anesthesia providers with this dataset is difficult; however, this study offers an area for potential improvement in health care disparities and patient outcomes specifically related to anesthesia practice.

STRATEGIES FOR ADDRESSING PEDIATRIC HEALTH CARE DISPARITIES

Recent demographic projections indicate that by the year 2020 more than half of the children living in the United States will be considered part of a minority race or ethnic group.[44] Furthermore, by the year 2044, a crossover is projected to occur whereby the non-Hispanic white population will comprise less than 50% of the nation's total population, making the United States a "majority-minority" nation (**Table 2**).[44] Given that ethnic/racial minorities have been shown to have poorer health outcomes and racial bias is one of the putative factors responsible for this, the subject of perioperative health care disparity is a timely one.

At the provider level, one of the standards put forth by the Department of Health and Human Services is to recruit, promote, and support a diverse workforce.[45] Studies have shown that a diverse health care workforce leads to better delivery of care to minority patients.[46] Although the number of female medical school graduates pursuing training in anesthesia has increased somewhat over the past several decades,[47] only 6% of practicing anesthesiologists were considered part of a minority group according to a

Table 2
Distribution of United States population by race/ethnicity in minors less than 18 years old and practicing anesthesiologists in the United States

Race/Ethnic Group	2014 Census Data,[44] %	2060 Projected Census Data,[44] %	Practicing US Anesthesiologists, 2013,[48] %
White	52.0	35.6	78.8
Black	13.8	13.2	2.4
Latino/Hispanic	24.4	33.5	3.4
Asian	4.7	7.9	11.3
Other	5.4	9.7	3.9

2013 report.[48] Future recruitment of minority medical school graduates to the field of anesthesia will be a key in improving health care outcomes for patients of all races and ethnicities. Racial and cultural dissonance between pediatric anesthesia care providers and the families they care for is a relatively unexplored topic. Given that racial concordance between provider and patients has been shown to increase care delivery, as well as satisfaction with care delivered,[49,50] there is a need for concerted efforts to increase the number of ethnic/racial minorities in the perioperative workforce. In addition, education surrounding cultural competency and linguistics is needed to narrow the health care outcomes gap between racial and ethnic minority groups.[46]

At the patient level, access to adequate health insurance coverage is imperative. When the Affordable Care Act was signed into law in 2010, nearly 32 million Americans were newly insured; 48% of these were considered part of a minority group.[51] Ensuring continued access to affordable health care is a key driver in eliminating racial disparities in health care outcomes. On a more local level, continued improvement in communication between health care providers and patients is needed. Shared decision making between parents of minority children and their provider will facilitate better care of these children, including making informed decisions during the stressful perioperative period.[52] Improved interactions between pediatric patients, their caregivers, and their physicians during all patient encounters can foster better communication and improved patient outcomes and satisfaction.

At a systems level, the US Secretary of Health and Human Services has called for improved data collections and reporting standards, especially with regard to reporting of race, ethnicity, sex, primary language, and disability status.[53] With improved data collection, more research into the causes for health disparities can be used. Accuracy of data collection begins during the hospital or clinic registration process. Patients and their families must be provided the opportunity to self-identify their race and ethnicity (or that of their child). Self-recording, as opposed to staff documentation, is critical, as a recent study showed that when staff members enter these data for patients, they often do so inaccurately.[54] In addition, proposals for institution of provider feedback regarding racial and ethnic disparities in health outcomes have been put forth. As an example, the Alliance for Innovation on Maternal Health provides feedback to staff and leadership regarding reduction of peripartum racial and ethnic disparities in order to better reflect on causes for such disparities and provide opportunities for disparity reduction.[55]

SUMMARY

Despite concerted efforts to decrease disparities in health care at the federal and state levels, health care disparities remain a pervasive problem. This critical area of research stands relatively unexplored in the pediatric perioperative setting, and more studies are needed. Results from the limited number of available studies are largely inconclusive because of their retrospective or observational design and inconsistencies in the definition of predictor and outcome variables. A complex combination of factors may be responsible for health care disparities at the patient, provider, and system levels, and it is critical for future investigators to distinguish differences in health outcomes because of race from disparities in health care based on race. The former may not be easily modifiable, whereas the latter may be morally and lawfully unconscionable. Providing suboptimal care based on race, ethnicity, gender, religion, or socioeconomic status is simply wrong and requires effort to correct and prevent. Although racial disparity appears to be relatively uncommon in the delivery of pediatric anesthesia care, one must continually assess their performance. Several opportunities exist in pediatric anesthesia to reduce disparities in health care delivery. From recruitment of minority physicians, to improved communication and cultural competency, better use of the electronic health care record, and provision of feedback to providers in a dashboard setting, anesthesiologists are uniquely poised to advance health equity and improve outcomes for arguably one of the most vulnerable populations in our country.

ACKNOWLEDGMENTS

The authors thank Shobha Malviya, MD and Jack Wheeler, PhD for assistance in editing the article.

DISCLOSURE

A.E. Baetzel, A. Holman, N. Dobija, and P.I. Reynolds have reported no conflicts of interest, commercial, financial, or otherwise. This review article was supported by no grants or any other funding. O.O. Nafiu has reported no conflicts of interest, commercial, financial, or otherwise. National Institute of General Medical Sciences (NIGMS) grant number K23 GM104354 supported Dr O.O. Nafiu's work and efforts.

REFERENCES

1. Gornick ME, Eggers PW, Reilly TW, et al. Effects of race and income on mortality and use of services among Medicare beneficiaries. N Engl J Med 1996;335(11): 791–9.
2. Smedley BD, Stith AY, Nelson AR, editors. Unequal treatment: confronting racial and ethnic disparities in healthcare. Institute of Medicine (US) Committee on understanding and eliminating racial and ethnic disparities in health care. Washington, DC: National Academies Press (US); 2003.
3. National Healthcare Disparities Report." U. S. Department of Health and Human Services Agency for Healthcare Research and Quality, dated July 2003. Available at: https://archive.ahrq.gov/qual/nhdr03/nhdr03.htm. Accessed May 20, 2019.
4. Blustein J. Medicare coverage, supplemental insurance, and the use of mammography by older women. N Engl J Med 1995;332:1138–43.
5. Ayanian JZ, Udvarhelyi IS, Gatsonis CA, et al. Racial differences in the use of revascularization procedures after coronary angioplasty. JAMA 1993;269: 2642–6.
6. Murphy MM, Simons JP, Ng SC, et al. Racial differences in cancer specialist consultation, treatment and outcomes for locoregional pancreatic adenocarcinoma. Ann Surg Oncol 2009;16:2968–77.

7. Greenwald AG, Banaji MR. Implicit social cognition: attitudes, self-esteem, and stereotypes. Psychol Rev 1995;102(1):4–27.
8. Dovido JF, Kawakami K, Gaertner SL. Implicit and explicit prejudice and interracial interaction. J Pers Soc Psychol 2002;82(1):62–8.
9. Johnson RL, Roter D, Powe NR, et al. Patient race/ethnicity and quality of patient-physician communication during medical visits. Am J Public Health 2004;94(12): 2084–90.
10. Paasche-Orlow M, Roter D. The communication patterns of internal medicine and family medicine physicians. J Am Board Fam Pract 2003;16(6):485–93.
11. Sabin J, Nosek BA, Greenwald A, et al. Physicians' implicit and explicit attitudes about race by MD race, ethnicity, and gender. J Health Care Poor Underserved 2009;20(3):896–913.
12. Nosek BA, Smyth FL, Hansen JJ, et al. Pervasiveness and correlates of implicit attitudes and stereotypes. Eur Rev Soc Psychol 2007;18:36–88.
13. Roter DL, Hall JA. Why physician gender matters in shaping the physician-patient relationship. J Womens Health 1998;7(9):1093–7.
14. Bertakis KD, Franks P, Azari R. Effects of physician gender on patient satisfaction. J Am Med Womens Assoc (1972) 2003;58(2):69–75.
15. Sabin JA, Rivara FP, Greenwald AG. Physician implicit attitudes and stereotypes about race and quality of medical care. Med Care 2008;46(7):678–85.
16. Bogart LM, Catz SL, Kelly JA, et al. Factors influencing physicians' judgments of adherence and treatment decisions for patients with HIV disease. Med Decis Making 2001;21(1):28–36.
17. Stevens GD, Shi L. Effect of managed care on children's relationships with their primary care physicians: differences by race. Arch Pediatr Adolesc Med 2002; 156(4):369–77.
18. Fiscella K, Franks P, Gold M, et al. Inequality in quality: addressing socioeconomic, racial, and ethnic disparities in health care. JAMA 2000;283:2579–84.
19. Flores G, Committee on Pediatric Research. Technical report–racial and ethnic disparities in the health and health care of children. Pediatrics 2010;125(4): e979–1020.
20. Jimenez N, Seidel K, Martin LD, et al. Perioperative analgesic treatment in Latino and non-Latino pediatric patients. J Health Care Poor Underserved 2010;21(1): 229–36.
21. Cepeda MS, Farrar JT, Roa JH, et al. Ethnicity influences morphine pharmacokinetics and pharmacodynamics. Clin Pharmacol Ther 2001;70(4):351–61.
22. Bond C, LaForge KS, Tian M, et al. Single nucleotide polymorphism in the human mu opioid receptor gene alters beta-endorphin binding and activity: possible implications for opiate addiction. Proc Natl Acad Sci U S A 1998;95(16):9608–13.
23. Sadhasivam S, Chidambaran V, Ngamprasertwong P, et al. Race and unequal burden of perioperative pain and opioid related adverse effects in children. Pediatrics 2012;129(5):832–8.
24. Balyan R, Zhang X, Chidambaran V, et al. OCT1 genetic variants are associated with postoperative morphine-related adverse effects in children. Pharmacogenomics 2017;18(7):621–9.
25. Nafiu OO, Chimbira WT, Stewart M, et al. Racial differences in the pain management of children recovering from anesthesia. Paediatr Anaesth 2017;27:760–7.
26. Rosenbloom JM, Senthil K, Long AS, et al. A limited evaluation of the association of race and anesthetic medication administration: a single-center experience with appendectomies. Paediatr Anaesth 2017;27:1142–7.

27. Goyal MK, Kuppermann N, Cleary SD, et al. Racial disparities in pain management of children with appendicitis in emergency departments. JAMA Pediatr 2015;169(11):996–1002.
28. Baetzel AE, Brown DJ, Koppera PK, et al. The adultification of black children in pediatric anesthesia. Anesth Analg 2019;129(4):1118–23.
29. Epstein R, Blake JJ, Gonzalez T. Girlhood Interrupted: the erasure of black girls' childhood. Washington, DC: The Georgetown Law Center of Poverty and Inequality; 2017.
30. Jablonski KA, Guagliardo MF. Pediatric appendicitis rupture rate: a national indicator of disparities in healthcare access. Popul Health Metr 2005;3:1–9.
31. Lee SL, Shekherdimian S, Chiu VY, et al. Perforated appendicitis in children: equal access to care eliminates racial and socioeconomic disparities. J Pediatr Surg 2010;45(6):1203–7.
32. Ponsky TA, Huang ZJ, Kittle K, et al. Hospital- and patient-level characteristics and the risk of appendiceal rupture and negative appendectomy in children. JAMA 2004;292:1977–82.
33. Smink DS, Fishman SJ, Kleinman K, et al. Effects of race, insurance status, and hospital volume on perforated appendicitis in children. Pediatrics 2005;115:920–5.
34. Guagliardo MF, Teach SJ, Huang ZJ, et al. Racial and ethnic disparities in pediatric appendicitis rupture rate. Acad Emerg Med 2003;10:1218–27.
35. Hayes SL, Riley P, Radley DC, et al. Reducing racial and ethnic disparities in access to care: has the Affordable Care Act made a difference? Issue Brief (Commonw Fund) 2017;2017:1–14.
36. Lathan CS, Neville BA, Earle CC. The effect of race on invasive staging and surgery in non-small-cell lung cancer. J Clin Oncol 2006;24(3):413–8.
37. Linnard-Palmer L, Kools S. Parents' refusal of medical treatment for cultural or religious beliefs: an ethnographic study of health care professionals' experiences. J Pediatr Oncol Nurs 2005;22(1):48–57.
38. Wahl TS, Goss LE, Morris MS, et al. Enhanced recovery after surgery (ERAS) eliminates racial disparities in postoperative length of stay after colorectal surgery. Ann Surg 2018;268(6):1026–35.
39. Raval MV, Heiss KF. Development of an enhanced recovery protocol for children undergoing gastrointestinal surgery. Curr Opin Pediatr 2018;30(3):399–404.
40. Rove KO, Edney JC, Brockel MA. Enhanced recovery after surgery in children: promising, evidence-based multidisciplinary care. Paediatr Anaesth 2018;28(6):482–92.
41. Gan TJ, Diemunsch P, Habib AS, et al, Society for Ambulatory Anesthesia. Consensus guidelines for the management of post-operative nausea and vomiting. Anesth Analg 2014;118:85–113.
42. Macario A, Chung A, Weinger MB. Variation in practice patterns of anesthesiologists in California for prophylaxis of post-operative nausea and vomiting. J Clin Anesth 2001;13:353–60.
43. Andreae MH, Gabry JS, Goodrich B, et al. Antiemetic prophylaxis as a marker of health care disparities in the national anesthesia clinical outcomes registry. Anesth Analg 2018;126(2):588–99.
44. Colby SL, Ortman JM. Projections of the size and composition of the U.S. Population: 2014 to 2060. Washington, DC: U.S. Census Bureau Public Information Office; 2015. Available at: https://www.census.gov/library/publications/2015/demo/p25-1143.html. Accessed May 20, 2019.

45. Stone J, Moskowitz GB. Non-conscious bias in medical decision making: what can be done to reduce it? Med Educ 2011;45:768–76.
46. Betancourt JR, Corbett J, Bondaryk MR. Addressing disparities and achieving equity: cultural competence, ethics and health-care transformation. Chest 2014;145(1):143–8.
47. Wong CA, Stock MC. The status of women in academic anesthesiology: a progress report. Anesth Analg 2008;107(1):178–84.
48. Baird MD, Daugherty L, Kumar KB, et al. The anesthesiologist workforce in 2013: a final briefing to the American Society of Anesthesiologists. Santa Monica (CA): Rand Corporation; 2014.
49. Poma PA. Race/ethnicity concordance between patients and physicians. J Natl Med Assoc 2017;109(1):6–8.
50. Street RL, O'Malley KJ, Cooper LA, et al. Understanding concordance in patient-physician relationships: personal and ethnic dimensions of shared identity. Ann Fam Med 2008;6:198–205.
51. Robert Wood Johnson Foundation. Disparities in health care persist. Robert Wood Johnson Foundation website. Available at: http://www.rwjf.org/content/dam/farm/reports/issue_briefs/2012/rwjf402390/subassets/rwjf402390_3. Accessed August 5, 2019.
52. King JS, Eckman MH, Moulton BW. The potential of shared decision making to reduce health disparities. J Law Med Ethics 2011;39(1):S30–3.
53. Gracia JN. Moment of opportunity: reducing health disparities and advancing health equity 2015. Available at: www.minorityhealth.hhs.gov. Accessed August 5, 2019.
54. Boehmer U, Kressin NR, Berlowitz DR, et al. Self-reported vs administrative race/ethnicity data and study results. Am J Public Health 2002;92:1471–2.
55. Lange EMS, Rao S, Toledo P. Racial and ethnic disparities in obstetric anesthesia. Semin Perinatol 2017;41(5):293–8.

Genetics and Gender in Acute Pain and Perioperative Opioid Analgesia

Albert Hyukjae Kwon, MD[1], Pamela Flood, MD, MA*

KEYWORDS

- Acute pain • Opioid analgesia • Gender • Sex • Genetic variability
- Single-nucleotide polymorphism • Pharmacogenetics

KEY POINTS

- Biological sex as a variable in experimental pain perception has been well studied and characterized.
- Translation of experimental pain studies to clinical acute pain and gender studies has yielded conflicting results.
- With affordable, high-throughput, genetic testing platforms, interindividual genetic variants have been studied in acute pain, opioid analgesic effects, and metabolism of opioid analgesics.
- Generalized use of such genetic testing modalities for acute pain has yet to prove its clinical value.

INTRODUCTION

Acute postoperative pain is a major clinical challenge given the large volume of inpatient and ambulatory surgeries and other procedures performed in the United States annually. In 2010, a combined estimate of 100 million surgical and nonsurgical procedures were performed in the United States.[1,2] Given the sheer number of procedures, perioperative outcomes and costs related to delivering patient care have major clinical and economic implications.

Under- or overtreatment of acute postoperative pain can lead to physical and psychological complications and patient dissatisfaction that negatively impacts long-term outcome. Undertreatment of pain can cause adverse physiologic effects, including tachycardia and increased cardiac metabolic demand that contribute to risk for a major adverse cardiac and neurologic events. Uncontrolled acute pain further impairs a

Department of Anesthesiology, Perioperative, and Pain Medicine, Stanford University School of Medicine, 300 Pasteur Drive, Room H3580, Stanford, CA 94305, USA
[1] Present address: New York Medical College, Westchester Medical Center, 100 Woods Road, Valhalla, NY 10595.
* Corresponding author.
E-mail address: pflood@stanford.edu

Anesthesiology Clin 38 (2020) 341–355
https://doi.org/10.1016/j.anclin.2020.01.003
anesthesiology.theclinics.com
1932-2275/20/

patient's postoperative recovery and rehabilitation, which in turn lengthens postanesthesia care unit and hospital stay and increases hospital readmission rates.[3] In contrast, overtreatment of acute pain may cause respiratory complications, delirium, oversedation, postoperative nausea and vomiting, urinary retention, and ileus. These risks can be translated into individual patient morbidity and mortality as well as increased economic cost to society.[4,5]

Identification of patient-specific and procedure-related factors predictive of these complications may guide perioperative pain management and improve patient outcomes. Because pain is a perceived, unpleasant sensory and emotional experience, the individual's pain perception is the basis of their treatment plan. Characterization of factors that are associated with pain experience is 1 strategy to identify new targets for treatment. Genetic differences and including sex have been associated with variability in pain perception, depending on experimental and clinical setting. Clearly, sex and genotype are not modifiable variables. However, sex is associated with many other variables, including hormonal differences that can be used to a patient's advantage for pain management.[6,7] Smaller genetic differences in a gene or regulatory pathway can also point to targets for intervention.

OVERALL GENETIC VARIABILITY IN PAIN PERCEPTION

Comparing differences in pain perception between monozygotic and dizygotic twins can help separate the role of genetics from the role of the environment. Twin studies have been used to evaluate the role of genetics using quantitative sensory testing. Although quantitative sensory testing may seem remote to acute and postoperative pain experience, it has the benefit of allowing for identification of a specific mechanism that can then be evaluated in the appropriate clinical model. For example, treatments effective in modulating response to heat and acid would be important to investigate in burn injury. Understanding the different aspects of pain perception, including the underlying physiology and pharmacology, may yield clinically important findings and treatment options.

Pain perception studies frequently quantify pain threshold and pain tolerance. It is important to note that pain threshold and tolerance are 2 different phenomena. Pain threshold is a measure of pain perception sensitivity, whereas pain tolerance is a measure of the maximum painful stimulus a person can endure. Clinically, pain tolerance may be of greater interest in patients with acute postoperative pain from surgery who need to participate in activities related to recovery. This aspect of the pain experience is impacted by physiologic and psychological factors.

In experimental pain paradigms, twin studies predict that approximately 50% of the variance in cold pressor pain sensitivity can be attributed to genetic factors.[8,9] Similarly, 25% to 53% of heat sensitivity variance was attributed to genetic factors.[8,10] Pain induced by injection of acid and ATP (modeling ischemic pain) has significant heritable component also.[10]

SEX AS A VARIABLE IN EXPERIMENTAL PAIN PERCEPTION

Several investigative approaches have been used to evaluate sex-related differences in pain. Research began in earnest in the 1980s and accelerated in the 1990s and 2000s.[11]

Pressure Pain Stimuli

Woodrow and colleagues[12] described one of the largest studies characterizing pain tolerance to pressure on the Achilles tendon in 41,119 subjects. They found that men have greater pain tolerance to pressure than women. Jensen and colleagues[13] tested pressure pain thresholds of cephalic muscles in 1000 randomly sampled subjects in Denmark and found a similar trend in relation to sex. This finding was replicated again in a study by Chesterton and colleagues[14] in a study of healthy volunteers in the United Kingdom where men had higher pressure pain thresholds in their first dorsal interosseous muscle compared with women. The finding of greater tolerance to pressure pain in men seems to be robust and is not dependent on the body part investigated.

Heat Pain Stimuli

Painful perception of heat stimuli has been characterized as a distinct noxious stimulus. Transduction of heat to a nociceptive signal is mediated by TRPV1 receptors on C nerve fibers. Capsaicin is a well-known agonist of this nociceptor.[15] Using a standard thermode that contacts an area of the skin, several studies have demonstrated both higher thermal pain threshold and tolerance in men compared with those in women.[16,17] Clinically, individual variation of heat pain perception correlated with clinical postsurgery pain scores and analgesic use after cesarean section in healthy women.[18]

Cold Pain Stimuli

Cold pressor task is commonly used to quantify cold pain perception. In the cold pressor task, subjects are asked to immerse a body part in cold water as the experimenter quantifies how pain is perceived. Multiple studies have consistently found that men have a higher pain tolerance in cold pressor tasks than women. The mechanism is unknown, but systemic inflammatory biomarkers have been linked to increased cold pain sensitivity in women.[19] Basic science studies have found that TRPM8 is the predominant thermoreceptor for cold temperatures.[20] This channel is also activated by menthol.[21] Although there is some interest in modulation of the TRPM8 receptor in human pain and a potential difference related to polymorphisms, there is no obvious clinical phenotype.

Electrical Stimuli

Robin and colleagues[22] demonstrated greater pain tolerance threshold in men than women in response to electrical stimulation. They also quantified affective dimensions of the pain experience and found significant correlation between anxiety score and the pain threshold of their research subjects. The finding of higher pain threshold to electrical stimuli in men has been replicated.[23] Interestingly, electrical stimuli delivered transcutaneously has also been shown to modulate pain perception. Transcutaneous electrical nerve stimulation can suppress pain with electrical stimuli.[24] This therapy is used clinically but the exact mechanism is not fully understood.

Ischemic Pain Stimuli

The submaximal effort tourniquet procedure is used to assess for ischemic pain onset and ischemic pain tolerance. This pain phenotype is a model for pain due to vascular insufficiency. Maixner and Humphrey[25] showed that the ischemic pain threshold is similar between men and women, but pain tolerance is greater in men. However, other studies have failed to show significant differences in ischemic pain between the 2 sexes.[26,27] Therefore, it is difficult to generalize Maixner and Humphrey's findings.

Inflammatory Pain Stimuli

Pain, particularly acute postoperative pain, commonly has an inflammatory component. The processes that are required for healing necessarily involve inflammation that can be modulated when it occurs in excess or for a prolonged period outside of that required for wound healing. Nonsteroidal anti-inflammatory drugs are useful for pain management after surgery. They have been shown to increase patient satisfaction, decrease opioid use, and minimize opioid-induced complications.[28] Iontophoresis of acid has been developed as a method to test acid-induced pain,[29] but this has not been used to study sex differences.

SEX HORMONES AND PAIN PERCEPTION IN WOMEN

Sex hormones have been a subject of investigation in explaining difference in pain perception between men and women. Women have different exposure to estrogen and testosterone compared with men throughout embryonic, child, and adult life. The differences serve critical roles not only in fetal development and physical changes during puberty, but also can affect activity of the central nervous system (CNS) and peripheral nervous system.

Pain perception to pressure stimulation, cold pressor pain, thermal heat stimulation, and ischemic muscle pain vary across a woman's menstrual cycle, during which higher pain thresholds are manifest during the follicular phase compared with the luteal phases.[30] Clinically significant findings of sex hormones affecting pain experience have been found in chronic pain conditions, such as rheumatoid arthritis, hormone-related migraines, fibromyalgia, and chronic fatigue syndrome.[31–33] There is weak evidence that postoperative pain is perceived more during the luteal phase. If replicated, painful elective surgery should perhaps be preferentially scheduled during the luteal phase in premenopausal women.

Oxytocin is a neuropeptide that has significantly more recognized roles in women, but it also plays a role in male physiology. In women, oxytocin has been shown to be important not only to uterine contraction during childbirth and lactation in the postpartum period but also to social bonding and promoting maternal behaviors.[34,35] The effects of oxytocin on pain and analgesia is gaining more attention. Oxytocin has analgesic effects at the spinal cord and peripheral nerves and has shown potential to be used to modulate experimental ischemic and cold pain stimuli.[7,36]

SEX AS A FACTOR IN POSTOPERATIVE ACUTE PAIN

Clinical trials are by their nature more complex than evaluation of a subject's response in a laboratory setting. A standardized stimulus administered to a highly selected volunteer is replaced by messy clinical reality. The benefit is that these studies are most directly referable and translatable to the clinical setting. Clinical studies that have evaluated sex differences in postoperative pain response have provided conflicting results. Several studies showed that women had higher intraprocedural or postoperative pain ratings than men in elective abdominal surgery,[37] unsedated colonoscopy,[38] gastric bypass surgery,[39] ultrasound-guided abdominal interventions,[40] lung cancer surgery,[41] cardiac surgery,[42] and total hip arthroplasty.[43] Interestingly, although women reported higher pain ratings, men required more morphine after elective abdominal surgery.[37] In contrast, some studies showed the opposite trend, where men reported higher postoperative acute pain ratings than women in excisional hemorrhoidectomy,[44] stapled hemorrhoidepexy,[45] and liver transplantation.[46] Numerous other studies have found no differences in postoperative pain perception and reporting between the sexes.[47–50] Given the wide variety of surgical type, study design, and overall conflicting results, it is difficult to draw conclusions and generalize a particular study's finding to all surgical scenarios.

SEX AND OPIOID ANALGESIA

Sex differences in sensitivity to analgesia and side effects of mu and kappa opioid agonists have been well established in humans and other animals. Activation by kappa opioid agonists—such as nalbuphine[51] and pentazocine[52]—have been associated with sex-related differences in analgesia after oral surgery. Sex difference in analgesia from mu opioid activation is less clear. A small study did not find differences in analgesic sensitivity to morphine (a classic mu opioid receptor agonist) between men and women, but did find differences in subjective side effects[53] Studies of opioid consumption according to sex have been mixed; however, these studies have been small with a high risk of bias. It is important to keep in mind that the absence of a positive effect in small studies does not prove the negative, but often reflects a lack of statistical power.

SINGLE GENE MUTATIONS—SINGLE-NUCLEOTIDE POLYMORPHISMS AND PAIN

The advent of high-throughput DNA screening has made identification of single-nucleotide polymorphisms (SNPs) not only possible but affordable. Companies have used "gene chips" that contain many small samples of DNA and allow for detection of many genetic differences or SNPs at one time. These chips are used to identify genetic differences in disease processes and drug response and are marketed directly to the public. They have also allowed for genetic association studies that link SNPs to specific phenotypes of acute and persistent postsurgical pain, and response to analgesic drugs.

The association of a wide variety of SNPs with pain and analgesia phenotypes after a wide variety of surgeries has been studied. In these studies, postoperative pain report, opioid analgesic use, and development of persistent postsurgical pain were assessed and genetic differences were evaluated. A partial list of genes and surgery types evaluated is found in **Table 1**. A more complete summary of genetic association studies is beyond the scope of this review but can be found in the review articles by Chidambaran and colleagues,[75] Elmallah and colleagues,[76] Fillingim and colleagues,[77] and Ren and colleagues.[78]

Recent advances have made gene chip analysis routine, whole human genome sequencing tractable, and likely soon economical. Thus, there are important caveats to keep in mind. These techniques are very powerful and have the possibility of finding important associations, in fact picking a needle out of a haystack. However, making conclusions from their results requires restraint and careful statistical consideration. If one attempts to identify an association at a P value of 0.05, 5% of the time the apparent association will be false. If one looks at 20 potential SNPs that have no association with an outcome, you are virtually assured to find 1 false-positive association. For this reason, the association must be very strong and replicated in another dataset.

With those limitations in mind, some pain-related outcomes have been mapped multiple times to several genes in multiple different gene association studies using different techniques. We discuss potentially pain-related SNPs in 4 pain-related genes that have been extensively studied: COMT, OPRM1, ABCB1, and MC1R.

COMT Gene

The COMT gene encodes a protein that catalyzes the transfer of a methyl group from S-adenosylmethionine in catecholamines and neurotransmitters, such as dopamine, epinephrine, and norepinephrine. The COMT enzyme plays a role in phase II

Table 1
Single-nucleotide polymorphism variants implicated in postoperative acute pain according to sex and surgery type

Gene	Chromosome	Surgery/Pain	Sex	References
MAOB	23	Tonsillectomy	Both	54
COMT	22	Third molar extraction Lumbar spine surgery Tonsillectomy Cesarean section Knee replacement	Both Both Both Female Both	55–59
IL1R2	2	Breast cancer surgery	Female	60
IL10	1	Breast cancer surgery	Female	61
OPRM1	6	Hysterectomy Cesarean section Thoracotomy Tonsillectomy	Female Female Both Both	60,62–64
ABCB1	7	Cesarean section Colorectal	Female Both	65,66
NTRK1	1	Ortho/Abd	Both	67
KCNA1 KCNJ3 KCNJ6 KCND2 KCNK9	12 2 21 7 8	Breast cancer surgery	Female	68
GCH1	14	Herniaotomy	Male	69
HCRTR2	6	Abdominal surgery	Both	70
SCN9A	2	Gynecologic laparoscopic surgery	Female	71
BDNF	11	Various with skin incision	Both	72
CTSG	14	Various with skin incision	Both	73
ADRB2	5	First-stage labor pain	Female	74

biotransformation reactions when detoxifying medications. The activity of the COMT enzyme plays a role in modulating catechol-dependent functions, such as cognition, cardiovascular function, and pain signal processing. Patients with COMT SNPs (rs6269, rs4633, rs4818, and rs4680) typically have lower metabolic activity of the COMT enzyme that is associated with lower postoperative pain scores, less opioid requirements, and a lower incidence of postsurgical persistent pain.[55–59] There are many common SNPs in the COMT gene that are in linkage disequilibrium and, as such, it is difficult to make mechanistic assumptions about the role of any particular SNP. However, low enzyme activity would be expected to result in a greater average amount of norepinephrine available at the synapse, facilitating descending inhibition. Drugs that inhibit norepinephrine metabolism, including serotonin–norepinephrine reuptake inhibitors are effective analgesics.

ABCB1 Gene

The ATP-binding cassette (ABC) transporters are membrane-associated active transporters of various molecules across the cell membrane. ABCB1 codes for P-glycoprotein, which is also well known for the active transport of many drugs into and out of the cell and across the blood-brain barrier.[79] As part of the blood-brain barrier it acts to actively transport morphine out of the CNS. Important in anesthesia, this active transport is the reason why in the CNS the activity of morphine takes longer to peak than that of other opioids. Two different studies identified an SNP in the ABCB1 gene, C3435T, which is associated with clinically relevant persistent pain after caesarian section and opioid sensitivity in abdominal surgical patients.[65,66] Patients homozygous for the C3435T allele required less fentanyl postoperatively after colorectal abdominal surgery.[65] Individuals who are homozygous for the C3435T allele have decreased drug efflux activity, which presumably allows for more opioids to accumulate in the CNS compared with the wild-type genotype. However, after cesarean section, Sia and colleagues[62] did not find an association between postoperative opioid use during the first 24 hours and ABCB1 genotype. This is perhaps not surprising as in the study by Sia and colleagues, all participants received morphine intrathecally on induction of surgical anesthesia for caesarian section. Intrathecal morphine used in spinal anesthesia bypasses the blood-brain barrier and metabolism by P-glycoprotein.

OPRM1 Gene

Opioid receptor agonists are currently the mainstay in the treatment of moderate to severe postoperative pain. There are 3 major subtypes of opioid receptors: mu, delta, and kappa. Commonly used opioid analgesic agents are divided into primarily 2 classes—mu and kappa—based on their predominant opioid receptor subtype activity (**Table 2**). The delta opioid receptor is the primary receptor for enkephalins, and its role in acute pain is debated. There is a fourth subtype of opioid-like receptor, the nociception/orphanin FQ receptor, which is thought to play a role in anxiety and stress that may be related to the addictive potential of opioids and other drugs.[80]

The opioid receptor mu 1 gene is intuitively relevant to acute pain as this is the principal target of most endogenous and exogenous opioid compounds. Although it is difficult to establish a causal role between OPRM1 SNPs and postsurgical acute pain, chronic pain, and substance abuse phenotypes, the association has been identified in multiple genomic studies. Many studies have looked for association between OPRM1 SNPS and acute postoperative pain after a variety of procedures and opioid requirement. The 2 outcomes are usually followed in the same trial as they can be difficult to separate. In extreme situations, a patient with more pain may use minimal opioid and report more pain. In contrast, a patient may have severe pain but take more opioid and thus report a low pain score but have high opioid use. Most studies find a combination of effects.

The OPRM1 A118G allele has been associated with greater pain scores and opioid requirement after hysterectomy and cesarean section in the Asian population.[62,63] However, in patients who had a thoracotomy, the OPRM1 A118G variant was not identified as being associated with increased pain. Other haplotype variants of OPRM1 gene were linked to increased acute postsurgical pain instead.[64] It is still unclear if type of surgery matters. In labor pain, the 304A/G polymorphism in the OPRM1 gene has been found to influence intrathecal fentanyl's median effective dose[49] when used for combined spinal-epidural for labor analgesia.[81]

MC1R Gene

It has been postulated that individuals who carry the mutation that results in red hair color require greater doses of opioid analgesics to achieve the same effect compared with dark haired counterparts. This seems surprising, but Mogil and colleagues[82] have identified variants of melanocortin-1 receptor gene in both mouse and humans that are associated with this phenotype. In humans, R151C, R160W, and D294H genetic variants cause loss of function when an individual is homozygous or compound

Table 2
Opioid agents, their routes of administration, and target receptor activity

Opioid Agent	Route of Administration	Mu	Kappa	Delta	Other Targets
Morphine	PO, IV, IM, SC, PR, IT, epidural	Agonist	Agonist	Agonist	–
Oxycodone	PO	Agonist	Agonist	Agonist	–
Oxymorphone	PO, IM, IV, SC, PR	Agonist	–	–	–
Hydrocodone	PO	Agonist	–	Agonist	–
Hydromorphone	PO, IV, IM, SC, PR, IT, epidural	Agonist	Agonist	Partial Agonist	–
Fentanyl	SL, TB, TD, IV, IN, IM	Agonist	–	Agonist	MRP1/ABCB1
Sufentanil	SL, IV, IM, IT, epidural	Agonist	–	–	–
Alfentanil	IV	Agonist	–	–	–
Remifentanil	IV	Agonist	–	–	–
Codeine	PO, IM, SC	Agonist	Agonist	Agonist	–
Tapentadol	PO	Agonist	–	–	Noradrenaline reuptake inhibitor
Levorphanol	PO, IV	Agonist	Agonist	Agonist	NMDA antagonist
Butorphanol	IV, IM, IN	Partial antagonist	Agonist	Agonist	–
Tramadol	PO	Agonist	–	–	Serotonin and noradrenaline reuptake inhibitor
Buprenorphine	TB, SL, TD	Partial agonist	Antagonist	–	–
Methadone	PO, IV	Agonist	–	Agonist	Serotonin and noradrenaline reuptake inhibitor NMDA antagonist Neuronal acetylcholine receptor subunit alpha-10 antagonist
Pentazocine	PO, IM, IV, SC	Antagonist	Agonist	–	Sigma nonopioid intracellular receptor 1 agonist
Meperidine	PO, IV, IM, SC	–	Agonist	–	–
Nalbuphine	IV, IM, SC	Antagonist	Agonist	Antagonist	–

heterozygous for these 3 variants.[83] These variants happen to be commonly manifest with red hair or fair skin.[84] Although it seems odd that mutations that regulate skin and hair pigmentation also affect opioid analgesia, the melanocortin-1 gene is expressed in glial cells and the ventral periaqueductal gray.[85,86]

METABOLIC PATHWAY GENETIC POLYMORPHISMS AND OPIOID ANALGESIA

The influence of individual variations in metabolism and opioid analgesic effects has produced a significant body of research. Although these findings are robust and repeatable, clinical consequences are less clear, except in the case of codeine (discussed below). There is a significant industry that has grown up around providing consumers with a report on their personal genetic polymorphisms related to drug metabolism that suggest what drugs they should and should not use. These services are not approved by the Food and Drug Administration and should not be used in the absence of medical advice.

Opioids are predominantly metabolized by the liver. Cytochrome P450 family enzymes carry out phase I and phase II biotransformation reactions. Some metabolites can still have activity at the target receptor until they are further metabolized or excreted. In contrast, when an opioid prodrug is metabolized, it becomes active. Codeine, for example, is metabolized to the active moiety, morphine, through CYP2D6. Then, morphine undergoes conjugation by UGT2B7 to morphine-6-glucuronide and morphine-3-glucuronide. Morphine-6-glucuronide has less but some residual opioid analgesic activity.

The liver enzymes CYP2D6 and UGT2B7 have numerous genetic variants described that affect enzymatic activity. Individuals who have genotypes that result in lower activity of the enzyme are called "poor metabolizers," whereas patient who carry at least 3 normal activity variant genes are called "ultrarapid metabolizers." Ultrarapid metabolizers who take codeine may quickly reach supratherapeutic levels of morphine that cause more side effects and the analgesic effect may be short lived.[87,88] Alternatively, poor metabolizers of codeine may not achieve a therapeutic level of morphine and may not receive any analgesic benefits. In respect to postoperative opioid analgesics, codeine is generally no longer used. Tramadol is also a prodrug metabolized by cytochrome P450 (CYP) enzymes CYP2D6 and CYP3A4 to more potent opioid analgesic metabolites. Tramadol's potency is also affected by genetics, with poor metabolizers experiencing little conversion to the active form and ultra-metabolizers experiencing the greatest opioid analgesic effects. Genetic variability in metabolism of oxycodone,[89,90] fentanyl,[91] tramadol,[92,93] and hydrocodone[89,94] has been reported. However, other than the above examples, there are not enough replicated studies to make specific recommendations for management of patients suspected to be ultrarapid or poor metabolizers.

In the future, recognizing interindividual differences in metabolism of opioids and other analgesic drugs may prove to be a practical strategy to predict an individual's response and appropriately adjust the pharmacotherapy. Computerized clinical decision support has been used to guide treatment in medical centers and private companies have offered such services to individuals.[95] However, evidence to support the use of a genetic report in postoperative opioid prescription beyond the recommendation to avoid codeine is still forthcoming.

CONCLUDING REMARKS

In the past 4 decades, basic and clinical studies have demonstrated the presence of sex differences and interindividual variation in pain perception and analgesic effect of opioids. With the exception of men typically reporting greater tolerance to several pain stimuli in healthy volunteer studies, there are few reproducible findings. In a similar time period, experimental pain and clinical acute pain outcome variability was studied by stratifying healthy and perioperative patient populations by ethnicity,[96,97] skin tone,[98] and socioeconomic and cultural backgrounds.[99] In some sense, stratifying research subjects by phenotype, may provide some information to identify the role of genetic variations associated with the phenotype in question.

With the development of affordable, high-throughput genetic assays, the focus seems to have shifted away from gender and ethnic background to interindividual genetic variations. The ability to rapidly characterize thousands of genes is very powerful, but this high-throughput approach also comes with a higher chance of false-positive findings. Important information may be gained from identifying multiple associations between SNPs in genes encoding proteins known to be important in pain pathways and pain phenotypes.

Interindividual pharmacokinetic differences may add clinical value in aiding appropriate selection and dosing of analgesics in the perioperative period. A panel of genetic tests that identify slow or ultrafast metabolizers may not be clinically helpful. However, an affordable, real-time, point of care test showing the serum concentration of an analgesic being administered with or without knowledge of a patient's metabolism genetic profile may hold greater clinical promise in appropriate dosing of medications.

The biological and psychosocial differences among individuals are multifaceted, complex, and likely beyond discovery using currently available tools. Differences identified on the basis of sex and other genetic factors are specific to the assessment or pain variety and are not currently generalizable.

DISCLOSURE

The authors have no conflict of interests to disclose regarding the topics discussed in this review article.

REFERENCES

1. Hall MJ, Schwartzman A, Zhang J, et al. Ambulatory surgery data from hospitals and ambulatory surgery centers: United States, 2010. Natl Health Stat Rep 2017;(102):1–14. Available at: https://www.cdc.gov/nchs/data/nhsr/nhsr102.pdf. Accessed August 25, 2019.
2. Centers for Disease Control and Prevention (CDC). NCCHS. National hospital discharge survey: 2010 table, procedures by selected patient characteristics—number by procedure category and age. Atlanta (GA): CDC; 2010. Available at: http://www.cdc.gov/nchs/nhds/nhds_tables.htm. Accessed August 25, 2019.
3. Kehlet H. Multimodal approach to control postoperative pathophysiology and rehabilitation. Br J Anaesth 1997;78(5):606–17.
4. Mörwald EE, Olson A, Cozowicz C, et al. Association of opioid prescription and perioperative complications in obstructive sleep apnea patients undergoing total joint arthroplasties. Sleep Breath 2018;22(1):115–21.
5. Ladha KS, Gagne JJ, Patorno E, et al. Opioid overdose after surgical discharge. JAMA 2018;320(5):502–4.
6. Al-tarrah K, Moiemen N, Lord JM. The influence of sex steroid hormones on the response to trauma and burn injury. Burns Trauma 2017;5:29.
7. Xin Q, Bai B, Liu W. The analgesic effects of oxytocin in the peripheral and central nervous system. Neurochem Int 2017;103:57–64.

8. Nielsen CS, Stubhaug A, Price DD, et al. Individual differences in pain sensitivity: genetic and environmental contributions. Pain 2008;136(1–2):21–9.
9. Angst MS, Phillips NG, Drover DR, et al. Pain sensitivity and opioid analgesia: a pharmacogenomic twin study. Pain 2012;153(7):1397–409.
10. Norbury TA, Macgregor AJ, Urwin J, et al. Heritability of responses to painful stimuli in women: a classical twin study. Brain 2007;130(Pt 11):3041–9.
11. Fillingim RB, King CD, Ribeiro-dasilva MC, et al. Sex, gender, and pain: a review of recent clinical and experimental findings. J Pain 2009;10(5):447–85.
12. Woodrow KM, Friedman GD, Siegelaub AB, et al. Pain tolerance: differences according to age, sex and race. Psychosom Med 1972;34(6):548–56.
13. Jensen R, Rasmussen BK, Pedersen B, et al. Cephalic muscle tenderness and pressure pain threshold in a general population. Pain 1992;48(2):197–203.
14. Chesterton LS, Barlas P, Foster NE, et al. Gender differences in pressure pain threshold in healthy humans. Pain 2003;101(3):259–66.
15. Zhang F, Jara-oseguera A, Chang TH, et al. Heat activation is intrinsic to the pore domain of TRPV1. Proc Natl Acad Sci U S A 2018;115(2):E317–24.
16. Feine JS, Bushnell MC, Miron D, et al. Sex differences in the perception of noxious heat stimuli. Pain 1991;44(3):255–62.
17. Fillingim RB, Maixner W, Kincaid S, et al. Sex differences in temporal summation but not sensory-discriminative processing of thermal pain. Pain 1998;75(1):121–7.
18. Pan PH, Coghill R, Houle TT, et al. Multifactorial preoperative predictors for post-cesarean section pain and analgesic requirement. Anesthesiology 2006;104(3):417–25.
19. Schistad EI, Stubhaug A, Furberg AS, et al. C-reactive protein and cold-pressor tolerance in the general population: the Tromsø Study. Pain 2017;158(7):1280–8.
20. Mckemy DD, Neuhausser WM, Julius D. Identification of a cold receptor reveals a general role for TRP channels in thermosensation. Nature 2002;416(6876):52–8.
21. Liu B, Fan L, Balakrishna S, et al. TRPM8 is the principal mediator of menthol-induced analgesia of acute and inflammatory pain. Pain 2013;154(10):2169–77.
22. Robin O, Vinard H, Vernet-maury E, et al. Influence of sex and anxiety on pain threshold and tolerance. Funct Neurol 1987;2(2):173–9.
23. Lund I, Lundeberg T, Kowalski J, et al. Gender differences in electrical pain threshold responses to transcutaneous electrical nerve stimulation (TENS). Neurosci Lett 2005;375(2):75–80.
24. Janko M, Trontelj JV. Transcutaneous electrical nerve stimulation: a microneurographic and perceptual study. Pain 1980;9(2):219–30.
25. Maixner W, Humphrey C. Gender differences in pain and cardiovascular responses to forearm ischemia. Clin J Pain 1993;9(1):16–25.
26. Campbell TS, Hughes JW, Girdler SS, et al. Relationship of ethnicity, gender, and ambulatory blood pressure to pain sensitivity: effects of individualized pain rating scales. J Pain 2004;5(3):183–91.
27. Edwards RR, Haythornthwaite JA, Sullivan MJ, et al. Catastrophizing as a mediator of sex differences in pain: differential effects for daily pain versus laboratory-induced pain. Pain 2004;111(3):335–41.
28. Gupta A, Bah M. NSAIDs in the treatment of postoperative pain. Curr Pain Headache Rep 2016;20(11):62.
29. Jones NG, Slater R, Cadiou H, et al. Acid-induced pain and its modulation in humans. J Neurosci 2004;24(48):10974–9.
30. Riley JL, Robinson ME, Wise EA, et al. A meta-analytic review of pain perception across the menstrual cycle. Pain 1999;81(3):225–35.

31. Cutolo M, Giusti M, Foppiani L, et al. The hypothalamic-pituitary-adrenocortical and gonadal axis function in rheumatoid arthritis. Z Rheumatol 2000;59(Suppl 2):II/65–9.
32. Ashkenazi A, Silberstein SD. Hormone-related headache: pathophysiology and treatment. CNS Drugs 2006;20(2):125–41.
33. Korszun A, Young EA, Engleberg NC, et al. Follicular phase hypothalamic-pituitary-gonadal axis function in women with fibromyalgia and chronic fatigue syndrome. J Rheumatol 2000;27(6):1526–30.
34. Yoshihara C, Numan M, Kuroda KO. Oxytocin and parental behaviors. Curr Top Behav Neurosci 2018;35:119–53.
35. Mitre M, Minder J, Morina EX, et al. Oxytocin modulation of neural circuits. Curr Top Behav Neurosci 2018;35:31–53.
36. Goodin BR, Anderson AJB, Freeman EL, et al. Intranasal oxytocin administration is associated with enhanced endogenous pain inhibition and reduced negative mood states. Clin J Pain 2015;31(9):757–67.
37. Periasamy S, Poovathai R, Pondiyadanar S. Influences of gender on postoperative morphine consumption. J Clin Diagn Res 2014;8(12):GC04–7.
38. Holme O, Bretthauer M, De lange T, et al. Risk stratification to predict pain during unsedated colonoscopy: results of a multicenter cohort study. Endoscopy 2013;45(9):691–6.
39. Zeidan A, Al-temyatt S, Mowafi H, et al. Gender-related difference in postoperative pain after laparoscopic Roux-En-Y gastric bypass in morbidly obese patients. Obes Surg 2013;23(11):1880–4.
40. Lindner A, Frieser M, Heide R, et al. Postinterventional pain and complications of sonographically guided interventions in the liver and pancreas. Ultraschall Med 2014;35(2):159–65.
41. Oksholm T, Rustoen T, Cooper B, et al. Trajectories of symptom occurrence and severity from before through five months after lung cancer surgery. J Pain Symptom Manage 2015;49(6):995–1015.
42. Bjørnnes AK, Rustøen T, Lie I, et al. Pain characteristics and analgesic intake before and following cardiac surgery. Eur J Cardiovasc Nurs 2016;15(1):47–54.
43. Petrovic NM, Milovanovic DR, Ignjatovic ristic D, et al. Factors associated with severe postoperative pain in patients with total hip arthroplasty. Acta Orthop Traumatol Turc 2014;48(6):615–22.
44. Selvaggi F, Pellino G, Sciaudone G, et al. Development and validation of a practical score to predict pain after excisional hemorrhoidectomy. Int J Colorectal Dis 2014;29(11):1401–10.
45. Zhao Y, Ding JH, Yin SH, et al. Predictors of early postoperative pain after stapled haemorrhoidopexy. Colorectal Dis 2014;16(6):O206–11.
46. Bianco T, Cillo U, Amodio P, et al. Gender differences in the quality of life of patients with liver cirrhosis related to hepatitis C after liver transplantation. Blood Purif 2013;36(3–4):231–6.
47. Choi GW, Kim HJ, Kim TW, et al. Sex-related differences in outcomes after hallux valgus surgery. Yonsei Med J 2015;56(2):466–73.
48. Grodofsky SR, Sinha AC. The association of gender and body mass index with postoperative pain scores when undergoing ankle fracture surgery. J Anaesthesiol Clin Pharmacol 2014;30(2):248–52.
49. Shin S, Min KT, Shin YS, et al. Finding the 'ideal' regimen for fentanyl-based intravenous patient-controlled analgesia: how to give and what to mix? Yonsei Med J 2014;55(3):800–6.

50. Theodoraki K, Staikou C, Fassoulaki A. Postoperative pain after major abdominal surgery: is it gender related? An observational prospective study. Pain Pract 2014;14(7):613–9.
51. Gear RW, Miaskowski C, Gordon NC, et al. The kappa opioid nalbuphine produces gender- and dose-dependent analgesia and antianalgesia in patients with postoperative pain. Pain 1999;83(2):339–45.
52. Gear RW, Gordon NC, Heller PH, et al. Gender difference in analgesic response to the kappa-opioid pentazocine. Neurosci Lett 1996;205(3):207–9.
53. Comer SD, Cooper ZD, Kowalczyk WJ, et al. Evaluation of potential sex differences in the subjective and analgesic effects of morphine in normal, healthy volunteers. Psychopharmacology (Berl) 2010;208(1):45–55.
54. Serý O, Hrazdilová O, Didden W, et al. The association of monoamine oxidase B functional polymorphism with postoperative pain intensity. Neuro Endocrinol Lett 2006;27(3):333–7.
55. Lee PJ, Delaney P, Keogh J, et al. Catecholamine-O-methyltransferase polymorphisms are associated with postoperative pain intensity. Clin J Pain 2011;27(2): 93–101.
56. Rut M, Machoy-mokrzyńska A, Ręcławowicz D, et al. Influence of variation in the catechol-O-methyltransferase gene on the clinical outcome after lumbar spine surgery for one-level symptomatic disc disease: a report on 176 cases. Acta Neurochir (Wien) 2014;156(2):245–52.
57. Sadhasivam S, Chidambaran V, Olbrecht VA, et al. Genetics of pain perception, *COMT* and postoperative pain management in children. Pharmacogenomics 2014;15(3):277–84.
58. Somogyi AA, Sia AT, Tan EC, et al. Ethnicity-dependent influence of innate immune genetic markers on morphine PCA requirements and adverse effects in postoperative pain. Pain 2016;157(11):2458–66.
59. Thomazeau J, Rouquette A, Martinez V, et al. Predictive factors of chronic post-surgical pain at 6 months following knee replacement: influence of postoperative pain trajectory and genetics. Pain Physician 2016;19(5):E729–41.
60. Stephens K, Cooper BA, West C, et al. Associations between cytokine gene variations and severe persistent breast pain in women following breast cancer surgery. J Pain 2014;15(2):169–80.
61. Lee MG, Kim HJ, Lee KH, et al. The influence of genotype polymorphism on morphine analgesic effect for postoperative pain in children. Korean J Pain 2016;29(1):34–9.
62. Sia AT, Lim Y, Lim EC, et al. Influence of mu-opioid receptor variant on morphine use and self-rated pain following abdominal hysterectomy. J Pain 2013;14(10): 1045–52.
63. Sia AT, Lim Y, Lim EC, et al. A118G single nucleotide polymorphism of human mu-opioid receptor gene influences pain perception and patient-controlled intravenous morphine consumption after intrathecal morphine for postcesarean analgesia. Anesthesiology 2008;109(3):520–6.
64. Ochroch EA, Vachani A, Gottschalk A, et al. Natural variation in the μ-opioid gene OPRM1 predicts increased pain on third day after thoracotomy. Clin J Pain 2012; 28(9):747–54.
65. Dzambazovska-trajkovska V, Nojkov J, Kartalov A, et al. Association of single-nucleotide polymorhism C3435T in the ABCB1 gene with opioid sensitivity in treatment of postoperative pain. Pril (Makedon Akad Nauk Umet Odd Med Nauki) 2016;37(2–3):73–80.

66. Sia AT, Sng BL, Lim EC, et al. The influence of ATP-binding cassette sub-family B member-1 (ABCB1) genetic polymorphisms on acute and chronic pain after intrathecal morphine for caesarean section: a prospective cohort study. Int J Obstet Anesth 2010;19(3):254–60.
67. Mamie C, Rebsamen MC, Morris MA, et al. First evidence of a polygenic susceptibility to pain in a pediatric cohort. Anesth Analg 2013;116(1):170–7.
68. Langford DJ, Paul SM, West CM, et al. Variations in potassium channel genes are associated with distinct trajectories of persistent breast pain after breast cancer surgery. Pain 2015;156(3):371–80.
69. Belfer I, Dai F, Kehlet H, et al. Association of functional variations in COMT and GCH1 genes with postherniotomy pain and related impairment. Pain 2015; 156(2):273–9.
70. Nishizawa D, Kasai S, Hasegawa J, et al. Associations between the orexin (hypocretin) receptor 2 gene polymorphism Val308Ile and nicotine dependence in genome-wide and subsequent association studies. Mol Brain 2015;8:50.
71. Duan G, Xiang G, Guo S, et al. Genotypic analysis of SCN9A for prediction of postoperative pain in female patients undergoing gynecological laparoscopic surgery. Pain Physician 2016;19(1):E151–62.
72. Tian Y, Liu X, Jia M, et al. Targeted genotyping identifies susceptibility locus in brain-derived neurotrophic factor gene for chronic postsurgical pain. Anesthesiology 2018;128(3):587–97.
73. Liu X, Tian Y, Meng Z, et al. Up-regulation of cathepsin G in the development of chronic postsurgical pain: an experimental and clinical genetic study. Anesthesiology 2015;123(4):838–50.
74. Terkawi AS, Jackson WM, Hansoti S, et al. Polymorphism in the ADRB2 gene explains a small portion of intersubject variability in pain relative to cervical dilation in the first stage of labor. Anesthesiology 2014;121(1):140–8.
75. Chidambaran V, Gang Y, Pilipenko V, et al. Systematic review and meta-analysis of genetic risk of developing chronic postsurgical pain. J Pain 2019. https://doi.org/10.1016/j.jpain.2019.05.008.
76. Elmallah RK, Ramkumar PN, Khlopas A, et al. Postoperative pain and analgesia: is there a genetic basis to the opioid crisis? Surg Technol Int 2018;32:306–14.
77. Fillingim RB, Wallace MR, Herbstman DM, et al. Genetic contributions to pain: a review of findings in humans. Oral Dis 2008;14(8):673–82.
78. Ren ZY, Xu XQ, Bao YP, et al. The impact of genetic variation on sensitivity to opioid analgesics in patients with postoperative pain: a systematic review and meta-analysis. Pain Physician 2015;18(2):131–52.
79. Thiebaut F, Tsuruo T, Hamada H, et al. Cellular localization of the multidrug-resistance gene product P-glycoprotein in normal human tissues. Proc Natl Acad Sci U S A 1987;84(21):7735–8.
80. Koob GF, Arends MA, Moal ML. Drugs, addiction, and the brain. Oxford: Academic Press; 2014.
81. Landau R, Kern C, Columb MO, et al. Genetic variability of the mu-opioid receptor influences intrathecal fentanyl analgesia requirements in laboring women. Pain 2008;139(1):5–14.
82. Mogil JS, Wilson SG, Chesler EJ, et al. The melanocortin-1 receptor gene mediates female-specific mechanisms of analgesia in mice and humans. Proc Natl Acad Sci U S A 2003;100(8):4867–72.
83. Schiöth HB, Phillips SR, Rudzish R, et al. Loss of function mutations of the human melanocortin 1 receptor are common and are associated with red hair. Biochem Biophys Res Commun 1999;260(2):488–91.

84. Rees JL, Birch-machin M, Flanagan N, et al. Genetic studies of the human melanocortin-1 receptor. Ann N Y Acad Sci 1999;885:134–42.
85. Wikberg JE. Melanocortin receptors: perspectives for novel drugs. Eur J Pharmacol 1999;375(1–3):295–310.
86. Xia Y, Wikberg JE, Chhajlani V. Expression of melanocortin 1 receptor in periaqueductal gray matter. Neuroreport 1995;6(16):2193–6.
87. Kirchheiner J, Schmidt H, Tzvetkov M, et al. Pharmacokinetics of codeine and its metabolite morphine in ultra-rapid metabolizers due to CYP2D6 duplication. Pharmacogenomics J 2007;7(4):257–65.
88. Voronov P, Przybylo HJ, Jagannathan N. Apnea in a child after oral codeine: a genetic variant—an ultra-rapid metabolizer. Paediatr Anaesth 2007;17(7):684–7.
89. Susce MT, Murray-carmichael E, De leon J. Response to hydrocodone, codeine and oxycodone in a CYP2D6 poor metabolizer. Prog Neuropsychopharmacol Biol Psychiatry 2006;30(7):1356–8.
90. Samer CF, Daali Y, Wagner M, et al. The effects of CYP2D6 and CYP3A activities on the pharmacokinetics of immediate release oxycodone. Br J Pharmacol 2010; 160(4):907–18.
91. Takashina Y, Naito T, Mino Y, et al. Impact of CYP3A5 and ABCB1 gene polymorphisms on fentanyl pharmacokinetics and clinical responses in cancer patients undergoing conversion to a transdermal system. Drug Metab Pharmacokinet 2012;27(4):414–21.
92. Stamer UM, Musshoff F, Kobilay M, et al. Concentrations of tramadol and O-desmethyltramadol enantiomers in different CYP2D6 genotypes. Clin Pharmacol Ther 2007;82(1):41–7.
93. Gan SH, Ismail R, Wan adnan WA, et al. Impact of CYP2D6 genetic polymorphism on tramadol pharmacokinetics and pharmacodynamics. Mol Diagn Ther 2007;11(3):171–81.
94. Stauble ME, Moore AW, Langman LJ, et al. Hydrocodone in postoperative personalized pain management: pro-drug or drug? Clin Chim Acta 2014; 429:26–9.
95. Miotto K, Cho AK, Khalil MA, et al. Trends in tramadol: pharmacology, metabolism, and misuse. Anesth Analg 2017;124(1):44–51.
96. Rahim-williams B, Riley JL, Williams AK, et al. A quantitative review of ethnic group differences in experimental pain response: do biology, psychology, and culture matter? Pain Med 2012;13(4):522–40.
97. Kim HJ, Yang GS, Greenspan JD, et al. Racial and ethnic differences in experimental pain sensitivity: systematic review and meta-analysis. Pain 2017;158(2): 194–211.
98. Yosipovitch G, Meredith G, Chan YH, et al. Do ethnicity and gender have an impact on pain thresholds in minor dermatologic procedures? A study on thermal pain perception thresholds in Asian ethinic groups. Skin Res Technol 2004;10(1): 38–42.
99. Clark WC, Clark SB. Pain responses in Nepalese porters. Science 1980; 209(4454):410–2.

The Flaw of Medicine

Addressing Racial and Gender Disparities in Critical Care

Ebony J. Hilton, MD[a,*], Kristina L. Goff, MD[b],
Roshni Sreedharan, MD[c], Nadia Lunardi, MD, PhD[a],
Mariam Batakji, MD[a], Dorothea S. Rosenberger, MD, PhD[d]

KEYWORDS

• Race • Gender • Health disparities • Minority physicians • Critical care

KEY POINTS

- Race has been identified as an independent risk factor associated with increased morbidity and mortality for some of the leading causes of acute critical illnesses, such as sepsis, acute respiratory distress syndrome, and cardiac arrest. In totality, African Americans have higher death rates than whites for all-cause mortality in all age groups less than 65 years old.
- Racial health disparities involve multiple factors with contributors both on the community and individual ends and within the hospital system itself.
- Gender concordance as well as racial concordance between physicians and patients have been associated with improved outcomes.
- Female physicians and those of minority race remain under-represented in critical care medicine. There is a paucity of systemic data pertaining to reasons behind this disparity, alluding to a need for additional studies targeting the recruitment, training, and retention patterns of the hospital system.

INTRODUCTION

The age of modern medicine has ushered in tremendous advancements and, with them, longevity of life. With early detection of diseases, groundbreaking research

Note: for terminology reasons, use of the sex-specific "male" and "female" in this article are used to differentiate between the 2 most common genotypes XX and XY and not for gender identification.

[a] University of Virginia Health System, PO Box 800710, Charlottesville, VA 22908, USA; [b] University of Texas Southwestern Medical Center, 3851 Beutel Court, Dallas, TX 75229, USA; [c] Case Western Reserve University School of Medicine, 9500 Euclid Avenue, Mail Code G-58, Cleveland, OH 44195, USA; [d] University of Utah School of Medicine, 30 North 1900 East, Room 3C444 SOM, Salt Lake City, UT 84132, USA
* Corresponding author.
E-mail address: eh3nf@hscmail.mcc.virginia.edu

Anesthesiology Clin 38 (2020) 357–368
https://doi.org/10.1016/j.anclin.2020.01.011
1932-2275/20/

leading to curative treatment options for once fatal conditions, and innovative medical devices that serve to all but replace failing organs, there has been a 1.6-fold increase in life expectancy over the past century in the United States.[1] The question is, Has everyone benefited from these developments equally? The presence of gender and racial health disparities suggests that there is work still left to be done. The first target of intervention may well be the medical establishment itself. With research suggesting that patient/physician race and gender concordance results in better outcomes, it becomes imperative to analyze the recruitment, training, retention, and promotion of medical providers reflective of the diverse population that is served.[2,3] The literature presented in this article identifies potential targets for interventions and areas for future exploration. With simple changes, the gap can and will be closed.

PRECISION MEDICINE IN THE INTENSIVE CARE UNIT: INFLUENCE OF BASIC SCIENCE ON HEALTH DISPARITIES

The process of drug development and research to explain pathophysiologic mechanisms prior to the utilization of new medications and modalities for the treatment of patients includes cell cultures, animal models, and different phases of clinical trials.

Classic cell/tissue and animal models use predominately male genotypes. From the perspective of a basic scientist, the all-male animal model assures the most homogenous patient group to explain mechanisms without significant fluctuations in sex hormone levels. Leaving out female cell lines and female animal models completely, however, and assuming that results from an all-male model can be extrapolated to women, is questionable science. The influence of sex hormones on disease and drug interaction at different times during the life span of a woman, including the menstrual cycle, pregnancy, and menopause, is largely unknown and cannot be ignored.

Basic scientists face limitations in choosing the appropriate animal model. For example, it is challenging to model female humans' menopause, when only approximately 4 other mammals (orcas, belugas, short-finned pilot whales, and narwhals) have physiologic menopause.[4] Rodents and other larger mammals do not develop menopause comparable to humans. Therefore, oophorectomy frequently is performed to synthesize a model for postmenopausal patients. Racial and ethnic confounding factors and epigenetic phenomena cannot be modeled with animals either. These only may be simulated, with significant limitations at best.

Hepatic metabolism and renal drug clearance models are based on body weight and muscle mass, which differ between men and women. The possible increased risk of undesirable side effects and drug clearance errors related to different muscle and fatty tissue distribution is substantial when based only on male models.[5] The Food and Drug Administration (FDA) released a safety announcement for zolpidem in 2013, recommending dose adjustment for women to 50% of the recommended dose for male patients, after a significantly higher rate of next-morning cognitive impairment in women compared with men, based on different pharmacokinetics and drug clearance.[6] Other drugs, such as aspirin, utilized for the prevention of myocardial infarction (MI) and stroke, also have been found to vary in their effectiveness and have gender-specific differences in application that need to be taken into consideration.[5]

Clinical trials often still do not allow enrollment of women of childbearing or perimenopausal age. This was routine practice until 1993, when the FDA published a revision of its 1977 guideline, renaming it "Guideline for the Study and Evaluation of Gender Differences in the Clinical Evaluation of Drugs."[7] This document acknowledges that the exclusion of women of childbearing potential completely leaves out approximately

50% of the population and assumes male sex equals female sex for results. Drugs frequently were approved for both sexes based on this assumption, often with a blanket safety warning for use during pregnancy.

The National Institutes of Health (NIH) Revitalizing Act of 1993 was enacted with the intention to change the practice of study participation. The NIH made it a requirement to include female patients as well as patients of all racial backgrounds represented within the general population in the United States in clinical trials and to analyze subgroups for significant differences as indicated.[7] Although this is a step in the right direction, caution is needed when assuming that results from trials in the United States, which reflect a racial population mix specific to the United States, apply to different racial-ethnic patient populations across Asia, Africa, South/Central America, Australia/Oceania, and Europe. One study result may not fit all.

Sex-specific differences seen in study participation, presentation, and outcome have been noticed in several areas of research, including cancer, traumatic brain injury, Alzheimer disease, and heart disease.[8–11] Variability in outcomes based on ethnic differences has been observed in transplant surgery, cardiac, and pulmonary disease.[12–14] For example, a recent publication by Silva and colleagues[12] highlights the importance of race-match for African American male liver recipients. Although differences in outcomes are noted, the exact pathophysiologic mechanisms of these sex and racial differences are not well understood.

One major improvement in identifying specific genotypes is gene sequencing for so-called single-nucleotide polymorphisms (SNPs), gene loci that help correlate clinical risk factors with specific genetic sequences. This practice is increasingly well known because testing for the breast cancer (BRCA) gene and its mutations/SNPs has led to the option of choosing preventive gynecologic surgeries in high-risk patients. It also is useful in creating chemotherapy protocols based on genetic profiles correlating with optimal drug response patterns. The following studies are all examples of an increasing number of investigations (cell, animal, and clinical) that shed light on sex-specific and race-specific differences. These investigations seek to identify specific genotypes and phenotypes that may be helpful in allowing for an individualized approach and precision medicine in a critical care unit.

Traumatic Brain Injury

Sports-related head injuries, with all severity levels of traumatic brain injury (TBI), have been reported with increasing frequency over the past decade. Consequently, the number of female TBI patients also has increased.[15,16] Most TBI animal models favored male animals. Research with regard to sex-specific outcomes after TBI is a work in progress. The role of sex hormones mostly is unclear, depending on the animal model chosen, as reported in a review of 50 TBI animal models by Rubin and Lipton in 2019.[17] Sex played a role in response to vasopressors to improve cerebral blood flow and, on a molecular level, in the evolution of post-TBI inflammatory response.[17,18]

Thoracic Aortic Surgery with Hypothermic Circulatory Arrest

Female sex is an independent risk factor for worse outcome after complex thoracic aortic surgery. Female patients had higher mortality and risk for postoperative stroke despite a lower incidence of coronary artery disease, better cardiac function, and shorter cross-clamp and total cardiopulmonary bypass times compared with male patients.[19]

Postoperative Delirium and the APOE4 Gene

The APOE4 gene is linked to Alzheimer disease. Female patients positive for APOE4 allele have a higher risk for Alzheimer disease compared with male patients. A longitudinal study published by Schenning and colleagues,[20] in 2019, however, demonstrated that male patients positive for APOE4 present with significantly worse postoperative cognitive decline compared with the overall male-female cohort, despite correction for age and comorbidities.

Race-Matching in Liver Transplants

Hepatocellular carcinoma (HCC), a highly aggressive tumor carrying a mean survival estimate of between 6 months and 20 months, is the most common primary tumor of the liver. Due to the aggressive nature of the disease and the side effects of alternative treatment options, liver transplantation often is utilized as the primary modality of therapy for patients with HCC. A recent study by Silva and colleagues,[12] in 2019, revealed African American liver transplant recipients with HCC had improved overall survival when matched with African American organ donors. This held true even while adjusting for comorbidities and disease characteristics.

Basic science research is fundamental in shaping the practice of modern clinical medicine. There are limitations, however, that need to be considered. Better understanding of how these limitations may contribute to the race-based and gender-based health disparities that exist will be paramount in improving care and closing these gaps.

GENDER IMPACT ON HEALTH DISPARITIES IN CRITICAL CARE

Gender and race have tremendous and wide-ranging impacts on health care delivery, with powerful implications for both health care providers and their patients. For many years, there has been evidence that gender affects, often negatively, the care and outcomes of female patients for a variety of reasons. Perhaps one of the most simplistic (and frustrating) illustrations of this is the dramatic discrepancy between the rates of bystander cardiopulmonary resuscitation (CPR) performed in public places on men (45%) versus women (39%), unfortunately translating into a 29% higher likelihood of survival to hospital discharge for men compared with women.[21]

Extensive work has been done to explore the ways gender has played a role in the world of primary and preventative care. It has been recognized that women more often fail to seek care or are nonadherent to treatment regimens due to cost or lack of resources (childcare, time, and transportation).[22] Women with chronic diseases, such as heart or renal failure, have been observed to receive fewer guideline-based diagnostic procedures, get less-invasive treatments, and be referred later for heart or kidney transplantation and/or dialysis. Women with chronic pain more likely are given sedatives as treatment, whereas men more often are prescribed pain medication, and women with rheumatoid arthritis are much less likely to be sent to see a specialist than are men.[23] But does the same hold true for critically ill patients?

MI is a common cause of critical illness and also is an area where gender effects have been heavily investigated. This most likely is due to the well-recognized differences in susceptibility, presentation, and outcomes between women and men. In general, the rate of MIs is declining in every demographic group except young women. Yet women who experience MI are, once again, more likely to receive less-invasive diagnostic and therapeutic interventions and have a higher mortality rate after their first MI.[23] Furthermore, female gender has long been recognized as an independent predictor of increased morbidity and mortality after coronary artery bypass surgery and, as such, is included as part of many of the risk-stratification scoring systems used by cardiothoracic surgeons.[24] The reasons behind these differences are complex and likely not generalizable.

To understand the impact of patient gender during critical illness, not only must the differences in patient biology and pathophysiology but also the factors that influence diagnosis and treatment strategies be understood. Do women present differently from men with certain illnesses? Do health care providers assess the severity of illness differently in women versus men, and can this affect intensive care unit (ICU) admission rates? Does gender play a role when patients and their families make decisions about aggressiveness of treatment, and do physicians offer the same interventions in the same way regardless of patient gender? Or are physicians' approaches subtly biased?

In looking at patients with varied forms of critical illness, potentially contradictory results begin to be seen. For example, at least in part because of the effects of sex hormones and the differences in the cytokine and other inflammatory response systems, premenopausal women cared for in the ICU after trauma or with sepsis fare better than their male counterparts. Looking at trauma patients, women develop fewer infections in the ICU, with lower rates of pneumonia and bacteremia.[25,26] These results have fueled research into the manipulation of sex hormones as a potential therapeutic strategy.

The FROG-ICU (French and European Outcome Registry in Intensive Care Unit) study, a trial conducted in France and Belgium and published in early 2019, looked at gender-related outcome differences across a large population of ICU patients and found remarkably similar demographic characteristics, clinical presentations, and illness severity between the 2 groups, with no difference in 28-day or 1-year survival rates.[27]

Although it is clear that gender plays a role in a variety of illnesses, it is difficult to make a compelling case that patient gender influences outcomes in the critically ill in a consistent manner. It is especially challenging to try to tease apart the matrix of factors that may contribute to any trends that may be identified. As women physicians gain a more secure footing in many medical specialties, including critical care medicine, however, researchers increasingly are investigating the other side of the coin. What, if any, differences in patient care can be associated with the gender of the health care provider?

Here again, the research is more robust in the nonacute setting. For example, in primary care environments, female physicians often have more patient-centric communication styles and focus more on both preventative care and psychosocial issues.[28] Elderly patients cared for by female physicians during their hospital admissions have lower mortality and readmission rates.[29]

Recently, the unique contributions of female physicians in the critical care setting were examined in 2 significant studies. A publication in the *Proceedings of the National Academy of Sciences*[3] journal garnered national attention in 2018. Greenwood and colleagues reported improved survival for patients presenting to emergency departments (EDs) with an acute MI when cared for by a female physician compared with a male physician. The impact of this difference was most pronounced for female patients. Of the various combinations, female patients cared for by male physicians were the least likely to survive. And the survival of female patients as a whole was positively correlated with the proportion of female physicians working in the department.[3]

In 2019, Meier and colleagues[30] published a study examining the relationship between physician gender and survival in patients who suffer in-hospital cardiac arrest. This retrospective analysis of more than 1000 cardiac arrests found that female code leadership was associated with an increased likelihood of achieving return of spontaneous circulation (76.8% vs 71.7%) and an increased rate of survival to discharge (37.3% vs 29.8%). The study also looked at the impact of gender concordance between physician and nursing leadership in codes and found that a female code leader and a female code nurse conferred survival benefit over a male code leader with either a male or female code nurse and over female code leaders paired with male code nurses (although this combination of gender concordance amongst physician and lead nurse during a code was quite rare, occurring only 7% of the time).[30]

Although the data represent complex and likely multifactorial associations, they do suggest a potential patient benefit derived from critical care provided by female physicians. They represent yet another facet of the interplay between gender and medicine. Seen as a whole, these findings implore the health care community to take a closer look at the impact gender has on patients, practices, and providers.

RACE IMPACT ON HEALTH DISPARITIES IN CRITICAL CARE

With regard to health care disparities, the topic cannot be addressed without confrontation of the history of medicine and its intersection with race. Throughout American history, there has been a marked phenomenon of increased mortality for patients of minority status, in particular those of African American lineage. This disparity continues into current times. The present-day age-adjusted death rate for the non-Hispanic black population is 1.2 times greater than for whites and, excluding mortality associated with suicide or unintentional trauma, African Americans have higher age-adjusted death rates for 8 of the 13 leading causes of death.[31]

Holding all things constant, including socioeconomic status, educational level, and access to resources, significant disparity remains for African Americans in conditions, such as infant and maternal mortality, death related to cardiovascular disease, and death related to the most common cancers.[32–34] African American children, in comparison to white children, are 2.2 times more likely to die before their first birthday. African American mothers are approximately 4 times more likely to die in the peripartum period than their white counterparts.[32,35]

Furthermore, contrary to common trends, improved socioeconomic status in the form of increased income level and higher attainment of education is not protective as it pertains to racial inequalities in health outcomes. For instance, an African American infant born to a mother with a doctorate degree is approximately 2 times more likely to die in infancy than a child born to a white mother with an eighth-grade education level.[36,37] This variance from the social determinants model, the association of increasing disparities along racial lines even with higher levels of socioeconomic status, also is noted in studies targeting conditions, such as heart attacks, stroke, and several commonly diagnosed cancers like breast, prostate, and lung cancers.[38]

Due to these findings, tremendous efforts have been geared toward understanding the factors that contribute to this gap in medical outcomes in the community as well as infractions within the medical institution. Through these studies, many factors have been suggested as leading to increased morbidity and mortality along racial lines, including the skewed presence of environmental toxins, food deserts leading to undernutrition and malnutrition, physiologic stressors within minority-populated communities, implicit and explicit racial bias among health care providers, and the inequality of resource utilization and availability within minority communities and the local hospitals serving them.[39–50] The totality of this 2-tier system is implicated not only as a contributor to the higher prevalence of diseases commonly treated within the primary care sector in minority communities (eg, hypertension, diabetes, and asthma) but also in regard to African Americans having worse outcomes for conditions carrying the highest morbidity and mortality within the critical care arena (eg, sepsis, cardiac arrest, and acute respiratory distress syndrome [ARDS]).[39,44–47,49]

Racial Health Disparities in Regard to Mortality Associated with Acute Critical Illnesses

In the United States, more than 5.7 million patients are admitted to the ICU annually, with an overall associated mortality rate upwards of 10% to 29%, with determinants of death largely age and severity of disease.[51,52] Although advancements have been achieved in earlier recognition and treatment of critical disease processes, there remains high mortality associated with certain diagnoses in the ICU, namely ARDS with 50% mortality, sepsis with upwards of 45% to 60%, and in-hospital versus out-of-hospital cardiac arrest, with 75% versus 88% mortality, respectively.[53–57]

Data also reveal that, although treatment strategies often are heavily protocolized, racial health disparities persist among these conditions, with many studies highlighting treatment bias in health care practice as a potential contributor.[58] Winchester and colleagues (2018)[47] demonstrated increased mortality rate associated with critical troponin levels. African Americans presenting with this finding, however, were statistically less likely to have either a consultation from a cardiologist or cardiac catheterization performed during their hospitalization in comparison to white patients with similar presentations. Additional studies reveal African Americans are more likely to have delayed admission to an ICU and altogether are less likely to be admitted to a cardiac care unit in comparison to whites, even after controlling for hospital and insurance plans.[59] Moreover, race has been noted as an independent risk factor associated with delayed cardiac arrest interventions, including defibrillation, conferring higher odds of death for African Americans after both in-hospital and out-of-hospital CPR.[46]

Similar disparities exist for ARDS and sepsis. Although there has been a steady decrease in overall mortality from these processes in recent years, African Americans continue to have higher mortality rates for both in comparison to whites.[44,45,60] Researchers present many factors contributing to these findings. With regard to sepsis, it has been established that delayed resuscitation and treatment of the infectious source results in higher morbidity and mortality.[61,62] This understanding led to the founding of the Surviving Sepsis Campaign in 2004, which resulted in the Surviving Sepsis guidelines, which provide optimal treatment pathways for all patients presenting with sepsis.[63] Despite these efforts, subsequent studies continue to show differences in care delivered to critically ill minority patients. Mayr and colleagues[64] (2010) reported that African Americans diagnosed with community-acquired pneumonia are less likely to receive guideline-concordant antibiotics within the recommended 4 hours from presentation in comparison to whites. This is noteworthy in that pneumonia is the most common source of infection associated with severe sepsis, and severe sepsis is the second leading cause of death in noncoronary ICUs, claiming the lives of more than 200,000 people per year in the United States alone.[51,65,66] An interesting study published recently examined outcomes of septic patients after New York State mandated that management follow established sepsis protocols. As would be expected, protocol completion rates increased and mortality rates declined. A closer look at these results revealed, however, that there was a greater protocol completion rate in white patients (14.0 percentage points) compared with black patients (5.3 percentage points).[67] It appeared that hospitals that took care of a larger proportion of black and minority patients struggled with consistent implementation of performance measures. This study highlights the disparities that exist in the care provided in largely minority versus nonminority hospitals and urges policy makers to be cognizant of the disparities that might arise. It is imperative to put appropriate measures in place when rolling out new mandates, so that all patients benefit from these efforts.

Additional studies, like that of Pines and colleagues[68] demonstrate African Americans having longer ED boarding times while awaiting ICU admission than white patients. Longer boarding time in the ED is directly associated with increased mortality rate for those admitted to the ICU and carries higher rates of ventilatory-associated pneumonia in trauma patients. Additionally, investigators question whether subtle inequalities in health care providers' interventions, for example, delays in diagnosis or treatment of conditions that cause acute lung injury or noncompliance with recommended low tidal volume ventilatory strategies, may factor into the higher mortality rates seen in African Americans diagnosed with ARDS. These inequalities warrant further investigational studies.[69,70]

Racial Health Disparities: The Role of the Physician

The complexities contributing to the racial health disparities, discussed previously, in the continuum of acute critical illness are vast, encompassing the patient, community, and potentially modifiable practices at the hospital level.[39,49,62,71] As physicians, abilities to influence the former 2 factors may be limited to those of an everyday citizen, but the absolute duty to eradicate the influence of the third factor is mandated in the Hippocratic oath that was pledged. Unfortunately, studies continue to reveal deviations in diagnosing practices as well as treatments offered to critically ill minority patients in comparison to majority patients with similar disease processes, throughout their hospital stays.[41,45–47,50,59,64,68,69,71] More and more, studies are investigating the influence of implicit and explicit biases among physicians and the impact not only on the patient experience but also on morbidity and mortality.[40–43] Physician bias may prove to be the most challenging modifiable risk factor leading to racial health disparities to eliminate.

Race-associated beliefs are developed along the entirety of a life span and become so interwoven in thought processes that recognition of those differences may be subconscious for some, that is, implicit bias.[43] Physicians are no different from the general population in this regard: studies demonstrate equal prevalence of implicit bias among health care providers in comparison to the average citizen, and, alarmingly, but not surprisingly, implicit bias is correlated directly with lower quality of care for targeted patients.[58] Only through the acknowledgment of racial health disparities can a conversation be sparked among physicians and other members of the health care team, allowing for individual and collective reflections and discourse that ultimately will improve the health care systems.

SUMMARY

Disparities exist and affect all facets of medicine. Although gender disparities have historically received more investigative efforts, race and ethnicity have more recently been shown to be integral components woven into the tapestry of disparity. The repercussions of these elements in the care provided for patients have been recognized over time. From the structure of basic science research models, which are the backbone of modern medicine, to the differential care provided to patients based on their gender, racial, and ethnic differences, these disparities are deeply ingrained in medicine. Recognition is the first step in addressing and eliminating the barriers that exist. Through this narrative, these concerns have been attempted to be brought to the forefront, to help physicians move forward from a state of subconscious bias and enable them to provide the best care they can to every patient they see.

DISCLOSURE

E.J. Hilton is a cofounder of a medical consulting firm, GoodStock Consulting, LLC, where the mission is based on addressing racial health disparities.

REFERENCES

1. Life expectancy at birth, at age 65, and at age 75, by sex, race, and Hispanic origin: United States, selected years 1900–2016. Center for Disease Control and Prevention. 2017. Available at: https://www.cdc.gov/nchs/data/hus/2017/015.pdf. Accessed July 22, 2019.
2. Cooper L, Powe N. Disparities in patient experiences, health care processes, and outcomes: the role of patient-provider racial, ethnic, and language concordance. The Commonwealth Fund. 2004. Available at: https://www.commonwealthfund.org/publications/fund-reports/2004/jul/disparities-patient-experiences-health-care-processes-and. Accessed July 22, 2019.
3. Greenwood BN, Carnahan S, Huang L. Patient-physician gender concordance and increased mortality among female heart attack patients. Proc Natl Acad Sci U S A 2018;115(34):8569–74.
4. Croft DP, Brent LJ, Franks DW, et al. The evolution of prolonged life after reproduction. Trends Ecol Evol 2015;30(7):407–16.
5. Whitley H, Lindsey W. Sex-based differences in drug activity. Am Fam Physician 2009;80(11):1254–8.
6. U S Food & Drug Administration. Drug Safety Communications. Risk of next-morning impairment after use of insomnia drugs; FDA requires lower recommended doses for certain drugs containing zolpidem Web site. 2018. Available at: https://www.fda.gov/media/84992/. Accessed June 29, 2019.
7. FDA guideline for the study and evaluation of gender differences in the clinical evaluation of drugs. Fed Regist 1993;58(139):39406–16.
8. Jagsi R, Motomura AR, Amarnath S, et al. Under-representation of women in high-impact published clinical cancer research. Cancer 2009;115(14):3293–301.
9. Mollayeva T, Colantonio A. Gender, sex and traumatic brain injury: transformative science to optimize patient outcomes. Healthc Q 2017;20(1):6–9.
10. Ferretti MT, Iulita MF, Cavedo E, et al. Sex differences in Alzheimer disease - the gateway to precision medicine. Nat Rev Neurol 2018;14(8):457–69.
11. Ko D, Rahman F, Schnabel RB, et al. Atrial fibrillation in women: epidemiology, pathophysiology, presentation, and prognosis. Nat Rev Cardiol 2016;13(6):321–32.
12. Silva JP, Maurina MN, Tsai S, et al. Effect of donor race-matching on overall survival for African-American patients undergoing liver transplantation for hepatocellular carcinoma. J Am Coll Surg 2019;228(3):245–54.
13. Leigh JA, Alvarez M, Rodriguez CJ. Ethnic minorities and coronary heart disease: an update and future directions. Curr Atheroscler Rep 2016;18(2):9.
14. Celedon JC, Roman J, Schraufnagel DE, et al. Respiratory health equality in the United States. The American thoracic society perspective. Ann Am Thorac Soc 2014;11(4):473–9.
15. Broshek DK, Kaushik T, Freeman JR, et al. Sex differences in outcome following sports-related concussion. J Neurosurg 2005;102(5):856–63.
16. Bazarian JJ, Blyth B, Mookerjee S, et al. Sex differences in outcome after mild traumatic brain injury. J Neurotrauma 2010;27(3):527–39.
17. Rubin TG, Lipton ML. Sex differences in animal models of traumatic brain injury. J Exp Neurosci 2019;13. 1179069519844020.

18. Curvello V, Hekierski H, Riley J, et al. Sex and age differences in phenylephrine mechanisms and outcomes after piglet brain injury. Pediatr Res 2017;82(1): 108–13.
19. Chung J, Stevens LM, Ouzounian M, et al. Sex-related differences in patients undergoing thoracic aortic surgery. Circulation 2019;139(9):1177–84.
20. Schenning KJ, Murchison CF, Mattek NC, et al. Sex and genetic differences in postoperative cognitive dysfunction: a longitudinal cohort analysis. Biol Sex Differ 2019;10(1):14.
21. Blewer AL, McGovern SK, Schmicker RH, et al. Gender disparities among adult recipients of bystander cardiopulmonary resuscitation in the public. Circ Cardiovasc Qual Outcomes 2018;11(8):e004710.
22. Women's Health Policy: Gender Differences in Health Care, Status, and Use: Spotlight on Men's Health. Henry J Kaiser Family Foundation. 2013 Kaiser Men's Health Survey and 2013 Kaiser Women's Health Survey Web site. 2015. Available at: https://www.kff.org/womens-health-policy/fact-sheet/gender-differences-in-health-care-status-and-use-spotlight-on-mens-health/. Accessed June 29, 2019.
23. Regitz-Zagrosek V. Sex and gender differences in health. Science & Society Series on Sex and Science. EMBO Rep 2012;13(7):596–603.
24. Blasberg JD, Schwartz GS, Balaram SK. The role of gender in coronary surgery. Eur J Cardiothorac Surg 2011;40(3):715–21.
25. Guidry CA, Swenson BR, Davies SW, et al. Sex- and diagnosis-dependent differences in mortality and admission cytokine levels among patients admitted for intensive care. Crit Care Med 2014;42(5):1110–20.
26. Vezzani A, Mergoni M, Orlandi P, et al. Gender differences in case mix and outcome of critically ill patients. Gend Med 2011;8(1):32–9.
27. Hollinger A, Gayat E, Feliot E, et al. Gender and survival of critically ill patients: results from the FROG-ICU study. Ann Intensive Care 2019;9(1):43.
28. Roter DL, Hall JA, Aoki Y. Physician gender effects in medical communication: a meta-analytic review. JAMA 2002;288(6):756–64.
29. Tsugawa Y, Jena AB, Figueroa JF, et al. Comparison of hospital mortality and readmission rates for medicare patients treated by male vs female physicians. JAMA Intern Med 2017;177(2):206–13.
30. Meier A, Yang J, Liu J, et al. Female physician leadership during cardiopulmonary resuscitation is associated with improved patient outcomes. Crit Care Med 2019;47(1):e8–13.
31. National Vital Statistics Report. Deaths: final data for 2017. National Center for Health Statistics. Available at: https://www.cdc.gov/nchs/data/nvsr/nvsr68/nvsr68_09-508.pdf. Accessed July 6, 2019.
32. Coy P. For black women, education is no protection against infant mortality. Bloomberg Businessweek 2018.
33. Vital signs: preventable deaths from heart disease and stroke. Center for Disease Control and Prevention. 2013. Available at: https://www.cdc.gov/dhdsp/vital_signs.htm. Accessed June 6, 2019.
34. Health Care and the 2008 elections: eliminating racial/ethnic disparities in health care: what are the options? The Henry J. Kaiser Family Foundation. 2008. Available at: https://www.kff.org/wp-content/uploads/2013/01/7830.pdf. Accessed June 6, 2019.
35. U.S. Department of Health and Human Services. Infant mortality and African Americans web site. 2017. Available at: https://minorityhealth.hhs.gov/omh/browse.aspx?lvl=4&lvlid=23. Accessed July 6, 2019.

36. Smith I, Bentley-Edwards K, El-Amin S, et al. Fighting at birth: eradicating black-white infant mortality. Oakland (CA): Duke University's Samuel DuBois Cook Center on Social Equity and Insight Center for Community Economic Development; 2018.
37. Kothari CL, Paul R, Dormitorio B, et al. The interplay of race, socioeconomic status and neighborhood residence upon birth outcomes in a high black infant mortality community. SSM Popul Health 2016;2:859–67.
38. Singh GK, Jemal A. Socioeconomic and racial/ethnic disparities in cancer mortality, incidence, and survival in the United States, 1950-2014: over six decades of changing patterns and widening inequalities. J Environ Public Health 2017;2017:2819372.
39. Mikati I, Benson AF, Luben TJ, et al. Disparities in distribution of particulate matter emission sources by race and poverty status. Am J Public Health 2018;108(4):480–5.
40. Green AR, Carney DR, Pallin DJ, et al. Implicit bias among physicians and its prediction of thrombolysis decisions for black and white patients. J Gen Intern Med 2007;22(9):1231–8.
41. Schulman KA, Berlin JA, Harless W, et al. The effect of race and sex on physicians' recommendations for cardiac catheterization. N Engl J Med 1999;340(8):618–26.
42. Hoffman KM, Trawalter S, Axt JR, et al. Racial bias in pain assessment and treatment recommendations, and false beliefs about biological differences between blacks and whites. Proc Natl Acad Sci U S A 2016;113(16):4296–301.
43. Jones CP. Levels of racism: a theoretic framework and a gardener's tale. Am J Public Health 2000;90(8):1212–5.
44. Bime C, Poongkunran C, Borgstrom M, et al. Racial differences in mortality from severe acute respiratory failure in the United States, 2008-2012. Ann Am Thorac Soc 2016;13(12):2184–9.
45. Jones JM, Fingar KR, Miller MA, et al. Racial disparities in sepsis-related in-hospital mortality: using a broad case capture method and multivariate controls for clinical and hospital variables, 2004-2013. Crit Care Med 2017;45(12):e1209–17.
46. Ehlenbach WJ, Barnato AE, Curtis JR, et al. Epidemiologic study of in-hospital cardiopulmonary resuscitation in the elderly. N Engl J Med 2009;361(1):22–31.
47. Winchester DE, Kline K, Estel C, et al. Associations between cardiac troponin, mortality and subsequent use of cardiovascular services: differences in sex and ethnicity. Open Heart 2018;5(1):e000713.
48. Rauscher GH, Allgood KL, Whitman S, et al. Disparities in screening mammography services by race/ethnicity and health insurance. J Womens Health (Larchmt) 2012;21(2):154–60.
49. Hilmers A, Hilmers DC, Dave J. Neighborhood disparities in access to healthy foods and their effects on environmental justice. Am J Public Health 2012;102(9):1644–54.
50. Fang P, He W, Gomez D, et al. Racial disparities in guideline-concordant cancer care and mortality in the United States. Adv Radiat Oncol 2018;3(3):221–9.
51. Critical Care Statistics. Society of Critical Care Medicine. Available at: https://www.sccm.org/Communications/Critical-Care-Statistics. Accessed July 6, 2015.
52. Barrett ML, Smith MW, Elixhauser A, et al. Utilization of intensive care services, 2011. HCUP Statistical Brief #185. Rockville (MD): Agency for Healthcare Research and Quality; 2014. Available at: http://www.hcup-us.ahrq.gov/reports/statbriefs/sb185-Hospital-Intensive-Care-Units-2011.pdf.

53. Wunsch H, Angus DC, Harrison DA, et al. Comparison of medical admissions to intensive care units in the United States and United Kingdom. Am J Respir Crit Care Med 2011;183(12):1666–73.
54. Elias KM, Moromizato T, Gibbons FK, et al. Derivation and validation of the acute organ failure score to predict outcome in critically ill patients: a cohort study. Crit Care Med 2015;43(4):856–64.
55. Daya MR, Schmicker RH, Zive DM, et al. Out-of-hospital cardiac arrest survival improving over time: Results from the Resuscitation Outcomes Consortium (ROC). Resuscitation 2015;91:108–15.
56. Dombrovskiy VY, Martin AA, Sunderram J, et al. Rapid increase in hospitalization and mortality rates for severe sepsis in the United States: a trend analysis from 1993 to 2003. Crit Care Med 2007;35(5):1244–50.
57. Monchi M, Bellenfant F, Cariou A, et al. Early predictive factors of survival in the acute respiratory distress syndrome. A multivariate analysis. Am J Respir Crit Care Med 1998;158(4):1076–81.
58. FitzGerald C, Hurst S. Implicit bias in healthcare professionals: a systematic review. BMC Med Ethics 2017;18(1):19.
59. Soto GJ, Martin GS, Gong MN. Healthcare disparities in critical illness. Crit Care Med 2013;41(12):2784–93.
60. Cochi SE, Kempker JA, Annangi S, et al. Mortality trends of acute respiratory distress syndrome in the United States from 1999 to 2013. Ann Am Thorac Soc 2016;13(10):1742–51.
61. Rivers E, Nguyen B, Havstad S, et al. Early goal-directed therapy in the treatment of severe sepsis and septic shock. N Engl J Med 2001;345(19):1368–77.
62. Vincent JL, Abraham E, Annane D, et al. Reducing mortality in sepsis: new directions. Crit Care 2002;6(Suppl 3):S1–18.
63. Dellinger RP, Carlet JM, Masur H, et al. Surviving Sepsis Campaign guidelines for management of severe sepsis and septic shock. Crit Care Med 2004;32(3):858–73.
64. Mayr FB, Yende S, D'Angelo G, et al. Do hospitals provide lower quality of care to black patients for pneumonia? Crit Care Med 2010;38(3):759–65.
65. Sepsis: data & reports. Center for Disease Control. Available at: https://www.cdc.gov/sepsis/datareports/index.html. Accessed June 6, 2019.
66. Mayr FB, Yende S, Angus DC. Epidemiology of severe sepsis. Virulence 2014;5(1):4–11.
67. Corl K, Levy M, Phillips G, et al. Racial and ethnic disparities in care following the New York State sepsis initiative. Health Aff (Millwood) 2019;38(7):1119–26.
68. Pines JM, Russell Localio A, Hollander JE. Racial disparities in emergency department length of stay for admitted patients in the United States. Acad Emerg Med 2009;16(5):403–10.
69. Chertoff J. Racial disparities in critical care: experience from the USA. Lancet Respir Med 2017;5(2):e11–2.
70. Erickson SE, Shlipak MG, Martin GS, et al. Racial and ethnic disparities in mortality from acute lung injury. Crit Care Med 2009;37(1):1–6.
71. Hamilton D. Working paper series: post-racial rhetoric, racial health disparities, and health disparity consequences of stigma, stress, and racism. Washington, DC: Washington Center for Equitable Growth; 2017.

Two Sides of the Same Coin

Addressing Racial and Gender Disparities Among Physicians and the Impact on the Community They Serve

Ebony J. Hilton, MD[a,*], Nadia Lunardi, MD, PhD[a],
Roshni Sreedharan, MD[b], Kristina L. Goff, MD[c],
Mariam Batakji, MD[a], Dorothea S. Rosenberger, MD, PhD[d]

KEYWORDS

- Racial bias • Gender bias • Female physicians • Minority physicians • Race
- Ethnicity • Gender • Academic medicine

KEY POINTS

- Race has been identified as an independent risk factor associated with increased morbidity and mortality for some of the leading causes of acute critical illnesses.
- Overall, African Americans have higher death rates than Caucasians for all-cause mortality in all age groups less than 65 years old.
- Racial health disparities involve multiple factors with contributors on both the community/individual end and within the hospital system itself.
- Both gender and racial concordance between physicians and patients have been associated with improved outcomes.
- Female physicians and those of minority race remain under-represented in critical care medicine. There is a paucity of systemic data pertaining to reasons behind this disparity.

Racial and gender disparities among licensed physicians in the United States have been widely prevalent, persisting long after the matriculation of Drs David Peck and Elizabeth Blackwell, the first African American and female physicians, respectively, to graduate from an American medical school.[1–4] Studies link this lack of diversity to poorer patient outcomes, which has bolstered the implementation of programs designed to recruit,

[a] University of Virginia Health System, PO Box 800710, Charlottesville, VA 22908, USA; [b] Case Western Reserve University School of Medicine, 9500 Euclid Avenue, Mail code G-58, Cleveland, OH 44195, USA; [c] University of Texas Southwestern Medical Center, 3851 Beutel Court, Dallas, TX 75229, USA; [d] University of Utah School of Medicine, 30 North 1900 East, Room 3C444 SOM, Salt Lake City, UT 84132, USA
* Corresponding author.
E-mail address: eh3nf@hscmail.mcc.virginia.edu

Anesthesiology Clin 38 (2020) 369–377
https://doi.org/10.1016/j.anclin.2020.01.001 **anesthesiology.theclinics.com**

train, and retain members of these minority groups in the medical field.[5,6] To better reflect and treat our increasingly diverse patient population, we must address the systemic obstacles that deter minorities from earning admission into medical school. Furthermore, factors hindering the successful appointment of minority physicians to leadership positions needs to be investigated to tackle them in a systematic fashion.

GENDER IMBALANCE IN CRITICAL CARE MEDICINE

Under-Representation of Female Physicians in Critical Care Medicine

The last 50 years have seen a dramatic increase in the number of women physicians. In the United States, Canada, Europe, and Australia, the percentage of women graduating from medical schools reached 50% during the 1990s and early 2000s.[1,2,7,8] As a result, one-half of the physician positions in several medical specialties are currently occupied by women. Although the number of female specialists in critical care medicine has also steadily increased, it has not grown proportionately to the number of women graduating from medical schools.[2] For example, 40% of critical care medicine specialists were women in the United States between 2011 and 2015.[8] In 2015, women comprised approximately 30% of the intensivists in Britain[10] and 19% of the critical care workforce in Australia.[7] A survey of the World Federation of Societies of Intensive and Critical Care Medicine from 2018 broadly estimated the number of female critical care medicine physicians to be 37 ± 11% (range, 26%–50%).[8]

Under-Representation of Female Physicians in Critical Care Medicine Leadership

Although approximately 30% of critical care medicine specialists are women in most developed countries, women comprised only 8% of the European Society of Intensive Care Medicine board and 7% of the council of the World Federation of Societies of Intensive and Critical Care Medicine in 2017.[8] Between 2000 and 2017, none of the presidents of the European Society of Intensive Care Medicine or the College of Intensive Care Medicine of Australia and New Zealand were women.[8] A review of invited lecturers at 4 leading critical care medicine symposia acknowledged that female faculty on average represented 22% of speakers in 2017, at best.[8] Only 8% of the editorial board members of the 5 highest ranked critical care journals were women.[9] Finally, a review of the authorship of critical care guidelines published between 2012 and 2016 found that only 13% of the authors were women.[10] A comprehensive database was used to look at the role of gender in faculty ranking in US medical schools. Even when adjusted for specialty, experience, research productivity, and age, women were significantly less likely to be full professors as compared with men.[11] This disparity in achieving faculty ranking in academic institutions trickles down into leadership opportunities as well. Even when taking into account medicine in general, although women account for about one-third of the full academic faculty in US medical schools, the percentage of women who are full professors (21%), chairs of departments (15%), or medical school deans (16%) are alarmingly low.[12]

Why More Female Physicians Are Needed in the Critical Care Medicine Workforce

There are at least 2 compelling reasons why gender equity should be actively pursued in critical care medicine. First, for the sake of diversity itself: men and women often bring different attitudes and perspectives to the care team, distinctive tactics to problem solving, and unique solutions. This diversity of approaches sharpens a team's performance, promotes innovation, and creates greater success.[13] Therefore, from a purely business standpoint, creating a diverse team enriched with representatives of different genders is a smart decision. Second, there is an advantage in the interest of improved patient outcomes. Several studies, largely based in non-acute settings, suggest there are differences in the way women and men practice medicine, and that such variations may have important implications for patient outcomes.[14–16] As an example, a recent study found that elderly hospitalized patients treated by female internists have lower 30-day mortality and readmission rates compared with those cared for by male internists.[17] Furthermore, they found that sicker patients were more likely to have a better outcome when they had a female physician. The findings from this particular study are consistent with results from prior investigations on process quality measures, showing that female physicians are more likely to adhere to clinical guidelines and evidence-based medicine, to practice patient-centered interviewing, and to offer prevention advice.[15,16] Two recent publications make the strong argument for improved patient outcomes when female providers lead the care team in acute settings too. A study from 2018 showed that patients with acute myocardial infarction are more likely to survive when cared for by female physicians.[18] Another report in 2019 reviewed outcomes after cardiac arrest based on the gender of the physician leading the resuscitation efforts, and found that patients whose resuscitation team was led by a female physician had a significantly higher likelihood of return of spontaneous circulation and survival to discharge.[19] In conclusion, there is growing evidence to support the notion that creating a nonhomogenous, gender-balanced workforce team is not only a savvy business decision, but also a requirement when the goal is to provide high-quality, effective care for all patients.

Reasons for the Under-Representation of Female Physicians in Critical Care Medicine

There is a paucity of systematic data evaluating the reasons behind the under-representation of women in critical care medicine. In a 2016 survey of Australia and New Zealand's female critical care medicine specialists, 37% of respondents felt disadvantaged as a female specialist in intensive care.[7] Only 50% of respondents stated that their work–life balance was satisfactory. The challenges of balancing a career in medicine with parenting included a lack of flexibility to attend to family responsibilities, difficulties arranging childcare, and the impact of maternity leave on their advancement.[7,11,20,21] Multiple studies show that, although female physicians are likely to have a partner who works full time, male physicians with children are more likely to have a partner who does not, placing them at an advantage compared with their female peers.[22–24] Although these issues have not been explicitly investigated within the specialty of critical care medicine, the high acuity demands of the intensive care unit are likely to pose even more challenges for female intensivists with children.

The survey mentioned elsewhere in this article also found that about 25% of respondents lamented gender-based discrimination in the intensive care unit and difficulties with academic advancement.[2] Several female intensivists commented on the limited numbers of women speaking at critical care medicine forums, attributing this to a lack of time to conduct research that would facilitate career advancement owing to familial obligations. A 2016 survey of the trainees of the College of Intensive Care Medicine of Australia and New Zealand[26] found that 12% experienced discrimination (defined as unjust or prejudicial treatment, especially on the grounds of race, age, or sex) and that discrimination was twice as high among women. Three percent of respondents reported sexual harassment (defined as the making of unwanted sexual advances or obscene remarks), the prevalence of which was 3 times higher in women compared with men.

Notably, there are no systematic investigations examining the reasons why female critical care medicine specialists are poorly represented in leadership positions. However, numerous studies have addressed the larger issue of under-representation of women in leadership roles in the field of medicine as a whole. For example, a study interviewing medical leaders in Australia to elicit their perspectives on the barriers to women advancing and taking on leadership roles was conducted in 2015.[20] The majority of interviewees noted several gender-related barriers impinging on the ability of women to achieve leading roles in academia. On an individual level, self-doubt and the tendency of women not to promote themselves as leaders may both play a role. At an organizational level, limited support for pathways that allow women to stay on a track of academic advancement despite an interruption in their career continues to be a challenge. Moreover, the pipeline theory of women not being in the system long enough still exists. On a cultural level, the assumption that family responsibilities lead women not to seek leadership roles, in addition to the perception that more "feminine" traits are stereotypically inconsistent with strong leadership, continue to be perpetuated. It is unclear whether and how these challenges apply to female physicians working in the intensive care unit, because no data pertaining to critical care medicine are available. However, there is no apparent reason why female intensivists should be uniquely exempt from the challenges lamented by a wide range of women across numerous other medical specialties.

Strategies to Remedy the Under-Representation of Female Physicians in Critical Care Medicine

The attainment of gender equality will require ad hoc and sustained efforts at the level of medical departments, hospitals and health care organizations, critical care medicine societies, boards of critical care medicine journals, and planning committees of intensive care meetings.

The first step should be regular publication of data on female representation in critical care medicine. This step will increase the visibility of the gender gap and help to evaluate the efficacy of strategies implemented to mitigate it.[25] Institutions should use and enforce a zero tolerance approach to gender-based discrimination in the workplace.[7] Mandatory institutional gender bias training may also prove helpful to increase awareness with regard to unconscious gender bias.[9] Additionally, systematic research on the reasons behind female under-representation is imperative.

At a hospital level, on-site childcare that accommodates early, long working hours, and child illness, as well as flexibility with regard to working through pregnancy and choosing accommodating shifts, should be available. On an institutional level, flexible academic advancement options, with part-time opportunities, time out for raising a family, a smooth reentry into clinical duty, and extended timelines to reach the criteria for promotion need to be incorporated into the structure of academic medicine. As eloquently pointed out by Dr Angell in her editorial commentary, "female physicians who work flexible times to raise their children are performing a highly useful function for society [therefore] choosing flexible work pathways should be not only possible, but respectable."[26]

Transparent selection processes should be enforced[20] and selection panels should be blinded to gender whenever possible. Gender-based quotas should be considered within departments, health care organizations, journal editorial boards, and critical care medicine scientific committees.[7] Quotas may help to increase the number of women in leadership roles with decision-making promotion responsibilities, which will in turn facilitate greater upward mobility of female peers and support the achievement of gender parity.

Institutions should foster mentoring and leadership training specifically tailored to women, as well as encourage participation in peer female support groups.[7] Because gender bias can negatively impact mentor–mentee relations, the effectiveness of junior female faculty mentorship should be evaluated and regularly compared against that of male peers.[27]

UNDER-REPRESENTATION OF ETHNIC MINORITY GROUPS AS PHYSICIANS

There is an abundance of literature that points toward better provision of health care and improved outcomes with the elimination of gender, racial, and ethnic disparities. When we look at factors affecting diversity in anesthesiology or medicine in general, the intersectionality of race and gender is an important factor to consider.

Where Does the Disparity Begin?

Ethnic minority groups face unique obstacles in pursuit of higher education that challenge the trajectory of success, including financial limitations, psychological stressors, and lack of exposure/mentorship in fields of interest. Studies show that, despite comparable educational achievement, African Americans with a 3.5 GPA or better are more likely to attend community college in comparison with Caucasians. Furthermore, African Americans are the only racial group more likely to discontinue enrollment in undergraduate studies, but despite doing so, still accumulate substantially more debt.[28] Besides financial pressures, minority college students report subjection to microaggression, overt racism, and social isolation as emotional stressors complicating their educational achievements.[29]

These complexities likely contribute to the skewed demographics of applicants accepted into medical school, as well as those of medical school graduates. Medical school admission rates differ along racial lines, with Caucasians having admission rates of 40% in comparison with lower rates of acceptance for African Americans at 34%. There is an even greater degree of disproportion when comparing medical school graduation rates, with Caucasians composing 51.2% in comparison with 5.7% for African Americans graduates.[30] Similar to college students, African American medical students and residents report psychological strain as they are exposed to environments in which they are in an even smaller minority, thereby increasing their exposure to race-related prejudices.[31,32] Perhaps the emotional cost is best evidenced by the fact that minority residents are 8 times more likely to take a leave of absence than their Caucasian counterparts and are 30% more likely to withdraw from residency.[32] These influences, when taken together, likely account, at least in part, for the disparities with regard to ethnic minorities among practicing physicians.

The Current State of Affairs

Women and ethnic minorities comprise 51% and 32% of the US general population respectively. These percentages put the data provided in the Association of American Medical Colleges Document on Diversity in the Physician Workforce from 2014 into perspective. Approximately 8.9% of physicians identify as African American, American Indian, Hispanic, or Latino. Although African Americans constitute 13% of our nation's population, they account for only about 4% of the physician workforce. Interestingly, among this group of young minority physicians, women constitute a greater percentage (52%) as compared with their male counterparts (48%).[30]

Looking specifically at the field of anesthesiology, Toledo and colleagues[33] published a survey evaluating the diversity in the demographics of the American Society of Anesthesiologists leadership. The results of this survey revealed that women (21%) and ethnic minorities (6%) were underrepresented in the American Society of Anesthesiologists leadership as compared with their representation within the general physician workforce (women 38%, ethnic minorities 8.9%). Similar results were found by Yu and colleagues[34] following retrospective analysis of the Association of American Medical Colleges data on faculty at US medical schools from 1997 to 2008. They focused on the influence of race and gender on the rate of academic advancement and leadership positions. Over a 12-year study period, they noted that 84.76% of professors, 88.26% of chairpersons, and 91.28% of deans were Caucasian, highlighting a gross disparity and underrepresentation of women and minorities in academic medicine. Although there was a minimal increase in the percentage of minority physicians in academic medicine over time, it is inadequate. In fact, they noticed that African American physicians have made the least progress over this time. This lack of progress is also evident in that ethnic minorities are also less likely to undergo promotion and more likely to receive lower compensation.[32] A systematic review conducted in 2014 puts forth evidence that racism, as well as funding and promotion disparities, in addition to a lack of mentorship, affect minority faculty members in academic medicine.[3] This finding further solidifies the notion that we need to implement proven pipeline strategies to increase the representation of these members. Rodriguez and colleagues[4] investigate another important concept of the under-represented minority in medicine responsibility disparity—commonly referred to as the minority tax. This term refers to the additional responsibilities in multiple areas, including efforts to create a diverse workplace, clinical responsibilities, mentorship, and promotion, that are conferred on the under-represented minority in medicine faculty in the name of diversity. These additional responsibilities tend to take time away from these faculty members, limiting their ability to engage in meaningful activities that could contribute to their promotion. Perhaps this reality contributes to the dwindling numbers of under-represented minority in medicine at the department chair level, with women of color representing only 3% in academic medicine.[30] This finding underlines the fact that diversity efforts in institutions have to be a unified initiative.

Why Do We Need More Minority Physicians in the Workforce?

A large body of evidence suggests that we need to have a physician workforce that demonstrates equity with respect to gender, race, and ethnicity. Several studies report that patients from ethnic minorities have lower levels of trust in providers as well as lower satisfaction with their health care. A research initiative, supported by The Commonwealth Fund, has shown that patient–physician race and ethnic concordance produce better outcomes of health care processes, better communication, and improved patient satisfaction scores.[5] Traylor and colleagues[35] demonstrated that race concordance for African American patients was associated with adherence to all their cardiovascular medications. Furthermore, in 2018 Alsan and colleagues[36] hypothesized that race concordance among African Americans could lower the mortality associated with heart disease by upwards of 19% for African American men. This conclusion was reached after finding these subjects sought more preventative services when treated by African American physicians. Patients have reported more participatory decision-making styles in physicians with whom they have race-concordant relationships. Moreover, there is strong evidence that shows that minority physicians are more likely to care for minority patients, patients in underserved areas or in places that have shortage of physicians, and patients with a socioeconomic disadvantage. In simple terms, patients relate better to physicians who come from a cultural background similar to their own. Having more minority physicians in the workforce would be invaluable in establishing more solid patient–doctor rapport and would have a great impact on health care outcomes in general.

What Can We Do?

Looking at the current state of racial disparity, it is clear that we must take an active effort to recruit, retain and advance these groups of physicians, with the goal of reducing health care disparity. The Association of American Medical Colleges has initiated several programs to increase diversity and to increase the representation of marginalized communities, including American Indians and Alaskan natives, who represent less than 0.5% of the physician workforce. Despite institutions and organizations making efforts to increase equity, the numbers of such faculty in academic medicine are disappointing. Kaplan and colleagues[6] explored the reasons behind difficulty in recruiting, retaining, and promoting racially and ethnically diverse faculty. They engaged senior faculty leaders, members in the Group on Diversity and Inclusion and the Group on Women in Medical Sciences at the institutions they surveyed. In addition to noting that the general climate was described as neutral or positive, a few common challenges were noted including the continued lack of a critical mass of minority faculty, the need for coordinated programmatic efforts for retention and promotion, and the need for a senior leader champion.

Strategies for Change

1. Early education (K–12) and medical school
   a. Early exposure of grade school and high school students to explore career options in the medical field
   b. Medical school curriculum including coursework in gender medicine, health disparities, and the impact on patient outcomes
2. Health care system
   a. Training for students and clinical and nonclinical staff to acknowledge and confront both implicit and explicit biases
   b. Cultural competency training for all health care professionals
   c. Development of diversity efforts engaging all clinicians
3. Support systems for minority students, residents, and faculty
   a. Mentorship and support for minority students, residents, and faculty
   b. Programmed efforts by appointment committees to advance minority faculty members
   c. Ensuring diverse selection committees for leadership positions
   d. Identification and elimination of psychological stressors identified by minority students, residents, and faculty
   e. Financial support, tuition relief, and expanded scholarships for socioeconomically underprivileged minorities

SUMMARY

The historical norms of the United States were based in the systematic oppression of racial minorities and women. These beliefs, once held as truths, had far-reaching consequences and helped to shape the demographics of practicing physicians we see today. Fortunately, we are able to learn from our past and, through the pooling of our minds, create a better future. With studies demonstrating improved patient outcomes with physician patient race and gender concordance, encouraging diversity should be the objective not only of minority physicians, but of all members of the medical community.[17–19,35,36]

DISCLOSURE

E. Hilton is a co-founder of a medical consulting firm, GoodStock Consulting, LLC, where our mission is based on addressing racial health disparities.

REFERENCES

1. Metaxa V. Is this (still) a man's world? Crit Care 2013;17(1):112.
2. Hawker FH. Female specialists in intensive care medicine: job satisfaction, challenges and work-life balance. Crit Care Resusc 2016;18(2):125–31.
3. Rodriguez JE, Campbell KM, Mouratidis RW. Where are the rest of us? Improving representation of minority faculty in academic medicine. South Med J 2014;107(12):739–44.
4. Rodriguez JE, Campbell KM, Pololi LH. Addressing disparities in academic medicine: what of the minority tax? BMC Med Educ 2015;15:6.
5. Cooper L, Powe N. Disparities in patient experiences, health care processes, and outcomes: the role of patient-provider racial, ethnic, and language concordance. New York: The Commonwealth Fund; 2004. Available at: https://www.commonwealthfund.org/publications/fund-reports/2004/jul/disparities-patient-experiences-health-careprocesses-and. Accessed July 22, 2019.
6. Kaplan SE, Gunn CM, Kulukulualani AK, et al. Challenges in recruiting, retaining and promoting racially and ethnically diverse faculty. J Natl Med Assoc 2018;110(1):58–64.
7. Modra L, Yong SA, Austin DE. Women in leadership in intensive care medicine. ICU Manag Pract 2016;16(3):174–6.
8. Venkatesh B, Mehta S, Angus DC, et al. Women in Intensive Care study: a preliminary assessment of international data on female representation in the ICU physician workforce, leadership and academic positions. Crit Care 2018;22(1):211.
9. Amrein K, Langmann A, Fahrleitner-Pammer A, et al. Women underrepresented on editorial boards of 60 major medical journals. Gend Med 2011;8(6):378–87.
10. Merman E, Pincus D, Bell C, et al. Differences in clinical practice guideline authorship by gender. Lancet 2018;392(10158):1626–8.
11. Jena AB, Khullar D, Ho O, et al. Sex Differences in academic rank in US Medical Schools in 2014. JAMA 2015;314(11):1149–58.
12. Lautenberger DDV, Raezer C, Sloane RA. The state of women in academic medicine. Washington, DC: AAMC; 2014.
13. Rock D, Grant H. Why diverse teams are smarter 2016. Available at: https://hbr.org/2016/11/why-diverse-teams-are-smarter. Accessed November 13, 2019.
14. Berthold HK, Gouni-Berthold I, Bestehorn KP, et al. Physician gender is associated with the quality of type 2 diabetes care. J Intern Med 2008;264(4):340–50.
15. Lurie N, Slater J, McGovern P, et al. Preventive care for women. Does the sex of the physician matter? N Engl J Med 1993;329(7):478–82.
16. Roter DL, Hall JA, Aoki Y. Physician gender effects in medical communication: a meta-analytic review. JAMA 2002;288(6):756–64.
17. Tsugawa Y, Jena AB, Figueroa JF, et al. Comparison of hospital mortality and readmission rates for Medicare patients treated by male vs female physicians. JAMA Intern Med 2017;177(2):206–13.
18. Greenwood BN, Carnahan S, Huang L. Patient-physician gender concordance and increased mortality among female heart attack patients. Proc Natl Acad Sci U S A 2018;115(34):8569–74.

19. Meier A, Yang J, Liu J, et al. Female physician leadership during cardiopulmonary resuscitation is associated with improved patient outcomes. Crit Care Med 2019;47(1):e8–13.
20. Bismark M, Morris J, Thomas L, et al. Reasons and remedies for under-representation of women in medical leadership roles: a qualitative study from Australia. BMJ Open 2015;5(11):e009384.
21. Jena AB, Olenski AR, Blumenthal DM. Sex differences in physician salary in US public medical schools. JAMA Intern Med 2016;176(9):1294–304.
22. Jolly S, Griffith KA, DeCastro R, et al. Gender differences in time spent on parenting and domestic responsibilities by high-achieving young physician-researchers. Ann Intern Med 2014;160(5):344–53.
23. Stamm M, Buddeberg-Fischer B. How do physicians and their partners coordinate their careers and private lives? Swiss Med Wkly 2011;141:w13179.
24. Holliday EB, Ahmed AA, Jagsi R, et al. Pregnancy and parenthood in radiation oncology, views and experiences survey (PROVES): results of a blinded prospective trainee parenting and career development assessment. Int J Radiat Oncol Biol Phys 2015;92(3):516–24.
25. Bonomo Y, Zundel S, Martin JH. Addressing unconscious bias for female clinical academics. Intern Med J 2016;46(4):391–3.
26. Angell M. Women in medicine: beyond prejudice. N Engl J Med 1981;304(19): 1161–2.
27. De Vries J. Mentoring for change. Melbourne (VIC): Universities Australia Executive Women & the LH Institute for higher education leadership and management; 2008.
28. Marcus J. Facts about race and college admission: political winds may shift, but racial factors in college success statistics don't. Hechinger Report. 2018. Available at: https://hechingerreport.org/facts-about-race-and-college-admission/. Accessed July 20, 2019.
29. Anderson M. For black Americans, experiences of racial discrimination vary by education level, gender. Washington, DC: Pew Research Center; 2019. Available at: https://www.pewresearch.org/fact-tank/2019/05/02/for-black-americans-experiences-of-racialdiscrimination-vary-by-education-level-gender/. Accessed July 22, 2019.
30. Current Trends in Medical Education. AAMC. Available at: https://www.aamcdiversityfactsandfigures2016.org/report-section/section-3/#. Accessed July 22, 2019.
31. Bullock SC, Houston E. Perceptions of racism by black medical students attending white medical schools. J Natl Med Assoc 1987;79(6):601–8.
32. Osseo-Asare A, Balasuriya L, Huot SJ, et al. Minority Resident Physicians' Views On The Role Of Race/Ethnicity In Their Training Experiences In The Workplace. JAMA Netw Open 2018;1(5):e182723.
33. Toledo P, Duce L, Adams J, et al. Diversity in the American Society of Anesthesiologists leadership. Anesth Analg 2017;124(5):1611–6.
34. Yu PT, Parsa PV, Hassanein O, et al. Minorities struggle to advance in academic medicine: a 12-y review of diversity at the highest levels of America's teaching institutions. J Surg Res 2013;182(2):212–8.
35. Traylor AH, Schmittdiel JA, Uratsu CS, et al. Adherence to cardiovascular disease medications: does patient-provider race/ethnicity and language concordance matter? J Gen Intern Med 2010;25(11):1172–7.
36. Alsan M, Garrick O, Graziani GC. Does diversity matter for health? Experimental evidence from Oakland. Working Paper 24787. Cambridge (MA): National Bureau of Economic Research; 2018.

Ethical Issues Confronting Muslim Patients in Perioperative and Critical Care Environments

A Survey of Islamic Jurisprudence

Andrew C. Miller, MD[a,b,*], Abba M. Khan, MD[b],
Karim Hebishi, MD[c], Alberto A. Castro Bigalli, MSc[d],
Amir Vahedian-Azimi, PhD[e]

KEYWORDS

• Ethics • Religion • Islam • Intensive care unit • Perioperative

KEY POINTS

- Some patients may have a desire to fast during the month of Ramadan, even when they are ill. Most scholars agree that infirm patients are exempt from fasting if they reasonably and justifiably fear that the fast will cause them significant loss or harm.
- Transplants, xenotransplants, and medications derived from animals considered unclean are controversial in the Muslim community, although many scholars view them as permissible. Counsel with an Islamic chaplain or local religious leader may be helpful.
- Do-not-resuscitate orders are controversial in the Muslim community, although some scholars view them as permissible if the intention is medical futility and not to hasten death. Counsel with an Islamic chaplain or local religious leader may be helpful.
- Postmortem examinations are controversial in the Muslim community. Autopsy for educational purposes is not permissible. Some scholars allow autopsy if the lives of other Muslims are at risk, or if required by law, but this may be distressing for the family.

Funding: None declared.

[a] Department of Emergency Medicine, Vidant Medical Center, East Carolina University Brody School of Medicine, 600 Moye Boulevard, Mailstop 625, Greenville, NC 27834, USA; [b] The MORZAK Collaborative, 600 Moye Boulevard, Mailstop 625, Greenville, NC 27834, USA; [c] Departments of Internal Medicine and Psychiatry, Vidant Medical Center, East Carolina University Brody School of Medicine, 600 Moye Boulevard, Mailstop 628, Greenville, NC 27834, USA; [d] East Carolina University Brody School of Medicine, 600 Moye Boulevard, Room 2S-20, Greenville, NC 27834, USA; [e] Trauma Research Center, Baqiyatallah University of Medical Sciences, P.O. Box 19575-174, Sheykh bahayi Stress, Vanak Square, Tehran, Iran

* Corresponding author. Department of Emergency Medicine, East Carolina University Brody School of Medicine, 600 Moye Boulevard, Mailstop 625, Greenville, NC 27834.

E-mail address: Taqwa1@gmail.com

Anesthesiology Clin 38 (2020) 379–401
https://doi.org/10.1016/j.anclin.2020.01.002
anesthesiology.theclinics.com

INTRODUCTION

As physicians encounter an increasingly diverse patient population, socioeconomic circumstances, religious values, and cultural practices may present opportunities and barriers to the delivery of quality care. Ethical dilemmas may arise when medical management conflicts with a patient's values, culture, religion, or legal considerations.[1] These challenges may manifest themselves as health disparities. Cultural competence and patient-centered care have been championed as means to reduce health care disparities.[1] In 2003, the Institute of Medicine called for cross-cultural training for all providers because of evidence that stereotyping, biases, and provider uncertainty contributed to unequal treatment.[2,3] This finding may be particularly true in perioperative and critical care settings, where patient beliefs may influence choice regarding (or interaction with) lifesaving or life-prolonging treatment regimens.[4,5] Medical professionals need an understanding of the rich and diverse array of beliefs, expectations, preferences, and behavioral makeup of the social cultures from which patients present to ensure that they are providing the best and most comprehensive care possible.[6]

BASICS OF ISLAM

Islam is a monotheistic faith that holds Muhammad ibn ʿAbdullah of seventh-century Mecca (modern Saudi Arabia) to be the final prophet from among a long line starting with Adam and including Abraham, Noah, Moses, and Jesus.[1] The followers of Islam are called Muslims. The Pew Research Center estimated that Muslims accounted for 23% of the world population (1.6 billion) in 2010.[7] The 2 largest sects are Sunni (80%–90%) and Shi'a (10%–20%). These groups share common core beliefs, including the Qur'an and legal structures (with some differences in legal sources); however, the fundamental difference relates to religious authority and political succession following the death of the Prophet Muhammad (صلى الله عليه وسلم).

FUNDAMENTALS OF ISLAMIC JURISPRUDENCE

Paramount to understanding how Islamic ethics and jurisprudence relate to medicine is an understanding of the concepts of halal (permissible or lawful), haram (prohibited), and makruh (discouraged but not legally forbidden). Often erroneously used interchangeably are the connected but not identical terms sharīʿah, sharīʿah law or Islamic law, and the discipline of fiqh (from the Arabic word meaning discernment). The word shara'a (Qur'an 45:18), from which the term sharīʿah is derived, is an overarching concept referring to a divinely ordained and immutable path for Muslims to follow in life in order to gain salvation in the hereafter.[8] However, comprehending what God wants from humans and fashioning this into moral principles and legal edicts requires human reasoning and discernment. Therefore, unlike sharīʿah, sharīʿah law is a human social construct undertaken by fuqaha (jurists) that is neither divine nor uniform and static through time. Thus, there are both consensus and diversity in the opinions of jurists in its interpretation and translation into law, even when using the same classical sources or usul al-fiqh (roots or fundamental principles of fiqh) as their framework for reasoning and opinions.[8] However, problems arise when the terms sharīʿah (divine made) and sharīʿah law (man-made derived through fiqh) are used interchangeably, giving a sense of divinity and immutability to the latter.[8]

Islamic jurisprudence, or fiqh, can be reduced to 4 foundational principles called usul al-fiqh. These sources (order of primacy) include (1) the Holy Qur'an, and (2) the sunnah, which consists of the traditions or inspired sayings, deeds, tacit approvals, character, and appearance of the Prophet Muhammad (صلى الله عليه وعلى آله وسلم) as recorded in a genre of literature known as hadith.[9–12] A ruling in the Qur'an or hadith may be conveyed either in text that is clear or in language that is open to different interpretations.[13] A single word in qur'anic text or hadith may have several different meanings, resulting in different legal consequences. A definitive text is one that is clear and specific; it has only 1 meaning and admits of no other interpretations. These texts are known as qat'i.[13] The second type of ruling is considered speculative (zanni), and independent legal reasoning (ijtihad) is required to understand the most suitable meaning.[13] Of note, the hadith differs significantly between the Sunni and Shi'a sects.[9]

To these were added (3) ijmāʿ (unanimous consensus of jurists) and (4) qiyās (precedent-based analogy or analogical reasoning).[9,14–16] On issues on which the aforementioned legal sources are ambiguous, jurists use secondary principles, although differences of opinion exist regarding their usage between the madhhab (schools of jurisprudence). Juristic principles, including ijtihad (independent legal reasoning),[14,15] istihsan (preferential reasoning of jurists), al-urf (local customary precedent), and al-masalih al-mursalah (public interest or welfare), among others, have allowed a degree of flexibility and accommodated a diversity of pragmatic legal rulings based on social context.[17] The rulings or fatwā (plural: fatawa) generated through ijtihad are case specific and not globally binding.[9,12,17] Disagreements (ikhtilaf) among jurists are seen in a positive light; legal texts record different juristic opinions on the same issue with a specific line of literature devoted to disagreements between jurists (ikhtilaf al-fuqaha).[8] This juristic ikhtilaf is key to understanding the development of the Islamic legal tradition and can provide an important juristic tool to interpreting sharīʿah law as it pertains to health and medicine.

Despite historical and current evidence to the contrary, there is an incorrect assumption among some Western writers that sharīʿah law is immutable and frozen in time, and its application is temporally and spatially uniform.[8] The reality is that although Muslims agree on matters of 'ibadaat (duties owed to God), when it comes to mu'amalat (matters connected to the temporal world), there may be consensus but also notable differences in the interpretation of sharīʿah law. The plurality of opinions between, and within, Muslim schools of jurisprudence in ascertaining the legal and the ethical is influenced by geographic and historical differences, cultural and societal diversity, prevailing customs, and the variety of political and administrative systems within which Muslims have existed.[8] However, under Islamic law, ijtihad is not reversible (al-ijtihad la yunqad), meaning that one ruling of ijtihad is not reversed by another of differing opinion.[13,18] Classical Muslim scholars have reminded followers that their opinion is a right one with the possibility of being wrong and others' opinions are wrong ones with the possibility of being right.[13] This advice may generate uncertainty or confusion for patients as it pertains to topics such as those discussed in this article, and explains why patients may have contrasting impressions of permissibility.

FASTING (SAWM)

Fasting (sawm) during the ninth month (Ramadan) of the Islamic lunar calendar is a religious obligation for able-bodied adult Muslims as prescribed in the Qur'an 2:186.[19] Fasting is obligatory for all adult Muslims who are of sound mind, not ill, and not traveling more than 80 km from their city of residence (Quran 2:184). Many things that come into or out of the body invalidate fasting, such as intentional eating or drinking, oral medications that reach the stomach, deliberate vomiting, and parenteral nutrition.[7]

In cases of sickness, the decision to fast depends on the nature and severity of the illness.[20] If a person has a temporary sickness or condition (including menses, pregnancy, postnatal bleeding, breast feeding), practitioners may not fast on the days they are indisposed but must fast after the month of Ramadan to compensate for the missed days.[7,20,21] If the person has an incurable sickness and is not expected to recover completely, that person is allowed to forego the fast and is obliged to feed the needy (or give an equivalent amount of money for 1 day's meals) for each fast missed (Quran 2:184).[20] The elderly who cannot tolerate fasting, the mentally disabled, and the sick for whom fasting would aggravate their condition or bring danger are exempt from fasting.[7,20,22–26] This exemption may be justified by Qur'an 2:195: "...and let not your own hands throw you into destruction."

Patients may be unsure whether their level of illness exempts them from fasting. This question is important, because many Muslim patients with chronic medical conditions (eg, diabetes) still choose to fast, and may discontinue or alter treatment regimens without physician consultation, thereby risking serious complications.[7] Some people who are unable to participate in the fast may have significant feelings of loss and may need emotional support.[27] Even those who are exempt may try to fast out of devotion and the desire to be a part of the shared experience of Ramadan.

A comprehensive discussion of all medical illnesses, medications, and procedures in the context of Ramadan is beyond the scope of this article; however, a summary of judicial rulings in the form of fatawa are provided in **Table 1**. All 13 identified fatawa (1 Sunni, 11 Shi'a, 1 joint Sunni and Shi'a) indicate that illness is a valid reason exempting a person from fasting.[22–26,28–35] Although specific verbiage may vary, the most common criteria are that the patient reasonably and justifiably fears that the fast will cause significant loss or harm (see **Table 1**).[29–32,35] Two indicate exemptions for patients prohibited to fast by a physician,[31,33] with 1 indicating that the physician should be religious and faithful.[33]

Remember that the fast may be more important to devout individuals than the treatment plan, so it is important to find a workable compromise, even if suboptimal. If a hospitalized patient does fast, there are things that clinicians can do to optimize care. If it is not therapeutic for the hospitalized patient to fast, explain the reason. If there are no contraindications and the patient desires to do so, the dietary department can provide a snack that can be eaten just before dawn.[27] When feasible, enteral medications may be scheduled during nonfasting hours.[7] Clinicians may reassure the patient that taking injections or having a blood test does not invalidate the fast.[20,36] Published recommendations of care modifications for diabetic patients are available.[7,19] In addition, clinicians may consider rescheduling elective procedures outside of Ramadan to avoid these complications.

CLEANLINESS AND PRAYER: STOMA AND URINARY CATHETERS

As in any religion, individual observance may vary; however, for many Muslims, performing the religious obligation of prayer is an important religious and cultural expression for maintaining health and preventing illness.[37] Although cleanliness is always valued by Muslims, this is especially true regarding prayer. Before prayer, each individual must perform ritual ablution (cleansing) to enter into a state of purity (wudhu).[27] This state is invalidated by voiding (eg, blood, flatulence, stool, urine).[38] An important dilemma for patients and health care providers may arise when a Muslim patient is counseled on issues including placement of a colostomy, cystectomy with placement of an incontinent urinary diversion, or even urinary catheters because of the belief by some that such conditions automatically invalidate their wudhu, thereby preventing

Table 1
Summary of Islamic fatawa regarding fasting during illness

Year	Source	Sect	Obligatory	Citation
1999	Ayatollah Al-udhma As-Sayyid Ali Al-Husaini as-Sistani	Shi'a	No	22,23
2000	Grand Ayatollah Hossein Vahid Khorasani (question no. 1752)	Shi'a	No	28
2002	Grand Ayatollah Hossein Ali Montazeri (question no. 343)	Shi'a	No	29
2005	Grand Ayatollah Lotfollah Safi Golpayegani (question no. 1753)	Shi'a	No	30
2006	Grand Ayatollah Mohammad Fazel Lankrani (questions no. 680)	Shi'a	No	31
2007	Grand Ayatollah Mohammad Reza Nekounam (question no. 666)	Shi'a	No	32
2009	Islamic Organization for Medical Sciences and the International Islamic Fiqh Academy of the Organization of Islamic Conference	Shi'a and Sunni	No	26
2010	Grand Ayatollah Seyed Ali Khamenei (question no. 751)	Shi'a	No	33
2012	Grand Ayatollah Naser Makarem Shirazi (question no. 564)	Shi'a	No	34
2013	Grand Ayatollah Ghorban Ali Mohaghegh Kabuli (question no. 1792)	Shi'a	No	35
2014	Sheikh Ahmed Kutty	Sunni	No	24
2016	Grand Ayatollah Seyed Ali Hosseini Khamenei	Shi'a	No	25
2019	Grand Ayatollah Nouri Hamadani	Shi'a	No	—

them from praying.[38] In 1 study of Egyptian patients, there was a clear relation between the impact of stoma on the performance of religious rituals and quality of life.[39] A clear ruling on this matter is lacking. However, in 1 survey of 134 imams (leaders of mosques in Sunni Islam) in the United Kingdom (response rate, 16.7%), greater than 90% answered that it is possible for a Muslim to perform ablution, pray, and enter a mosque with a urinary stoma.[38] Most imams (86.6%) also stated that refusal of a urinary stoma was not justified by religious teachings.[38] When asked whether patients should choose the option of a neobladder despite this surgery having greater risk, 57.5% of respondents stated that they were either unsure or agreed with this alternative.[38]

TRANSFUSION

Transfusion of blood products is generally accepted by Islamic scholars.[40–45] The act of blood donation and subsequent transfusion is considered by some to be morally virtuous, increasing to the status of sadiqah jariyah (ongoing charity), with the donor acquiring good deeds as long as the recipient benefits from the transfusion.[44] Although many fatawa are unconditional, others apply conditions including patient need, donor free will (not compelled), and that the transfusion will not endanger the donor's health.[44] Transfusion between the sexes and between Muslims and non-Muslims is generally permitted.[40–44] Appreciation in the form of money to the blood donor is not encouraged.[46] A summary of judicial rulings in the form of fatawa is provided in **Table 2**. All 17 identified fatawa (8 Sunni, 9 Shi'a) indicate that blood transfusion is permissible for Muslims.[29,31,34,40–43,45–52]

TRANSPLANTATION

The topic of transplantation has been one of the most contentious discussions in Islamic medical ethics in recent decades. For many, it places at odds 2 prominent Islamic principles: (1) the importance of maintaining and improving human health and well-being, and (2) the duty to respect the inviolability of the dead.[53] Thus, organ donation rates are lower in Muslim-majority countries.[54]

Although the Qur'an and hadith do not specifically address transplants, they serve as important lenses through which jurists view the issue. A first element in the theological argument is the idea of the sacredness of life (Qur'an 5:32). As a general rule, a human body should be respected, and deforming or degrading it is not permissible because each organ will be questioned as to its use and treatment on the day of judgment (Qur'an 17:36,70). Furthermore, in a hadith of the Prophet Muhammad (صلى الله عليه وعلى آله وسلم), he rebuked a man who broke a bone of a corpse that he found in a cemetery, stating: "the sin of breaking the bones of a dead man is equal to the sin of breaking the bones of a living man."[55,56]

These injunctions may suggest that organ transplants/donation cannot be allowed, but there is more to consider. Several principles from the Islamic jurisprudential

Table 2
Summary of Islamic fatawa regarding the permissibility of blood transfusion

Year	Source	Sect	Permissible	Citation
1959	Sheikh Hassan Mamoon, Grand Mufti, Egypt (fatwā no. 1065)	Sunni	Yes	—
1982	Fatwā Committee National Council of Islamic Religious Affairs Malaysia	Sunni	Yes	46
1999	Grand Ayatollah Mohammad Taghi Behjat (question no. 15)	Shi'a	Yes	52
2000	Grand Ayatollah Seyed Ali Mohammad Dastgheib (question no. 2973)	Shi'a	Yes	47
2001	Islamweb.net (fatwā no. 83172)	Sunni	Yes	40
2002	Grand Ayatollah Hossein Ali Montazeri	Shi'a	Yes	29
2003	Mufti Ebrahim Desai	Sunni	Yes	41
2004	Grand Ayatollah Seyed Ali Sistani (question no. 63)	Shi'a	Yes	48
2006	Grand Ayatollah Abolghasem Khoi (question 439)	Shi'a	Yes	49
2006	Grand Ayatollah Mirza Javad Tabrizi (addendum to the answer of the Ayatollah Khoi)	Shi'a	Yes	49
2006	Grand Ayatollah Mohammad Fazel Lankrani (questions no. 422–423)	Shi'a	Yes	31
2006	Islamweb.net (fatwā no. 91247)	Sunni	Yes	42
2008	Main Khalid Al-Qudah (fatwā no. 76784)	Sunni	Yes	50
2012	Grand Ayatollah Naser Makarem Shirazi (question no. 346)	Shi'a	Yes	34
2013	Grand Ayatollah Seyed Ali Hosseini Khamenei (question 12,036)	Shi'a	Yes	51
2015	Mufti Ebrahim Desai (fatwā no. 32245)	Sunni	Yes	43
2015	Mufti Muhammad ibn Adam al-Kawthari	Sunni	Yes	45

tradition do allow for transplants/donation of organs. These principles are the necessity-breaks-the-law principle (darura), the principle of working for the public interest or well-being of society (al-masalih al-mursalah), and the principle of altruism (al-ithar). Darura allows for exceptions to general rules, thereby making the prohibited lawful. The principles of al-masalih al-mursalah and al-ithar may be seen as arguments that overrule the individual in favor of the whole of society.[44]

Significant disagreement between jurists (ikhtilaf al-fuqaha) exists in transplantation fatawa. A summary of rulings in provided in **Table 3**. Of the 41 identified fatawa on transplantation, 23 were Sunni (13 permissible, 7 conditional, 3 prohibited), 17 were Shi'a (5 permissible, 11 conditional, 1 prohibited), and 2 were jointly Sunni and Shi'a (1 permissible, 1 conditional). In total, 35 of 40 (87.5%) identified fatawa permit organ donation in some capacity (see **Table 3**). Autologous transplants are widely accepted if performed for medical (ie, not cosmetic) purposes, success is likely, and there is no mortality risk of the surgery.[44] Allogeneic transplants are more restricted, with some proposed requirements including (1) donor has full mental capacity, (2) donor consent (may be granted postmortem by closest relatives),[57] (3) adult (preferable >21 years),[57,58] (4) the organ or tissue is medically determined to be life-saving or able maintain the recipient's quality of life without suitable alternative, (5) recipient benefit exceeds donor harm, and some fatawa stipulate (6) live donation only of nonvital (ie, self-renewing) or nonsingular organs such as hematopoietic cells, skin, kidney, lung, and possibly liver.[44] Transplant of gonads is forbidden, although transplant of other internal sex organs (eg, uterus) may be permissible.[44] Xenotransplantation is discussed later.

Given the large number of rulings on the topic, any individual local religious leader's topic knowledge may vary significantly, and public awareness of these fatawa is suboptimal.[8,59–65]

XENOTRANSPLANTATION AND MEDICATIONS DERIVED FROM ANIMALS CONSIDERED UNCLEAN

In modern medicine, many medications and therapeutic products are derived (at least in part) from animal-based products. Sometimes, the products are derived from animals considered unclean by Muslims (eg, porcine, canine). This issue is addressed by the Quran 2:173: "He has only forbidden to you dead animals, blood, the flesh of swine, and that which has been dedicated to other than Allah. But whoever is forced [by necessity], neither desiring [it] nor transgressing [its limit], there is no sin upon him. Indeed, Allah is Forgiving and Merciful."

The permissibility of medications or xenografts derived from animals considered unclean may be the source of considerable anxiety for some patients. Although a complete listing is beyond the scope of this article, common examples include anticoagulants (eg, daltaparparin, defibrotide, enoxaparin, heparin)[66,67]; insulin (eg, hypurin porcine)[67]; tissue augmentation and substitution materials (eg, Surgibone, collagen)[68]; tissue reconstructive materials (eg, pericardial patch, artificial skin)[68]; hemostatic materials (eg, Angio-Seal hemostatic puncture closure device)[68]; prostheses, blood vessels and biologic materials (eg, porcine valves and dermis, vascular grafts)[68,69]; sutures and ligatures (eg, plain and chromic gut sutures)[68]; vaccines (eg, Fluenz Tetra nasal spray)[67,70]; and venom-based products.[71] This question has been adjudicated on several occasions (**Table 4**). In 1995, the Islamic Organization of Medical Sciences (IOMS) along with the Eastern Mediterranean Regional Office of the World Health Organization deliberated on the use of "judicially prohibited and impure substances in foodstuffs and medicines."[72] In relation to biotransformation (istihalah), the IOMS

Table 3
Islamic fatawa regarding the permissibility of transplants

Year	Source	Sect	Permissible	Notes	Citation
1959	Sheikh Hassan Mamoon, Grand Mufti, Egypt (fatwā no. 1084)	Sunni	Conditional	Deceased donor corneal transplants	98
1966	Sheikh Hureidi, Grand Mufti, Egypt (fatwā no. 993)	Sunni	Yes	Extended prior ruling to other organs	99
1966	Mufti Mohammad Shafi (1897–1976; Pakistan)	Sunni	No	—	
1969	International Islamic Conference (Malaysia)	Sunni	Yes	—	100
1972	Algiers Supreme Islamic Council	Sunni	Yes	—	100
1973	Islamic Religious Council of Singapore	Sunni	No	—	—
1973	Sheikh Khater, Grand Mufti, Egypt	Sunni	Conditional	Allowed harvesting skin from unidentified corpses	101
1978	Imam Nawawi (631–671 H/AD 1233–1272)	Sunni	Conditional	Bone and teeth	102,103
1979	Saudi Grand Ulama in 1978 (decree no. 66)	Sunni	Conditional	Deceased donor corneal transplants	—
1979	Grand Mufti Gad al Haq, Grand Mufti, Egypt (fatwā no. 1323)	Sunni	Conditional	Live and deceased donor transplants if donated freely. Organ harvesting from unidentified corpse requires magistrate order	—
1980	Kuwaiti Ministry of Charitable Endowments (fatwā no. 132/79)	Sunni	Yes	Live and deceased donor transplants	—
1982	The Supreme Council of Ulama in Riyadh (fatwā no. 99)	Sunni	Yes	Sanctioned autografts unanimously; live and cadaveric transplants by majority	58
1985	Islamic Religious Islamic Council of Singapore	Sunni	Yes	—	53
1987	Islamic Fiqh Academy of the Muslim World League (decree no. 2, 10th session)	Sunni	Yes	Endorsed all prior fatawa on organ transplants	104
1988	Fourth International Conference of Islamic Jurists (resolution no. 1)	Shi'a and Sunni	Yes	Endorsed all prior fatawa on organ transplants; clearly rejected organ trafficking; stressed altruism	105
1990	Sixth International Conference of Islamic Jurists (decrees No. 56/5/6; 58/8/6)	Shi'a and Sunni	Conditional	Discussed transplants from embryos, in vitro fertilization projects, nerve tissue (including xenografts), anencephalic donors, and prohibited gonad transplants	106

1997	Sheikh Mohammed Metwali al-Sharawi	Sunni	No	—	—
1999	Ayatollah Al-udhma As-Sayyid Ali Al-Husaini as-Seestani	Shi'a	Yes	Live and deceased donor transplants, and xenografts from animals considered unclean	23
1999	Grand Ayatollah Mohammad Taghi Behjat (question no. 24)	Shi'a	Conditional	Deceased donor transplant is permissible if donor is non-Muslim, and it is lifesaving for recipient	52
2000	Grand Ayatollah Hossein Vahid Khorasani (question no. 2894)	Shi'a	Conditional	Deceased donor transplant is only permissible if lifesaving. If performed, then diyah must be paid[a]	28
2000	Grand Ayatollah Seyed Ali Mohammad Dastgheib (question no. 2969)	Shi'a	Conditional	Deceased donor transplants in permissible, but diyah must be paid[a]	47
2000	Islamweb.net (fatwā no. 82240)	Sunni	Yes	Live and deceased donor transplants, and xenografts with exception of porcine	107
2001	Sheikh Ahmad Kutty	Sunni	Yes	—	108
2001	Grand Ayatollah Hossein Nouri Hamadani (question no. 899)	Shi'a	Conditional	It is lawful for Muslims to receive transplants from non-Muslim donors if the donor is of the 'Ahl al-Kitāb[b]	93
2002	Grand Ayatollah Mohammad Ibrahiim Jannati (question no. 2991)	Shi'a	Conditional	Deceased donor transplant if lifesaving	94
2002	Grand Ayatollah Hossein Ali Montazeri (question no. 276)	Shi'a	Conditional	Deceased donor transplant from Muslim donor	29
2002	Islamweb.net (fatwā no. 84780)	Sunni	Yes	—	109
2003	Islamic Fiqh Academy of the Muslim World League (decree no. 3; 17th session)	Sunni	Conditional	Permits using leftover preembryos for stem cell research and treatment of serious ailments	110
2003	Islamweb.net (fatwā no. 85514)	Sunni	Yes	—	111
2003	Grand Ayatolah Mohammad Asef Mohseni (question no. 156)	Shi'a	Conditional	Permissible if donor is Muslim and it is lifesaving	112
2004	Grand Ayatollah Seyed Ali Sistani (question no. 85)	Shi'a	Yes	If lifesaving for recipient	48
2005	Grand Ayatollah Youssef Sanei (question no. 246)	Shi'a	Yes	Permissible among and between Muslims and non-Muslims	83
2006	Grand Ayatollah Mirza Javad Tabrizi	Shi'a	No	—	49
2006	Grand Ayatollah Mohammad Fazel Lankrani (question no. 375)	Shi'a	Conditional	Permissible if lifesaving for recipient, and donor is not approached after a life-threatening or unbearable loss	31

(*continued on next page*)

Table 3
(continued)

Year	Source	Sect	Permissible	Notes	Citation
2007	Grand Ayatollah Mohammad Reza Nekounam (question no. 240)	Shi'a	Yes	Permissible among and between Muslims and non-Muslims	32
2008	Main Khalid Al-Qudah (fatwā no. 76784)	Sunni	Yes	—	50
2009	European Council for Fatwā and Research (second collection, resolution 2/6)	Sunni	Yes	If done within the prescribed limits of the Shari'ah	113
2010	Grand Ayatollah Seyed Ali Khamenei (question no. 1292)	Shi'a	Conditional	Deceased donor transplant if donor gave prior consent, the donor's death is not hastened, and the transplant is lifesaving	33
2012	Grand Ayatollah Naser Makarem Shirazi (questions no. 282, 283)	Shi'a	Conditional	Permitted if saves recipient from death or major illness	34
2013	Grand Ayatollah Seyed Ali Hosseini Khamenei (question 12,009)	Shi'a	Conditional	If donor is non-Muslim and it is lifesaving	51
2016	Islamweb.net (fatwā no. 332080)	Sunni	Conditional	Xenograft (including porcine) is permissible if no pure alternative exists and it is the only remedy	114

[a] Under Islamic law, diyah is the financial compensation paid to the victim or heirs of a victim in the cases of murder, bodily harm, or property damage.
[b] 'Ahl al-Kitāb, or People of the Book, is an Islamic term that refers to Jews, Christians, Sabians, and sometimes members of other religious groups, such Zoroastrians.

Table 4
Summary of Islamic fatawa regarding the permissibility of using medical products and xenografts derived in part or completely from animals considered unclean (eg, Porcine, gelatin)

Year	Source	Sect	Permissible	Notes	Citation
1984	National Fatwa Committee of Malaysia	Sunni	Conditional	Gelatin use in medicine is permissible in case of emergency. If a halal element may replace the gelatin, then use of gelatin is forbidden	115
2004	Islamic Fiqh Academy of India	—	Conditional	Permits use of gelatin-containing products if nonporcine products are not available	73
2010	Egyptian Fatwā Council	Sunni	Conditional	Permits use of biotransformed products with preferred nonporcine products. Permits use of porcine heart valves in cases of extreme medical need (lifesaving) and nonavailability of nonporcine alternatives	74
2013	European Council for Fatwā and Research	Sunni	Undetermined	Undetermined opinion; awaiting final decision after further investigation	76
2015	International Islamic Fiqh Academy	Sunni	Conditional	May use porcine products in cases of extreme medical need and nonavailability of nonporcine alternatives	75

recommended that "transformation of a substance into another substance with different characteristics, changes substances that are judicially impure or are found in an impure environment into pure substances, and changes substances that are prohibited into lawful and permissible substances."[72]

A fatwā from the World Fatwā and Management System in Malaysia states that such haram products may be permissible where 3 conditions are fulfilled:

1. The medicine containing haram ingredients (alcohol as stated in the question, but it would apply to porcine also) must be necessary for the life of the person who takes it
2. That it was recommended by a knowledgeable and trustworthy Muslim physician
3. That there were no other halal or lawful alternatives available

Other rulings, including those by the Islamic Fiqh Academy of India (2004),[73] Egyptian Fatwā Council (2010),[74] and the International Islamic Fiqh Academy (2015),[75] have rendered conditional approval in cases of extreme medical need where nonporcine products of the same efficacy are not available (see **Table 4**).[73,74,76–78] Meanwhile, others have asserted that medicine should not be categorized as food or drink, and thus should be excluded from the rules applying to consumption of haram items.[77] However, support for this is not unanimous. In 2013, the European Council for Fatwā & Research reached an undetermined opinion.[75]

The role of physicians is to act in the best interests of our patients with respect to their cultural beliefs. When possible, clinicians are encouraged to prescribe non–porcine-based substitutes or equivalents. In the rare cases in which there is no suitable alternative, discuss this with the patient (or surrogate) and allow the patient to make an informed decision.

DO-NOT-RESUSCITATE STATUS

Do not resuscitate (DNR) is a medical order to withhold nonbeneficial resuscitation to allow natural death to take place.[79] The Islamic perspective regarding DNR orders is a "moving target."[79] In a survey of 461 Muslim physicians in the United States and other countries, only 66.8% of the respondents thought that DNR is allowed in Islam.[80] From the Islamic perspective, the law of practicing medical procedures is based on the principle of intention (al-umur bi maqasidiha). Namely, is the intention to withhold medical intervention with consent and because of medical futility, or is it to alleviate pain by hastening death?

The Qur'an does not directly address the DNR order; however, several hadith serve as important lenses through which jurists view the issue. For example, in Sahih Al-Bukhari (hadith no. 575), it is recorded that Prophet Muhammad (صلى الله عليه وعلى آله وسلم) said: "None of you should wish for death because of a calamity befalling him but if he must wish for death, he should say: 'O Allah! Keep me alive as long as life is better for me and let me die if death is better for me'." In another hadith narrated by Usamah bin Sharik and recorded in Sahih Al-Bukhari, the Prophet Muhammad (صلى الله عليه وعلى آله وسلم) said: "For Allah does not create any disease but He also creates with it the cure."

Of the 7 identified fatawa (5 Sunni, 2 Shi'a) on the topic of DNR orders (**Table 5**), DNR was ruled as permissible by 5,[81–85] and prohibited by 2.[32,86] For example, the Islamic Religious Council of Singapore (2006) ruled that:

It is permissible by Islamic law for a sane individual to make pledge to refuse life supporting treatment when terminally ill. It can be assumed that he or she decides to be patient and more willing to die naturally believing that death cannot be avoided at a certain point.[82]

Moreover, the Iftaa' Department of the Hashemite Kingdom of Jordan (decision no. 117; 2006) ruled:

There is no prohibition in Islam to refrain from putting a cancer patient on life support or respirator or dialysis if the medical and treatment team have confirmed and are certain that there is no hope of benefit for the patient in these measures, on the condition that this report is prepared by a medical team consisting of not less than three physicians, being specialists, fair, and trustworthy.[84,87]

In addition, the Administration of the Islamic Research and Ifta in the Kingdom of Saudi Arabia (fatwā no. 12086; 1998) delineated 6 situations in which a DNR order is permissible and stated that:

If three knowledgeable and trustworthy physicians agree that the patient's condition is hopeless, the life-supporting machines can be withheld or withdrawn. The family members' opinion is not included in the decision-making as they are unqualified to make such decisions.[79,81,88,89]

This statement is contrasted by the Grand Ayatollah Mohammad Reza Nekounam, who ruled (question no. 283; 2007) that:

Table 5
Summary of Islamic fatawa regarding the permissibility of advanced medical directives and do-not-resuscitate orders

Year	Source	Sect	Permissible	Notes	Citation
1988	Administration of Islamic Research and Ifta, Kingdom of Saudi Arabia	Sunni	Yes	—	81
2005	Islamic Religious Islamic Council of Singapore	Sunni	Yes	—	82
2005	Grand Ayatollah Youssef Sanei (question no. 291)	Shi'a	Yes	It is not obligatory for physicians to treat patients who do not hope to be cured, so refraining from continuing treatment is permissible, but it is not permissible to take medicines that help accelerate death	83
2006	Iftaa' Department of the Hashemite Kingdom of Jordan	Sunni	Yes	—	84
2006	Dr Hatem al-Haj	Sunni	No	If the cardiopulmonary resuscitation will save the person's life, and that person is not in a vegetative condition, then it is not allowable to request a DNR order	86
2007	Grand Ayatollah Mohammad Reza Nekounam (question no. 283)	Shi'a	No	Discontinuation of treatment is not permitted for those who do not hope for a cure. Physicians should not shorten the usual and conventional treatment or take action to help the premature death	32
2017	Mufti Ebrahim Desai	Sunni	Yes	—	85

Discontinuation of treatment is not permitted for those who do not hope for a cure. The physician should not shorten the usual and conventional size of the treatment.[32]

The idea that medical staff may unilaterally determine DNR status may seem unusual or concerning. In the United States, this is in part caused by the increase in patients' (or surrogates') right to request treatments from which physicians thought they would receive no medical benefit that followed the legal cases of Wanglie (1991) and Baby K (1994), in which the courts ruled in favor of this right. However, the pendulum has begun to swing in the opposite direction. In 1999, the Texas legislature passed the Texas Advance Directives Act. This law established a legally sanctioned extrajudicial process for resolving disputes about end-of-life decisions if the physician feels ethically unable to agree to patients' or surrogate's request. This law has become a model for other states (eg, Virginia HB 226; New York S07156) and for individual hospitals seeking to make changes in statutory regulations and institutional policies regarding end-of-life treatment decisions.

More discussion is needed to clarify the origin, scope, circumstances, intention (nia), and resultant permissibility of DNR orders for Muslims. Situations in which the physician believes that resuscitation is futile should be handled on a case-by-case basis through a predefined process that includes multiple safeguards to ensure that patients' rights are fully protected. The authors advise that the physician thoroughly explain to the patient or surrogate the reasons for the medical futility determination and document this discussion in the medical record. Entering a DNR order over the objection of a patient or surrogate should be reserved for rare or extreme circumstances after thorough attempts to settle or successfully appeal disagreements have been tried and have failed. In some cases, reaching out to an Islamic chaplain or local religious leader for patient counsel may be beneficial.

BURIAL AND POSTMORTEM EXAMINATION

Islam teaches that human beings should always maintain their dignity, even in disease and misfortune. The human body, living or dead, should be venerated likewise. After death, the body is thought to belong to God and should not be cut or harmed in any way, and modesty should be maintained as in life.[27] The dead are treated reverently and are buried quickly. The Islamic teaching of a quick burial without embalming may conflict with local laws. If the family is not sure how to proceed, seek assistance from an Islamic chaplain or local religious leader.[27]

For these reasons, postmortem examination is generally not performed unless required by law.[27] Under such circumstances, family and loved ones may experience significant distress over permissibility of the postmortem examination. However, performing postmortems need not be tantamount to mutilation of the corpse or an act of disrespect.

The authors identified 16 fatawa on postmortem examination (**Table 6**). Postmortem examination was determined to be permissible by 5,[32,83,90–92] conditional by 8,[22,23,31,33,34,47,93,94] and prohibited by 4.[28,48,49,51] The first fatwā to address this topic was issued in 1952 by Hasanayn Muhammad Makhluf, Chief Mufti of Egypt (1945–1990), in which he concluded that, although postmortems are permissible, they must be performed only when necessary and not too often. Doctors should be God fearing and should "know that God is All-seeing, Almighty and All-guiding."[90] Several subsequent fatawa have applied conditions to postmortem examinations, ruling that autopsy is not permissible for educational purposes but is only permissible if the life of another Muslim depends on it and the autopsy of a non-Muslim would not provide the answer.[22,23,28,33,34,47,93,94] Others have added that consent should be granted by the deceased in their wills (or by their heirs),[83] and 1 indicated need for requisite approval from a religious leader.[31]

In cases in which a patient or surrogate is opposed to autopsy on religious grounds, an alternative may be a virtual autopsy (virtopsy). Virtopsy is a forensic radiological imaging approach developed in Switzerland and used in the United Kingdom and other countries.[95] It relies on noninvasive methods, including computed tomography and MRI, is noninvasive, and is associated with reduced time per autopsy.[95,96] Although discernment of the cause of death may be limited with such techniques, virtopsy provides an alternative that may be more palatable compared with traditional postmortem examination.[97]

Table 6
Summary of Islamic fatawa regarding the permissibility of autopsy

Year	Source	Sect	Permissible	Notes	Citation
1952	Hasanayn Muhammad Makhluf, Chief Mufti of Egypt	Sunni	Yes	—	90
1999	Ayatollah Al-udhma As-Sayyid Ali Al-Husaini as-Seestani	Shi'a	Conditional	Not permissible for education. Permissible if the life of another Muslim depends on it	22,23
2000	Grand Ayatollah Seyed Ali Mohammad Dastgheib (question no. 2966)	Shi'a	Conditional	Permissible if the life of another Muslim depends on it and autopsy of non-Muslim would not provide the answer	47
2000	Grand Ayatollah Hossein Vahid Khorasani (question no. 2891)	Shi'a	No	—	28
2001	Grand Ayatollah Hossein Nouri Hamadani (question no. 892)	Shi'a	Conditional	Permissible if autopsy of non-Muslim would not provide the answer	93
2002	Grand Ayatollah Mohammad Ibrahiim Jannati (question no. 3002)	Shi'a	Conditional	Permissible if the life of another Muslim depends on it and autopsy of non-Muslim would not provide the answer	94
2004	Islamweb.net (fatwā no. 87495)	Sunni	Yes	—	91
2004	Grand Ayatollah Seyed Ali Sistani (question no. 55)	Shi'a	No	—	48
2005	Grand Ayatollah Youssef Sanei (question no. 277)	Shi'a	Yes	Permissible with consent granted by the deceased in the will or by the heir	83
2006	Grand Ayatollah Abolghasem Khoi (question 233)	Shi'a	No	If performed, then diyah must be paid	49
2006	Grand Ayatollah Mohammad Fazel Lankrani (questions no. 15, 16, 20)	Shi'a	Conditional	Autopsy of a Muslim is permissible only under special circumstances and should have permission from a religious ruler	31
2007	Grand Ayatollah Mohammad Reza Nekounam (question no. 269)	Shi'a	Yes	If rational and respectful	32
2008	Mufti Ebrahim Desai (fatwā no. 16282)	Sunni	Yes	Permissible in cases of necessity when it is required by law or in criminal cases	92
2010	Grand Ayatollah Seyed Ali Khamenei (question no. 1292)	Shi'a	Conditional	If new information discovered is needed to save the life of people threatened by a disease	33

(continued on next page)

Table 6
(continued)

Year	Source	Sect	Permissible	Notes	Citation
2012	Grand Ayatollah Naser Makarem Shirazi (question no. 42)	Shi'a	Conditional	Permitted if (1) the obtained information is the only way to save the life of another Muslim, (2) autopsy of a non-Muslim would not provide the necessary information, and (3) the doctor does not do more than is necessary	34
2013	Grand Ayatollah Seyed Ali Hosseini Khamenei (question 12,018)	Shi'a	No	—	51

SUMMARY

It is important that health care providers be sensitive to the religious and cultural framework that guides their patients' health care decisions. Islamic jurisprudence is complicated and welcoming of divergent opinions. As it pertains to critically ill and perioperative patients, some Muslim patients may have strong, religiously rooted convictions on procedures affecting cleanliness, prayer, and fasting; the permissibility of transplants, xenografts, and medications from animals considered unclean; DNR orders; and decisions on postmortem examinations. By understanding how faith may affect the health care decisions of Muslims, providers may optimize their care in a culturally respectful manner.

CONFLICTS OF INTEREST

None declared.

REFERENCES

1. Padela AI, del Pozo PR. Muslim patients and cross-gender interactions in medicine: an Islamic bioethical perspective. J Med Ethics 2011;37(1):40–4.
2. Smedley BD, Stith AY, Nelson AR, editors. Unequal treatment: confronting racial and ethnic disparities in health care. Washington, DC: National Academies Press; 2003.
3. Nelson A. Unequal treatment: confronting racial and ethnic disparities in health care. J Natl Med Assoc 2002;94(8):666–8.
4. Bashar FR, Vahedian-Azimi A, Salesi M, et al. Spiritual health and outcomes in muslim ICU patients: a nationwide cross-sectional study. J Relig Health 2018; 57(6):2241–57.
5. Farzanegan B, Elkhatib THM, Elgazzar AE, et al. Impact of religiosity on delirium severity among critically ill Shi'a Muslims: a prospective multi-center observational study. J Relig Health 2019. https://doi.org/10.1007/s10943-019-00895-7. Available at: http://link.springer.com/10.1007/s10943-019-00895-7.
6. Hammoud MM, White CB, Fetters MD. Opening cultural doors: Providing culturally sensitive healthcare to Arab American and American Muslim patients. Am J Obstet Gynecol 2005;193(4):1307–11.
7. Abolaban H, Al-Moujahed A. Muslim patients in Ramadan: a review for primary care physicians. Avicenna J Med 2017;7(3):81–7.
8. Moazam F. Sharia law and organ transplantation: through the lens of Muslim jurists. Asian Bioeth Rev 2011;3(4):316–32.
9. Miller AC. Opinions on the legitimacy of brain death among Sunni and Shi'a scholars. J Relig Health 2016;55(2):394–402.
10. Miller AC, Ziad-Miller A, Elamin EM. Brain death and islam: the interface of religion, culture, history, law, and modern medicine. Chest 2014;146(4):1092–101.
11. Babgi A. Legal issues in end-of-life care: perspectives from Saudi Arabia and United States. Am J Hosp Palliat Care 2009;26(2):119–27.
12. Weiss B. Interpretation in Islamic Law: the theory of ijtihad. Am J Comp Law 1978;26(2):199.
13. Hosen N. Hilal and Halal: how to manage Islamic pluralism in Indonesia. Asian J Comp Law 2012;7(1):1–18.
14. Hallaq WB. A history of Islamic legal theories: an introduction to Sunni Usul al-Fiqh. 1st edition. Cambridge (England): Cambridge University Press; 1997.

15. Khallaf AW. Science of the roots of Islamic jurisprudence. Dubai (United Arab Emirates): Dar Al Qalam Publishing and Distribution; 1978 [in Arabic].
16. Arozullah AM, Kholwadia MA. Wilāyah (authority and governance) and its implications for Islamic bioethics: a Sunni Māturīdi perspective. Theor Med Bioeth 2013;34(2):95–104.
17. Vogel FE. Islamic law and the legal system of Saudi: studies of Saudi Arabia. Leiden (the Netherlands): Brill; 2000.
18. Miller AC. Opinions on the legitimacy of death declaration by neurological criteria from the perspective of 3 abrahamic faiths. Medeniyet Med J 2019; 34(3):305–13.
19. Beshyah SA. Fasting during the month of Ramadan for people with diabetes: Medicine and Fiqh united at last. Ibnosina J Med Biomed Sci 2009;1(2):58–60.
20. Laway BA, Ashraf H. Basic rules of Ramadan: a medico-religious perspective. J Pak Med Assoc 2015;65(5 Suppl 1):S14–7.
21. Firouzbakht M, Kiapuor A, Jamali B, et al. Fasting in pregnancy: a survey of beliefs and manners of Muslim women about Ramadan fasting. Ann Trop Med Pub Health 2013;6(5):536–40.
22. Al-Sistani A. Question & answer: Nos. 01126, 02655. The official website of the office of His Eminence Al-Sayyid Ali Al-Husseini Al-Sistani. Available at: sistani.org/english/qa. Accessed October 8, 2019.
23. Al-Hakim AH. A code of practice for Muslims in the West: in accordance with edict of Ayatollah Al-udhma As-Sayyid Ali Al-Husaini as-Seestani. London: Imam Ali Foundation; 1999. Available at: https://www.sistani.org/english/book/46/2060/. Accessed October 8, 2019.
24. Kutty A. Ask the scholar: fasting during illness 2014. Available at: askthescholar.com https://askthescholar.com/answerdetails?qId=1691. Accessed October 8, 2019.
25. Khamenei SAH. 122 religious inquiries on Ramadan and fasting answered by Imam Khamenei. Khamenei.IR 2016. Available at: http://english.khamenei.ir/news/5715/122-religious-inquiries-on-Ramadan-and-fasting-answered-by-Imam. Accessed October 8, 2019.
26. Islamic Organization for Medical Sciences and the International Islamic Fiqh Academy of the Organization of Islamic Conference. 19th session, decree 183(19/9) on "Diabetes and Ramadan". United Arab Emirates. 2009.
27. Lawrence P, Rozmus C. Culturally sensitive care of the muslim patient. J Transcult Nurs 2001;12(3):228–33.
28. Khorasani A. According to the fatwa of Hussein Vahid Khorasani. Al-Masala's explanation. Qom (Iran): Baqar al-Alum school publication; 2000 [in Farsi].
29. Montazeri H. Medical rulings. 1st edition. Qom (Iran): Sayeh publishing; 2002 [in Farsi].
30. Golpayegani LS. Al-Masala's explanation. 39th edition. Qom (Iran): Samen al-Hajj publications; 2004 [in Farsi].
31. Khodadadi G. Doctors and infirmities in accordance with the fatwa of Ayatollah Fazel Lankrani. 1st edition. Imam Atari Jurisprudence Center; 2006 [in Farsi].
32. Nekounam MR. In: Medical rulings for physicians and patients. 1st edition. Qom Shafag: Zohor Publications; 2007 [in Farsi].
33. Khamenei SA. Forced elasticity. 2nd edition. Qom (Iran): Edalat Payam Publishing; 2010 [in Farsi].
34. Shirazi M. [Medical rulings], issue 3. Qom (Iran): Publication of Imam Ali bin Abi Talib; 2012 [in Farsi].
35. Kabuli G. Interpretation of the Prophet's messenger. 15th edition. Qom (Iran): The Darshan of Islam; 2013 [in Farsi].

36. Lambat I. Circumstances when a fast is not broken. Available at: http://www.crescentsofbrisbane.org/Files/Iqbal Lambat Ramadan/Week 2/What breaks a fast.pdf. Accessed February 8, 2019.
37. Luna LJ. Transcultural nursing care of Arab muslims. J Transcult Nurs 1989;1(1):22–6.
38. Miah S, Mangera A, Osman NI, et al. Islam and the urinary stoma: a contemporary theological and urological dilemma. Eur Urol Focus 2019;5(2):301–5.
39. Hussein AM, Fadl SA. Quality of life in Egyptian stoma patients. Egypt J Surg 2001;20(3):597–607.
40. Donating blood to non-Muslims: fatwa no. 83172. Available at: Islamweb.net https://www.islamweb.net/en/fatwa/83172/donating-blood-to-non-muslims. Accessed October 8, 2019.
41. Desai E. Blood transfusion and organ transplants 2003. Available at: Albalagh.net http://www.albalagh.net/qa/blood_transfusion_transplant.shtml. Accessed October 8, 2019.
42. Transfusing blood taken from a non-Muslim: fatwa no. 91247. Available at: Islamweb.net https://www.islamweb.net/en/fatwa/91247/transfusing-blood-taken-from-a-non-muslim. Accessed October 8, 2019.
43. Desai E. Fatwa no. 32245. Ask Imam Islam. Q&A with Mufti Ebrahim Desai 2015. Available at: http://www.askimam.org/public/question_detail/32245. Accessed October 8, 2019.
44. Van den Branden S, Broeckaert B. The ongoing charity of organ donation. Contemporary English Sunni fatwas on organ donation and blood transfusion. Bioethics 2011;25(3):167–75.
45. Al-Kawthari M. ibn A. Is blood donation permissible?. Available at: www.sunnipath.com http://www.themodernreligion.com/misc/hh/blood-donation.html. Accessed August 16, 2019.
46. No restrictions on organ, blood donation between Muslims and non-Muslims, FT Mufti says. Malaymail 2017. Available at: https://www.malaymail.com/news/malaysia/2017/02/13/no-restrictions-on-organ-blood-donation-between-muslims-and-non-muslims-ft/1313453. Accessed August 16, 2019.
47. Dastgheib Shirazi A. Interpretation of the Prophet's messenger. 3rd edition. Shiraz (Iran): Publications Office of Sayed Ali Mohammad Dastgheib; 2000 [in Farsi].
48. Alsistani SA. Al-Masa'il al-Mutaqibi: Al-Abadat and Deals. 9th edition. Qom (Iran): Ayatollah al-Sayyid Ali al-Sistani School of Sama'ah; 2004 [in Farsi].
49. Khoi A. Jurisprudence of al-Shariah and al-Masa'il al-Tubiyyah My Sarat al-Jinna. Qom (Iran): Dar al-Sadiq al-Shehideh; 2006 [in Farsi].
50. Al-Qudah MK. Organ donation and blood transfusion: Fatwa no. 76784. Assem. Muslim Jurists Am 2008. Available at: https://www.amjaonline.org/fatwa/en/76781/organ-donation-blood-transfusion. Accessed October 8, 2019.
51. Khamenei SAH. Emphasis is on Khomeini, vol. 10. Tehran (Iran): Research Institute for the Regulation of Publication of Imam Khomeini's Works; 2013 [in Farsi].
52. Behjat MT. Explanatory Treatise I. 40th edition. Qom (Switzerland): Shafaq Publications; 1999 [in Farsi].
53. Nasir NM. Organ donation and transplantation. In: Fatwas of Singapore. Majlis Ugama Islam Singapura; 2017. Available at: https://muisfatwa.pressbooks.com/chapter/organ-donation-and-transplantation/.
54. Rasheed SA, Padela AI. The interplay between religious leaders and organ donation among Muslims. Zygon 2013;48(3):635–54.

55. Sunan Abi Dawud, Book of Funerals, Hadith No. 3207, Sunnah.com. Available at: https://sunnah.com/search/?q=break+the+bones+Abi+dawud. Accessed February 19, 2020.
56. Ahmed Z, Al-Musnad min Masā'il Aḥmad B. Ḥanbal: an important work. Islam Stud 1981;20(2):97–110.
57. Albar M. Organ transplantation: a Sunni Islamic perspective. Saudi J Kidney Dis Transpl 2012;23(4):817.
58. Supreme Council of Ulama in Riyadh. Fatwa No. 99 dated 6/11/1402H (25 August 1982). International Islamic Juristic Academy in Makkah (of Muslim World League) no. 26. Riyadh, Kingdom of Saudi Arabia; 1982.
59. Hafzalah M, Azzam R, Testa G, et al. Improving the potential for organ donation in an inner city Muslim American community: the impact of a religious educational intervention. Clin Transplant 2014;28(2):192–7.
60. Eshraghian A. Religion, tradition, culture, and solid organ transplantation. Crit Care Med 2013;41(7):e134.
61. Raza M, Hedayat KM. Some sociocultural aspects of cadaver organ donation: recent rulings from Iran. Transplant Proc 2004;36(10):2888–90.
62. Mohsin N, Militsala E, Budruddin M, et al. Attitude of the Omani population toward organ transplantation. Transplant Proc 2010;42(10):4305–8.
63. al-Faqih SR. The influence of Islamic views on public attitudes towards kidney transplant donation in a Saudi Arabian community. Public Health 1991;105(2):161–5.
64. Tarhan M, Dalar L, Yildirimoglu H, et al. The view of religious officials on organ donation and transplantation in the Zeytinburnu District of Istanbul. J Relig Health 2014. Available at: http://www.ncbi.nlm.nih.gov/pubmed/24658689.
65. Padela AI, Zaganjor H. Relationships between Islamic religiosity and attitude toward deceased organ donation among American Muslims: a pilot study. Transplantation 2014;97(12):1292–9.
66. Zainal N, Satar J, Mohd Subri I, et al. Porcine based anticoagulant in pregnancy revisited: analysis and discussion of national fatwa in aligned with Istihalah Fiqh concept in clinical practice. Journal of Fatwa Management and Research 2019;13(1):549–63.
67. Ogden J. Religious constraints on prescribing medication. Prescriber 2016;27(12):47–51.
68. Easterbrook C, Maddern G. Porcine and bovine surgical products: Jewish, Muslim, and Hindu perspectives. Arch Surg 2008;143(4):366–70.
69. Dayton MT. Porcine and bovine surgical products: Jewish, muslim, and hindu perspectives-invited critique. Arch Surg 2008;143(4):370.
70. Padela AI, Furber SW, Kholwadia MA, et al. Dire necessity and transformation: entry-points for modern science in Islamic bioethical assessment of porcine products in vaccines. Bioethics 2014;28(2):59–66.
71. Rusmil MRA, Othman L, Mohamad CAC. The use of venom and venom-derived products in medicine and cosmetics: the ethical issues from Islamic perspective. Int Med J Malaysia 2018;17(1):1–6.
72. Nordin MM, Rani MFA, Yusoff Y. The permissibility of judicially prohibited and impure substances in medicines. KPJ Med J 2016;6(1):57–9.
73. Islamic Fiqh Academy of India. Fourteenth Jurisprudence Symposium, Decision no 60 (3/14): Gelatin material. 2004. Available at: http://ifa-india.org/arabic.php?do=home&pageid=arabic_seminar14. Accessed August 16, 2019.

74. Egyptian Fatwa Council. Fatwa no. 11808. 2010. Available from: http://dar-alifta.org/AR/ViewResearch.aspx?sec=fatwa&ID=11808. Accessed August 16, 2019.
75. International Islamic Fiqh Academy. Decision no. 210 (6/22): Decision on Istihala and consumption in supplementary substances in food and medicine 2015. Available at: http://www.iifa-aifi.org/3988.html. Accessed August 16, 2019.
76. European Council for Fatwa and Research. Resolution no. 3/23: On istihala and consumption 2013. Available at: https://www.e-cfr.org/-بشأن-الاستحالة-والاستهلاك/. Accessed August 16, 2019.
77. Question no. 6515. 2005. Available at: IslamiCity.com; https://www.islamicity.org/qa/action.lasso.asp?-db=services&-lay=Ask&-op=eq&number=6515&-format=detailpop.shtml&-find. Accessed August 19, 2019.
78. Al-Munajjid MS. Question no.130815: Permissibility of haraam things in the case of necessity and the conditions governing that. Islam Question and Answer. 2009. Available at: https://islamqa.info/en/answers/130815/permissibility-of-haraam-things-in-the-case-of-necessity-and-the-conditions-governing-that. Accessed August 19, 2019.
79. Albar MA, Chamsi-Pasha H. Do-not-resuscitate orders: Islamic viewpoint [Internet]. In: Fadel HE, editor. FIMA Yearbook 2016. Encyclopedia of Islamic medical ethics - Part III. Medical care at the end of life. Amman (Jordan): Jordan Society for Islamic Medical Sciences; 2016. p. 111–7.
80. Saeed F, Kousar N, Aleem S, et al. End-of-life care beliefs among Muslim physicians. Am J Hosp Palliat Care 2015;32(4):388–92.
81. Administration of Islamic Research and Ifta. Fatwa No. 12086 issued on 30.6.1409 (Hijra). Riyadh (Saudi Arabia): Kingdom of Saudi Arabia; 1988.
82. Pejabat Mufti Majlis Ugama Islam Singapura. Isu Arahan Awal Perubatan (Advance Medical Directive). Singapore: Islamic Religious Council of Singapore; 2006.
83. Sainei J. Medical estates: special medical rulings, special patient rulings. 8th edition. Qom (Iran): Maysam Tamar Publications; 2005 [in Farsi].
84. Hileel AM, Al-Khusaawinah A al-K, Ghaythan YA, et al. Decision Number (117): ruling on removing life support equipment from a patient who has no hope of recovery (18/9/1427 AH). The Hashemite Kingdom of Jordan; 2006. Available at: http://aliftaa.jo/DecisionEn.aspx?DecisionId=236#.XU5a8OhKiUI.
85. Ibrahim S, Desai E. Fatwa no. 35732. Ask Imam Islam. Q&A with Mufti Ebrahim Desai 2017. Available at: http://www.askimam.org/public/question_detail/35732. Accessed October 8, 2019.
86. Al-Haj H. Do not resuscitate: fatwa no. 2193. Assembly of Muslim Jurists of America 2006. Available at: https://www.amjaonline.org/fatwa/en/2193/do-not-resuscitate. Accessed October 8, 2019.
87. Malek MM, Rahman NM, Hasan MS. Do not resuscitate (DNR) order: Islamic views. Al-Qantatir: International Journal of Islamic Studies 2018;9(1):35–43.
88. Saiyad S. Do not resuscitate: a case study from the islamic viewpoint. Journal of the Islamic Medical Association of North America 2009;41(3):109–13.
89. Gouda A, Al-Jabbary A, Fong L. Compliance with DNR policy in a tertiary care center in Saudi Arabia. Intensive Care Med 2010;36(12):2149–53.
90. Rispler-Chaim V. Postmortem examinations in Egypt. In: Masud MK, Messick B, Powers DS, editors. Islamic legal interpretation. Cambridge (England): Harvard University Press; 1996. p. 278–85.
91. Examining the dead: fatwa no. 87495. Available at: Islamweb.net https://www.islamweb.net/en/fatwa/87495/examining-the-dead. Accessed October 8, 2019.

92. Desai E. Fatwa no. 16282. Ask imam Islam. Q&A with Mufti Ebrahim Desai 2008. Available at: http://www.askimam.org/public/question_detail/16282. Accessed October 8, 2019.
93. Hamadani HN. 1st edition. One Thousand and one jurisprudence Problems (Estafa's Collection), vol. 2. Qom (Iran): The Promised Mehdi Institute; 2001 [in Farsi].
94. Jannati MI. Interpretation of the Prophet's messenger. 1st edition. Qom (Iran): Cultural Institute of Ijtihad - Ansarien; 2002 [in Farsi].
95. Mohammed M, Kharoshah MA. Autopsy in Islam and current practice in Arab Muslim countries. J Forensic Leg Med 2014;23:80–3.
96. Roberts ISD, Benamore RE, Benbow EW, et al. Post-mortem imaging as an alternative to autopsy in the diagnosis of adult deaths: a validation study. Lancet 2012;379(9811):136–42.
97. Ben Taher M, Pearson J, Cohen M, et al. Acceptability of post-mortem imaging among Muslim and non-Muslim communities. Br J Radiol 2018;91(1091): 20180295.
98. Fatwa of Sheikh Hassan Maamoon (No. 1065, 9 June 1959). In: Dar Allfta Almisryah, Al-Fatwa Allslamiyah. Cairo (Egypt): The Supreme Islamic Council, Ministry of Endowment; 1982. p. 2552.
99. Fatwa of Sheikh Hureidi (No. 993; 1966). In: Dar Allfta Almisryah, Al-Fatwa Allslamiyah. Cairo (Egypt): The Supreme Islamic Council, Ministry of Endowment; 1982. p. 2278–82.
100. Abu Zaid B. Attashrith AlGothmani Wanagel Watta'weed Allnsani. In: Majalat Majmah AlFiqh Allslami. Jeddah (Saudi Arabia): Organization of the Islamic Conference; 1988. p. 145–6.
101. Fatwa of Sheikh Khater. In: Dar Allfta Almisryah, Al-Fatwa Allslamiyah. Cairo (Egypt): The Supreme Islamic Council, Ministry of Endowment; 1973. p. 2505–7.
102. AlNawawi MS. Minhag Attalibin. Beirut (Lebanon): Dar AlFikir; 1978.
103. AlNawawi MS. Almajmooh Shareh AlMohzab. Cairo (Egypt): AlFajalah Press.
104. Fiqh Academy of the Organization of Islamic Conference and the International Islamic Juristic Academy of the Muslim World League. Decree no 2, 10th session. Makkah Al Mukarramah, Kingdom of Saudi Arabia: 1987.
105. Fiqh Academy of the Organization of Islamic Conference and the International Islamic Juristic Academy of the Muslim World League. Fourth international conference of Islamic Jurists, resolution no. 1. Jeddah, Kingdom of Saudi Arabia: 1988.
106. Fiqh Academy Decree and Recommendations for the 6th Conference of Islam Jurists, Decrees No. 56/5/6 and 58/8/6. Jeddah, Kingdom of Saudi Arabia. 14-20 March 1990. Available at: http://www.iifa-aifi.org/cs. Accessed December 20, 2016]. [in Arabic].
107. Organ transplantation: fatwa no. 82240. Available at: Islamweb.net https://www.islamweb.net/en/fatwa/82240/organ-transplantation. Accessed October 8, 2019.
108. Kutty A. Ask the scholar: organ transplantation 2001. Available at: askthescholar.com https://askthescholar.com/answerdetails?qId=7035. Accessed October 8, 2019.
109. Muslims donating body organs: fatwa no. 84780. Available at: Islamweb.net https://www.islamweb.net/en/fatwa/84780/?Option=FatwaId. Accessed October 8, 2019.
110. Islamic Jurisprudence Council, Muslim World League. Fatwa No. 3. In: Book of Resolutions 17th session. Makkah (Saudi Arabia): Muslim World League; 2003. p. 33–5.

111. Receiving organs for transplantation: Fatwa no. 85514. 2003. Available at: Islamweb.net; https://www.islamweb.net/en/fatwa/85514/receiving-organs-for-transplantation. Accessed October 8, 2019.
112. Mohseni MA. Al-fiqh and medical issues. 1st edition. Qom (Iran): Qom Bookstore Institute; 2003.
113. European Council for Fatwa and Research. The Sixth Ordinary Session of the European Council for Fatwa and Research. Resolutions and Fatwas, Second Collection, Resolution 2/6. Dublin, Ireland. 8 Aug to 1 Sept, 2000. Available at: https://www.e-cfr.org/sixth-ordinary-session-european-council-fatwa-research/. Accessed February 19, 2020. [in Arabic].
114. Transplanting body part from pig to human. Fatwa no. 332080. 2016. Available at: Islamweb.net; https://www.islamweb.net/en/fatwa/332080/transplanting-body-part-from-pig-to-human. Accessed October 8, 2019.
115. Halim MA, Salleh MMM, Kashim MIAM, et al. Halal pharmaceuticals: Legal, Shari'ah issues and fatwa of drug, gelatine and alcohol. Int J Asian Soc Sci 2014; 4(12):1176–90.

Gender Differences in Postoperative Outcomes After Cardiac Surgery

Allison J. Bechtel, MD, Julie L. Huffmyer, MD*

KEYWORDS

• Coronary artery bypass graft surgery • Gender differences • Mitral valve surgery
• Aortic valve surgery • Transcatheter aortic valve replacement • Cardiac rehabilitation

KEY POINTS

- Women have increased risk for morbidity and mortality following cardiac surgery.
- Women present with a significantly different preoperative risk profile than men; they are older, and have hypertension, diabetes, as well as overweight or underweight BMI.
- Residual/untreated CAD after CABG is more common in women, and secondary prevention of CAD progression and treatment should be highlighted.
- Women presenting for transcatheter aortic valve replacement (TAVR) are older and more frail, have higher risk for intraoperative bleeding and vascular complications, but tend to have improved mid- and long-term mortality compared to men.
- Adherence to cardiac surgery rehabilitation programs is challenging, and solutions should focus on flexibility of scheduling, family support, and group exercise.

INTRODUCTION

Cardiovascular disease is the leading cause of death in the United States and was responsible for 840,000 deaths in the year 2016.[1] Although that number is staggering, over the last 13 years the overall death rate from cardiovascular disease has declined in the United States. For women, heart disease, defined in the broadest sense, remains the principal cause of death, claiming the lives of nearly 300,000 women in 2017, which is nearly one in five deaths of women.[2] Indeed some form of heart disease is responsible for death in African American and white US women, whereas American Indian and Alaskan Native women die of heart disease and cancer at nearly equal rates.[3] For Hispanic and Asian or Pacific Islander women, heart disease is the second leading cause of death behind cancer.[3] Coronary heart disease affects roughly 6% of women older than age 20 in the white, black, and Hispanic ethnicities.[1] The Society of

Department of Anesthesiology, University of Virginia Health, PO Box 800710, Charlottesville, VA 22908-0710, USA
* Corresponding author.
E-mail addresses: jh3wd@hscmail.mcc.virginia.edu; as4sk@hscmail.mcc.virginia.edu

Anesthesiology Clin 38 (2020) 403–415
https://doi.org/10.1016/j.anclin.2020.01.007 anesthesiology.theclinics.com

Thoracic Surgeons (STS) database, which collects population and outcome data on adult patients undergoing cardiac surgery in the United States, recorded that nearly 160,000 patients underwent isolated coronary artery bypass graft (CABG) surgery in 2016.[4,5] Heart transplant surgery accounted for 3244 cardiac surgical procedures in 2017, 28.4% were women, but survival in men and women was similar: approximately 90%.[6] Overall as the population ages and women tend to live longer than men, fewer men than women undergo CABG surgery.[7] For the purposes of this review, gender differences in postoperative outcomes following cardiac surgery was considered while keeping in mind that most of the references included information on the sex of the patient (the genetic trait with accompanying hormonal and anatomic differences) instead of the gender of the patient (personal identity and behaviors).[8]

HISTORY

In 1996, the European Heart Journal published a prospective study of more than 2000 patients who underwent CABG surgery that evaluated the morbidity and mortality at 2 years in relation to the patient's gender.[9] Approximately 80% of the patients undergoing surgery were men, but female patients presenting for surgery were more likely to have hypertension, diabetes, congestive heart failure (CHF), renal dysfunction, and obesity.[9] Postoperative complications that occurred more often in women included neurologic deficit, pneumothorax, myocardial ischemia, and requirement for mechanical assist devices.[9] In the subsequent multivariate analysis, although female sex was a risk factor for increased mortality at 30 days following the surgery, mortality at 2 years was not increased in women.[9] The survival benefit of undergoing CABG procedure because of significant coronary artery disease (CAD) seems to be equal for men and women at 2 years.[9] The Australasian Society of Cardiac and Thoracic Surgeons Cardiac Surgery Database Program found a similar ratio of male to female (22.2% women) patients a decade later in their evaluation of 20,000 patients.[10] Women again were more likely to have CHF, hypertension, diabetes, and cerebrovascular disease.[10] Although univariate analysis revealed increased 30-day and late mortality in women, multivariate analysis failed to retain this difference in mortality.[10] Women were less likely to develop acute renal failure and deep sternal wound infections, but were more likely to receive a blood transfusion.[10] There is an important link between the preoperative characteristics of patients presenting for cardiac surgery and the resultant postoperative complications and outcomes. Between the 1990s and early 2000s, there was no change in the preoperative characteristics of women compared with men.[9,10] A single-center, retrospective study in the Netherlands of nearly 18,000 patients undergoing CABG recently showed that the preoperative profile of men and women were significantly different with women more often having hypertension, diabetes, underweight status with body mass index less than 20 kg/m^2, and overweight status with body mass index greater than 30 kg/m^2.[11] This significant gender difference in the preoperative risk profile has persisted with little change over the past 25 years.

GENDER DIFFERENCES IN CARDIAC SURGERY

Patients undergoing cardiac surgery are at risk for postoperative complications, such as bleeding, infection, myocardial ischemia, cerebrovascular accident, and renal failure.[12] **Table 1** presents the differences based on gender with regard to biologic factors and clinical risk factors for men and women having cardiac surgery.

Men and women suffer from the same types of complications, but there seems to be an impact of gender leading to a higher rate of complications, increased severity, and overall increase in morbidity and mortality in women.[30] A Swedish study of 110,742

Table 1
Gender differences in patients presenting for cardiac surgery

Category	Women	Men
Biologic factors		
Age	Live longer; present with CAD later[13] If early MI/CAD, poor prognosis with increased mortality[14,15]	Present earlier with CAD
Vascular biology	Smaller coronary arteries, 10%–15% smaller LAD and left main coronary artery[16,17] more thrombogenicity	Larger target coronary arteries
Location of CAD	LAD most common	LAD most common At risk for multivessel, diffuse involvement, but collaterals extensive[18]
Steroid biology	Exposure to estrogen restricts (delays) atherosclerosis; estrogen contributes to slower CAD, better long-term response to vessel injury[19,20]	With aging and low androgens/ testosterone, increased risk for CAD, upregulated inflammation[21]
Pattern of presentation (angiography)	Less obstructive CAD; symptoms more attributable to coronary artery spasm, plaque rupture/ erosion; microvascular disease[22]	Obstructive, macrovascular CAD[22]
Clinical risk factors by gender	Urgent surgery with need for preoperative IABP support[23] Coexistent CHF; lower NYHA classification[23] Diabetes mellitus, COPD[25,26] Peripheral vascular disease[24] Smaller body surface area[28] Severe/unstable angina[29] Lower preoperative hematocrit[23]	Lower ejection fraction[24] Multivessel CAD; repeat surgery[18] Renal failure/CKD[27] Smoking history[27] Previous MI[27]

Abbreviations: CKD, chronic kidney disease; COPD, chronic obstructive pulmonary disease; IABP, intra-aortic balloon pump; LAD, left anterior descending; MI, myocardial infarction; NYHA, New York Heart Association.

CABG patients (21.3% women) evaluated social factors, sex, and mortality risk and found an increased mortality in men and women with low education, low income, and unmarried status, but the impact of marital status was magnified for women compared with men.[31] The authors attributed this difference to preoperative factors, such as antidepressant use and alcohol dependence, and postoperative factors including social support that were increased in women.[31] Ter Woorst and colleagues[11] found early mortality after CABG to be significantly higher in women than in men. Women tended to be older, and have lower hemoglobin and creatinine than men.[11]

The impact of gender on postoperative outcomes following cardiac surgery is significant and warrants an additional point on the EUROSCORE, a risk stratification tool used in cardiac surgery based on a prospective database from eight European countries.[32] The STS in the United States has a National Cardiac Surgery Registry and its database also includes female gender as an independent risk factor for adverse postcardiac surgery outcomes.[33] Both scoring systems are similar when predicting mortality for patients having isolated CABG surgery, but the EUROSCORE may more accurately predict mortality in female patients because of its reduced number of variables captured (18, instead of the 40–50 variables in the STS scoring system).[33]

Acute kidney injury (AKI) following cardiac surgery is a significant complication that portends an increased morbidity and mortality. A meta-analysis of studies from 1978 to 2015 identified 64 studies with data on more than 1 million patients undergoing cardiac surgery. When the analysis was refined to well-established, more current diagnostic criteria (eg, Acute Kidney Injury Network [AKIN] criteria, or RIFLE criteria), 29 studies were included with 120,000 patients, but there was no significant sex-related difference in AKI risk.[34] When the multivariate analysis was further restricted to using only AKIN criteria, risk for AKI was significantly lower in women compared with men.[34]

GENDER DIFFERENCES IN POSTOPERATIVE OUTCOMES AFTER CORONARY ARTERY BYPASS GRAFT SURGERY

It is inevitable that a discussion on postoperative outcomes following cardiac surgery must account for not only gender, but preoperative risk factors, clinical presentation and urgency, and surgical complexity. An early STS-based, multivariate analysis in the late 1990s showed that women had significantly higher mortality compared with equally matched men in low- and medium-risk categories but in the high-risk group, there was no significant difference between men and women.[29] In the early 2000s, a large database study of nearly 16,000 patients undergoing isolated CABG found that Q-wave myocardial infarction (MI), postoperative inotrope requirement, and prolonged ventilatory support were more common in women; however, female sex was not associated with increased mortality.[35]

Women presenting for CABG surgery were often older and required urgent or emergent surgery and were more likely to have vein grafts compared with arterial grafts.[27,36] Postoperatively, women were more likely to be admitted to the hospital in the first year after surgery and in the years that followed because of unstable angina and CHF, along with significant decline in physical function and increase in depression.[27,37,38] In addition, several studies have proposed that women presenting for cardiac surgery have a lower body surface area and smaller coronary arteries and may have higher mortality.[10,27,36,39] As a result, these smaller coronary arteries may be more difficult to bypass effectively and the grafts may be more likely to fail postoperatively.

Increased female mortality after CABG seems to be most significant for the first year after surgery, after which the risk for mortality approaches the risk for male mortality, becoming equal at 4 years post-CABG.[25] Although there is known increased risk for readmission in women, late MI is thought to be related to reduced graft patency, smaller target coronary size, fewer grafts, and decreased use of arterial graft conduit.[36] Male patients were more likely to have bilateral internal mammary artery use and multiple artery revascularization (three arteries).[37] This concept of residual/untreated coronary disease in women who end up with increased late admissions highlights the need for secondary prevention of CAD progression and aggressive management after CABG.

The development of new-onset postoperative atrial fibrillation is a common complication following cardiac surgery and is associated with increased intensive care unit and hospital length of stay and perioperative morbidity and mortality and long-term survival.[38] Postoperative atrial fibrillation seems to affect women less frequently than men and has less deleterious effects. Filardo and colleagues[40] evaluated 9203 patients in the STS database and found a 27.4% incidence of atrial fibrillation in women as compared with 32.8% in men; women had significantly lower risk of developing atrial fibrillation after CABG but also had significantly shorter first and longest atrial fibrillation duration.

Minimally invasive direct CABG procedures have the purported benefit of decreased perioperative morbidity especially with surgeons experienced in this surgical procedure.[41] Postoperative poor wound healing following minimally invasive direct CABG procedures is a complication that is seen more often in female patients compared with male patients and may be related to older age and diabetes with longer surgical procedures.[42]

Off-pump CABG surgery has been touted as being potentially beneficial to patients in high-risk cohorts because it avoids the morbidity associated with aortic manipulation, cross-clamping, global myocardial ischemia, and the systemic inflammation associated with the cardiopulmonary bypass machine.[43] Meta-analysis of data from high-volume centers showed that women having off-pump CABG surgery seemed to have improvement in outcomes (significantly decreased death, stroke, and MI) compared with women who underwent on-pump CABG.[44] However, during off-pump CABG surgery, women had higher risk of death, stroke, and adverse myocardial events.[44]

Not surprisingly, women who present with CAD and undergo percutaneous coronary intervention with coronary stent placement instead of CABG present with the same set of comorbidities as for CABG compared with men.[45] In the EXCEL trial, sex was not an independent predictor of adverse outcomes after revascularization for left main CAD; however, there was trend in women undergoing percutaneous coronary intervention toward worse outcomes, potentially related to associated comorbid conditions and periprocedural complications, such as MI.[45] Another large study in patients having percutaneous coronary intervention versus CABG showed similar primary outcome (composite of death from any cause, MI, or stroke) in men and women.[46]

GENDER DIFFERENCES IN POSTOPERATIVE OUTCOMES AFTER VALVE REPLACEMENT SURGERY

From 2003 to 2014, data from the National Inpatient Sample Files were used to evaluate the gender differences in outcomes of more than 24,000 patients following either mitral or aortic valve surgery. Increased all-cause mortality, stroke, or MI were noted in women compared with men, with improved outcomes overall; however, men had a more substantial reduction in the mortality rate.[47]

Patients undergoing mitral valve repair may sustain a return to normal life expectancy but there continues to be a discrepancy in outcomes between men and women. This difference may be caused by women being referred for surgery later in the disease process when they are older with more comorbidities.[48] Of 3761 patients undergoing minimally invasive mitral valve surgery, improved long-term survival in men compared with women was reported with 1-, 5-, and 10-year survival rates of 96%, 89%, and 72%, respectively, in men compared with 92%, 82%, and 58% in women.[49]

The Cardiothoracic Surgical Trials Network evaluated patients with severe ischemic mitral regurgitation comparing mitral valve replacement and repair on long-term outcomes at 2 years. Following mitral valve surgery, women had significantly increased all-cause mortality compared with men and were found to have an increased risk for major adverse cardiovascular and cerebrovascular events and decreased functional status and quality of life after 2 years.[50,51] There was no difference in left ventricular remodeling in men and women following surgery that could help explain these findings.[52] In the Netherlands, of 3411 patients having isolated mitral valve surgery from 2007 to 2011, women were more likely to be older, have higher EUROSCORE, and pulmonary hypertension and were more likely to undergo mitral valve replacement versus repair.[53] Despite these differences, there was no significant difference in short-term mortality between men and women.[54]

Patients undergoing open aortic valve replacement (AVR) have a decrease in their life expectancy following surgery by approximately 1.9 years with additional decreases in younger patients.[55] Studies in patients undergoing AVR have revealed similar gender differences in preoperative characteristics as those undergoing CABG procedures with women being older and more likely to have hypertension, diabetes, chronic obstructive pulmonary disease (COPD), atrial fibrillation or flutter, and anemia.[56] In a study of 28,237 propensity-matched pairs, women undergoing AVR incurred increased in-hospital mortality, vascular complications, and blood transfusions.[56] Similar results were found in the Italian OBSERVANT Registry with women presenting for surgery with risk factors of increased age and frailty score and decreased body weight and hemoglobin levels.[57] Following surgical AVR women had increased 30-day mortality and increased risk for blood transfusion.[57] This same study evaluated men and women undergoing transcatheter aortic valve replacement (TAVR) as well and reported increased risk for major vascular complications and blood transfusions in women compared with men.[50]

A large-scale review of patients undergoing TAVR with the CoreValve (Medtronic, Minneapolis, MN), a self-expanding valve, evaluated gender differences and mortality and complications.[51] This is an especially important area of study because even in low- and intermediate-risk patients there are similar mortality rates with demonstration of noninferiority between TAVR and surgical AVR with lower rates of myocardial ischemia and AKI in patients undergoing TAVR.[53] Women are older, more frail, with fewer comorbid medical problems including CAD, stroke, and CHF than corresponding male patients.[58] Comparing men and women, there is no difference in 30-day or 1-year mortality after TAVR.[51] However, women are at higher risk for intraoperative complications related to bleeding and vascular complications.[51,59,60] A meta-analysis of 16 TAVR studies showed a significantly better midterm ($\geq$6 months) overall survival in women compared with men.[57] This benefit to women undergoing TAVR has also been shown with reduced mortality at 1 year, thought to be related to less severe residual aortic insufficiency and lower overall cardiovascular mortality.[60] Risk factors for increased mortality following TAVR include renal failure, diabetes, peripheral artery disease, and COPD rather than gender.[59]

There are less data available on gender differences following tricuspid valve surgery even though women make up greater than 60% of patients. Pfannmueller and colleagues[58] report a series of 92 patients undergoing tricuspid valve surgery and there was no significant gender difference in 30-day mortality or 5-year survival.

GENDER DIFFERENCES IN POSTOPERATIVE OUTCOMES AFTER LEFT VENTRICULAR ASSIST DEVICES

The incidence of CHF after age 65 is approximately 10 per 1000 people, and after 20 years of age, men are more affected than women (2.5% vs 1.8%); however, mortality for women (58.2%) is much greater than that of men (41.8%).[61] Heart failure with preserved ejection fraction is a growing entity in the United States in men and women, and although survival has increased for patients with heart failure who have reduced ejection fraction, survival for the group of patients with heart failure with preserved ejection fraction has not seen this same increase.[62] Risk factors for development of heart failure with preserved ejection fraction are different based on gender with women having hypertension, chronic kidney disease, and obesity and men having history of myocardial ischemia, atrial fibrillation, and COPD.[63]

Regardless of indication for left ventricular assist device (LVAD) therapy, postoperative outcomes may be impacted by preoperative status of the patient coming to the operating room for LVAD placement. Women are less likely to receive LVAD therapy than men and are more likely to present in cardiogenic shock and receive an LVAD with a smaller pump.[64] Postoperatively, women are likely to require longer ventilatory support and inotropic support.[64] The increased intensive care unit length of stay may also be caused by the increased risk for right ventricular failure.[64,65] One year after LVAD placement, women were more likely to have worse overall survival, significant late bleeding complications, arrhythmias, and right ventricular failure.[64,66] In addition, women may be at higher risk for stroke (hemorrhagic and ischemic) depending on the type of the device (increased risk in the HeartMate II compared with the HeartMate 3 [Thoratec Corporation, Pleasanton, CA]).[66,67]

GENDER DIFFERENCES IN POSTOPERATIVE OUTCOMES AFTER HEART TRANSPLANT

Most heart transplant recipients internationally are men (75%).[68] The United Network for Organ Sharing waitlist for heart transplant reflects similar numbers with women making up approximately 25% of the waitlist patients.[68,69] Women often spend less time on the waiting list because of worse heart failure status leading to more urgent action for women on the waiting list.[70] In addition, women who are listed at the highest level of urgency for heart transplant, status 1A and 1B, are more likely to die on the waiting list before receiving a heart transplant.[67] Postoperative outcomes seem to be different depending on gender, but results from different registries of heart transplant recipients are conflicting. United Network for Organ Sharing registry data reveal decreased survival at 5 years for women compared with men, whereas the International Society of Heart and Lung Transplantation registry data favor improved long-term survival for women.[71,72] Gender does not seem to be protective for the development of microvasculopathy following heart transplantation.[70] Female heart transplant recipients may be more likely to develop rejection, MI, cardiac allograft vasculopathy, and end-stage renal disease.[73]

Sex of the donor and recipient in heart transplantation surgery deserves additional attention. There does not seem to be increased risk of rejection based on sex of the donor, but there is increased risk for rejection leading to death in female recipients.[70] A recent meta-analysis showed minimal gender effects on 1-year mortality after heart transplant; however, female donor to male recipient sex mismatch showed significant association with 1-year mortality.[68] This topic is discussed in greater detail Susan M. Walters and colleagues' article, "Perioperative Considerations Regarding Sex in Solid Organ Transplantation," elsewhere in this issue.

POSTOPERATIVE REHABILITATION AND QUALITY OF LIFE

It has been well-established in the literature that women and men cope with illness differently and in the recovery process from surgery.[69,74] For women, encouragement from adult children to attend rehabilitation programs and the goal of health promotion seem to be more powerful motivators than for men.[75] Illness behavior is defined by differences in the way that groups of patients think about, process, and confront medical illnesses. Modica and colleagues[76] examined illness behavior in a cross-sectional cohort of 1323 patients in cardiac rehabilitation after cardiac surgery and found that denial was more prevalent among men, but disease conviction, dysphoria, anxiety, and depression were significantly more prevalent in women. For men and women preoperative symptoms of depression and anxiety have been shown to minimally impact mortality. However, depression at 1 year after CABG has been associated with increased mortality at similar rates for men and women; women with postoperative anxiety symptoms had increased 11-year post-CABG mortality.[77] This highlights the need to screen for and aggressively treat psychiatric symptoms and illness in patients presenting for cardiac surgery.

Most quality of life studies after cardiac surgery have examined the outcomes of men. Emery and colleagues[69] evaluated quality of life in men and women after heart surgery using several well-validated scales looking at mental, physical, and medical outcomes, and social support. The authors found that women with cardiac disease who had surgery showed significantly lower quality of life compared with men, over the course of a 12-month follow-up time period. Social support, especially the sense of belonging to a group, was found to be especially important for women who had surgery. Thus, for women, postcardiac surgery social (group) support may be even more important than for men. Kendel and colleagues[74] found that women who presented for CABG with significantly lower physical function and 1 year after CABG showed similar improvement in health-related quality of life as men, but still reported worse functional capacity than their male counterparts.

Adherence to cardiac surgery rehabilitation programs is challenging, and solutions for women should aim to focus on sex differences, such as offering flexibility of scheduling, family support, use of exercises for women that use group activities (eg, dancing, exercise as a community, and incorporation of exercise into lifestyle modification).[78]

SUMMARY

It is clear that there are differences in postoperative outcomes following cardiac surgery for women compared with men. These differences seem to be multifactorial including biologic differences, age and disease severity at time of surgery, preexisting comorbidities, intraoperative complexities, and postoperative rehabilitation. Future research should seek to promote earlier referrals for cardiac surgery, investigate modifications to surgical techniques for women, and identify postoperative rehabilitation programs specifically designed for women.

DISCLOSURE

The authors have no commercial, funding conflicts of interest, or funding sources.

REFERENCES

1. Benjamin EJ, Muntner P, Alonso A, et al. Heart disease and stroke statistics-2019 update: a report from the American Heart Association. Circulation 2019;139(10): e56–528.
2. Underlying Cause of Death, 1999-2017 Results Form. Centers for Disease Control and Prevention, National Center for Health Statistics. Underlying Cause of Death 1999-2017 on CDC WONDER Online Database. 2018. Available at: https://wonder.cdc.gov/controller/datarequest/D76;jsessionid=65D0457421103F145B7E77B0312580E8. Accessed August 7, 2019.
3. Heron M. Deaths: leading causes for 2016. Natl Vital Stat Rep 2018;67(6):1–77.

4. Adult Cardiac Surgery Database: Executive Summary: 10 Years: STS Period Ending 06/30/2017. 2017. Available at: https://www.sts.org/sites/default/files/documents/ACSD2017Harvest3_ExecutiveSummary.pdf. Accessed August 7, 2019.
5. HCUPnet: a tool for identifying, tracking, and analyzing national hospital statistics. HCUPnet: Healthcare Cost and Utilization Project. Available at: https://hcupnet.ahrq.gov/. Accessed August 7, 2019.
6. Organ Procurement and Transplantation Network Data. Organ Procurement and Transplantation Network. 2019. Available at: https://optn.transplant.hrsa.gov/data/. Accessed August 7, 2019.
7. Shimizu T, Miura S, Takeuchi K, et al. Effects of gender and aging in patients who undergo coronary artery bypass grafting: from the FU-Registry. Cardiol J 2012;19(6):618–24.
8. Clayton JA, Tannenbaum C. Reporting sex, gender, or both in clinical research? JAMA 2016;316(18):1863–4.
9. Brandrup-Wognsen G, Berggren H, Hartford M, et al. Female sex is associated with increased mortality and morbidity early, but not late, after coronary artery bypass grafting. Eur Heart J 1996;17(9):1426–31.
10. Saxena A, Dinh D, Smith JA, et al. Sex differences in outcomes following isolated coronary artery bypass graft surgery in Australian patients: analysis of the Australasian Society of Cardiac and Thoracic Surgeons cardiac surgery database. Eur J Cardiothorac Surg 2012;41(4):755–62.
11. Ter Woorst JF, van Straten AHM, Houterman S, et al. Sex difference in coronary artery bypass grafting: preoperative profile and early outcome. J Cardiothorac Vasc Anesth 2019. https://doi.org/10.1053/j.jvca.2019.02.040.
12. Olivencia L, Macias I, Fernandez MD, et al. Postoperative cardiac surgery. Gender Differences. Intensive Care Med 2011;37(Supplement 2):S59.
13. Abramov D, Tamariz MG, Sever JY, et al. The influence of gender on the outcome of coronary artery bypass surgery. Ann Thorac Surg 2000;70(3):800–5 [discussion: 806].
14. Humphries KH, Gao M, Pu A, et al. Significant improvement in short-term mortality in women undergoing coronary artery bypass surgery (1991 to 2004). J Am Coll Cardiol 2007;49(14):1552–8.
15. Vaccarino V, Abramson JL, Veledar E, et al. Sex differences in hospital mortality after coronary artery bypass surgery. Circulation 2002;105(10):1176–81.
16. O'Connor NJ, Morton JR, Birkmeyer JD, et al. Effect of coronary artery diameter in patients undergoing coronary bypass surgery. Northern New England Cardiovascular Disease Study Group. Circulation 1996;93(4):652–5.
17. Sheifer SE, Canos MR, Weinfurt KP, et al. Sex differences in coronary artery size assessed by intravascular ultrasound. Am Heart J 2000;139(4):649–53.
18. Kyriakidis M, Petropoulakis P, Androulakis A, et al. Sex differences in the anatomy of coronary artery disease. J Clin Epidemiol 1995;48(6):723–30.
19. Walsh BW, Schiff I, Rosner B, et al. Effects of postmenopausal estrogen replacement on the concentrations and metabolism of plasma lipoproteins. N Engl J Med 1991;325(17):1196–204.
20. Mendelsohn ME. Nongenomic, ER-mediated activation of endothelial nitric oxide synthase: how does it work? What does it mean? Circ Res 2000;87(11):956–60.
21. Channer KS, Jones TH. Cardiovascular effects of testosterone: implications of the "male menopause"? Heart 2003;89(2):121–2.
22. Hansen KW, Soerensen R, Madsen M, et al. Developments in the invasive diagnostic-therapeutic cascade of women and men with acute coronary

syndromes from 2005 to 2011: a nationwide cohort study. BMJ Open 2015;5(6): e007785.

23. Aldea GS, Gaudiani JM, Shapira OM, et al. Effect of gender on postoperative outcomes and hospital stays after coronary artery bypass grafting. Ann Thorac Surg 1999;67(4):1097–103.
24. Blankstein R, Ward RP, Arnsdorf M, et al. Female gender is an independent predictor of operative mortality after coronary artery bypass graft surgery: contemporary analysis of 31 Midwestern hospitals. Circulation 2005;112(9 Suppl): I323–7.
25. Guru V, Fremes SE, Tu JV. Time-related mortality for women after coronary artery bypass graft surgery: a population-based study. J Thorac Cardiovasc Surg 2004; 127(4):1158–65.
26. Mehta RH, Honeycutt E, Shaw LK, et al. Clinical and angiographic correlates of short- and long-term mortality in patients undergoing coronary artery bypass grafting. Am J Cardiol 2007;100(10):1538–42.
27. Woods SE, Noble G, Smith JM, et al. The influence of gender in patients undergoing coronary artery bypass graft surgery: an eight-year prospective hospitalized cohort study. J Am Coll Surg 2003;196(3):428–34.
28. Peduzzi P, Kamina A, Detre K. Twenty-two-year follow-up in the VA cooperative study of coronary artery bypass surgery for stable angina. Am J Cardiol 1998; 81(12):1393–9.
29. Edwards FH, Carey JS, Grover FL, et al. Impact of gender on coronary bypass operative mortality. Ann Thorac Surg 1998;66(1):125–31.
30. Fox AA, Nussmeier NA. Does gender influence the likelihood or types of complications following cardiac surgery? Semin Cardiothorac Vasc Anesth 2004;8(4): 283–95.
31. Nielsen S, Giang KW, Wallinder A, et al. Social factors, sex, and mortality risk after coronary artery bypass grafting: a population-based cohort study. J Am Heart Assoc 2019;8(6):e011490.
32. Nashef SA, Roques F, Michel P, et al. European system for cardiac operative risk evaluation (EuroSCORE). Eur J Cardiothorac Surg 1999;16(1):9–13.
33. Ad N, Barnett SD, Speir AM. The performance of the EuroSCORE and the Society of Thoracic Surgeons mortality risk score: the gender factor. Interact Cardiovasc Thorac Surg 2007;6(2):192–5.
34. Neugarten J, Sandilya S, Singh B, et al. Sex and the risk of AKI following cardiothoracic surgery: a meta-analysis. Clin J Am Soc Nephrol 2016;11(12):2113–22.
35. Koch CG, Weng Y, Zhou SX, et al. Prevalence of risk factors, and not gender per se, determines short- and long-term survival after coronary artery bypass surgery. J Cardiothorac Vasc Anesth 2003;17(5):585–93.
36. Hessian R, Jabagi H, Ngu JMC, et al. Coronary surgery in women and the challenges we face. Can J Cardiol 2018;34(4):413–21.
37. Jabagi H, Tran DT, Hessian R, et al. Impact of gender on arterial revascularization strategies for coronary artery bypass grafting. Ann Thorac Surg 2018; 105(1):62–8.
38. El-Chami MF, Kilgo P, Thourani V, et al. New-onset atrial fibrillation predicts long-term mortality after coronary artery bypass graft. J Am Coll Cardiol 2010;55(13): 1370–6.
39. Fisher LD, Kennedy JW, Davis KB, et al. Association of sex, physical size, and operative mortality after coronary artery bypass in the Coronary Artery Surgery Study (CASS). J Thorac Cardiovasc Surg 1982;84(3):334–41.

40. Filardo G, Ailawadi G, Pollock BD, et al. Postoperative atrial fibrillation: sex-specific characteristics and effect on survival. J Thorac Cardiovasc Surg 2019. https://doi.org/10.1016/j.jtcvs.2019.04.097.
41. Smith NJ, Miles B, Cain MT, et al. Minimally invasive single-vessel left internal mammary to left anterior descending artery bypass grafting improves outcomes over conventional sternotomy: a single-institution retrospective cohort study. J Card Surg 2019. https://doi.org/10.1111/jocs.14144.
42. Gofus J, Vobornik M, Sorm Z, et al. Female sex as a risk factor in minimally invasive direct coronary artery bypass grafting. Scand Cardiovasc J 2019;53(3):141–7.
43. Dhurandhar V, Saxena A, Parikh R, et al. Comparison of the safety and efficacy of On-Pump (ONCAB) versus Off-Pump (OPCAB) coronary artery bypass graft surgery in the elderly: a review of the ANZSCTS database. Heart Lung Circ 2015;24(12):1225–32.
44. Puskas JD, Kilgo PD, Kutner M, et al. Off-pump techniques disproportionately benefit women and narrow the gender disparity in outcomes after coronary artery bypass surgery. Circulation 2007;116(11 Suppl):I192–9.
45. Serruys PW, Cavalcante R, Collet C, et al. Outcomes after coronary stenting or bypass surgery for men and women with unprotected left main disease: the EXCEL trial. JACC Cardiovasc Interv 2018;11(13):1234–43.
46. Park H, Ahn J-M, Yoon Y-H, et al. Effect of age and sex on outcomes after stenting or bypass surgery in left main coronary artery disease. Am J Cardiol 2019. https://doi.org/10.1016/j.amjcard.2019.05.061.
47. Wong SC, Yeo I, Bergman G, et al. The influence of gender on in-hospital clinical outcome following isolated mitral or aortic heart valve surgery. Cardiovasc Revasc Med 2019;20(6):468–74.
48. McNeely C, Vassileva C. Mitral valve surgery in women: another target for eradicating sex inequality. Circ Cardiovasc Qual Outcomes 2016;9(2 Suppl 1):S94–6.
49. Seeburger J, Eifert S, Pfannmüller B, et al. Gender differences in mitral valve surgery. Thorac Cardiovasc Surg 2013;61(1):42–6.
50. Onorati F, D'Errigo P, Barbanti M, et al. Different impact of sex on baseline characteristics and major periprocedural outcomes of transcatheter and surgical aortic valve interventions: results of the multicenter Italian OBSERVANT Registry. J Thorac Cardiovasc Surg 2014;147(5):1529–39.
51. Forrest JK, Adams DH, Popma JJ, et al. Transcatheter aortic valve replacement in women versus men (from the US CoreValve trials). Am J Cardiol 2016;118(3):396–402.
52. Giustino G, Overbey J, Taylor D, et al. Sex-based differences in outcomes after mitral valve surgery for severe ischemic mitral regurgitation: from the cardiothoracic surgical trials network. JACC Heart Fail 2019;7(6):481–90.
53. Ueshima D, Fovino LN, D'Amico G, et al. Transcatheter versus surgical aortic valve replacement in low- and intermediate-risk patients: an updated systematic review and meta-analysis. Cardiovasc Interv Ther 2019;34(3):216–25.
54. Mokhles MM, Siregar S, Versteegh MIM, et al. Male-female differences and survival in patients undergoing isolated mitral valve surgery: a nationwide cohort study in the Netherlands. Eur J Cardiothorac Surg 2016;50(3):482–7.
55. Glaser N, Persson M, Jackson V, et al. Loss in life expectancy after surgical aortic valve replacement: SWEDEHEART study. J Am Coll Cardiol 2019;74(1):26–33.
56. Chaker Z, Badhwar V, Alqahtani F, et al. Sex differences in the utilization and outcomes of surgical aortic valve replacement for severe aortic stenosis. J Am Heart Assoc 2017;6(9). https://doi.org/10.1161/JAHA.117.006370.

57. Takagi H, Umemoto T. All-Literature Investigation of Cardiovascular Evidence (ALICE) group. Better midterm survival in women after transcatheter aortic valve implantation. J Cardiovasc Surg (Torino) 2017;58(4):624–32.
58. Pfannmueller B, Eifert S, Seeburger J, et al. Gender-dependent differences in patients undergoing tricuspid valve surgery. Thorac Cardiovasc Surg 2013;61(1): 37–41.
59. Katz M, Carlos Bacelar Nunes Filho A, Caixeta A, et al. Gender-related differences on short- and long-term outcomes of patients undergoing transcatheter aortic valve implantation. Catheter Cardiovasc Interv 2017;89(3):429–36.
60. Saad M, Nairooz R, Pothineni NVK, et al. Long-term outcomes with transcatheter aortic valve replacement in women compared with men: evidence from a meta-analysis. JACC Cardiovasc Interv 2018;11(1):24–35.
61. Go AS, Mozaffarian D, Roger VL, et al. Heart disease and stroke statistics–2013 update: a report from the American Heart Association. Circulation 2013;127(1): e6–245.
62. Greiten LE, Holditch SJ, Arunachalam SP, et al. Should there be sex-specific criteria for the diagnosis and treatment of heart failure? J Cardiovasc Transl Res 2014;7(2):139–55.
63. Lam CSP, Carson PE, Anand IS, et al. Sex differences in clinical characteristics and outcomes in elderly patients with heart failure and preserved ejection fraction: the Irbesartan in Heart Failure with Preserved Ejection Fraction (I-PRESERVE) trial. Circ Heart Fail 2012;5(5):571–8.
64. Magnussen C, Bernhardt AM, Ojeda FM, et al. Gender differences and outcomes in left ventricular assist device support: the European Registry for Patients with Mechanical Circulatory Support. J Heart Lung Transplant 2018;37(1):61–70.
65. Weymann A, Patil NP, Sabashnikov A, et al. Gender differences in continuous-flow left ventricular assist device therapy as a bridge to transplantation: a risk-adjusted comparison using a propensity score-matching analysis. Artif Organs 2015;39(3):212–9.
66. Daoud D, Cheema FH, Morgan JA, et al. Sex-related differences in outcomes of thoracic organ transplantation and mechanical circulatory support. Tex Heart Inst J 2018;45(4):240–2.
67. Hsich EM. Sex differences in advanced heart failure therapies. Circulation 2019; 139(8):1080–93.
68. Foroutan F, Alba AC, Guyatt G, et al. Predictors of 1-year mortality in heart transplant recipients: a systematic review and meta-analysis. Heart 2018;104(2): 151–60.
69. Emery CF, Frid DJ, Engebretson TO, et al. Gender differences in quality of life among cardiac patients. Psychosom Med 2004;66(2):190–7.
70. Melk A, Babitsch B, Borchert-Mörlins B, et al. Equally interchangeable? How sex and gender affect transplantation. Transplantation 2019;103(6):1094–110.
71. Chambers DC, Yusen RD, Cherikh WS, et al. The Registry of the International Society for Heart and Lung Transplantation: thirty-fourth adult lung and heart-lung transplantation report-2017; focus theme: allograft ischemic time. J Heart Lung Transplant 2017;36(10):1047–59.
72. Weiss ES, Allen JG, Patel ND, et al. The impact of donor-recipient sex matching on survival after orthotopic heart transplantation: analysis of 18 000 transplants in the modern era. Circ Heart Fail 2009;2(5):401–8.
73. Peled Y, Lavee J, Arad M, et al. The impact of gender mismatching on early and late outcomes following heart transplantation. ESC Heart Fail 2017;4(1):31–9.

74. Kendel F, Dunkel A, Müller-Tasch T, et al. Gender differences in health-related quality of life after coronary bypass surgery: results from a 1-year follow-up in propensity-matched men and women. Psychosom Med 2011;73(3):280–5.
75. Lieberman L, Meana M, Stewart D. Cardiac rehabilitation: gender differences in factors influencing participation. J Womens Health 1998;7(6):717–23.
76. Modica M, Ferratini M, Spezzaferri R, et al. Gender differences in illness behavior after cardiac surgery. J Cardiopulm Rehabil Prev 2014;34(2):123–9.
77. Geulayov G, Novikov I, Dankner D, et al. Symptoms of depression and anxiety and 11-year all-cause mortality in men and women undergoing coronary artery bypass graft (CABG) surgery. J Psychosom Res 2018;105:106–14.
78. Galati A, Piccoli M, Tourkmani N, et al. Cardiac rehabilitation in women: state of the art and strategies to overcome the current barriers. J Cardiovasc Med (Hagerstown) 2018;19(12):689–97.

Role of Gender and Race in Patient-Reported Outcomes and Satisfaction

Natalie Kozlov, MD, Honorio T. Benzon, MD*

KEYWORDS

• Outcome domains • Measurement tools • Race • Socioeconomic status • Gender
• Outcomes • Patient satisfaction

KEY POINTS

- The recommended outcome domains reflect the multidimensionality of pain perception. For chronic pain research, the recommended outcome domains include(1) pain; (2) physical conditioning; (3) emotional functioning; (4) participant ratings of global improvement and satisfaction with treatment; (5) symptoms and adverse events; and (6) participant disposition (including adherence to the treatment regimen and reasons for premature withdrawal from the trial). Appropriate measurement tools for chronic pain research have been recommended for each of the outcome domains.
- Similar to chronic pain, studies on acute pain should examine not only pain and its management, and adverse events from the intervention, but also physical and emotional components and patient satisfaction. Similar to chronic pain, measurement tools are available for each of the outcome measures in postoperative pain.
- Lower socioeconomic status is associated with greater difficulty accessing care, poor communication with health care providers, limited shared decision-making, delays in health care delivery, poor satisfaction with care, and poor unadjusted and adjusted outcomes.
- Minority groups (blacks, Hispanics, Asians) have greater difficulty with access to and use of health care.
- Compared with men, women have inferior outcomes with regard to health-related quality of life after medical (myocardial, atrial fibrillation) and surgical (vascular, orthopedic) interventions.

The role of gender, race, and socioeconomic status in patient outcomes and satisfaction has been of interest to investigators, health policy makers, and the public. The results are reflected in patient-reported outcomes using measurement tools representing the outcome domains. Patient satisfaction involves several facets of

Department of Anesthesiology, Northwestern University Feinberg School of Medicine, Feinberg Pavilion, Suite 5-704, 251 E. Huron Street, Chicago, IL 60611, USA
* Corresponding author.
E-mail address: h-benzon@northwestern.edu

Anesthesiology Clin 38 (2020) 417–431
https://doi.org/10.1016/j.anclin.2020.01.012 anesthesiology.theclinics.com

health care delivery and the relief of pain, a multidimensional sensation. In this article, the authors analyze the outcome domains and vetted measurement tools related to pain and satisfaction and discuss the results of studies on the role of socioeconomic status, race, and gender on patients' outcomes and satisfaction.

OUTCOME DOMAINS AND TOOLS TO REFLECT THE MULTIDIMENSIONALITY OF PAIN

Pain, per the International Association for the Study of Pain definition, is multifaceted. It involves sensory as well as emotional components. It is for this reason that the Initiative on Methods, Measurement, and Pain Assessment in Clinical Trials (IMMPACT) group recommended 6 core outcome measures to be considered when designing chronic pain clinical trials, which include the following **(Box 1)**:

1. Pain;
2. Physical conditioning;
3. Emotional functioning;
4. Participant ratings of global improvement and satisfaction with treatment;
5. Symptoms and adverse events; and,
6. Participant disposition (including adherence to the treatment regimen and reasons for premature withdrawal from the trial).[1,2]

The IMMPACT group recommended measurement tools for the aforementioned outcome domains for chronic pain studies. These include the numerical rating scale, analgesic use, or the categorical rating for pain intensity, and spontaneously noted adverse events for the symptoms and adverse events domain. Either the Multidimensional Pain Inventory Interference Scale or the Brief Pain Inventory interference items

Box 1
Recommended core outcome measures for clinical trials of chronic pain treatment efficacy and effectiveness

Pain
- 11-point (0–10) numerical rating scale of pain intensity
- Usage of rescue analgesics
- Categorical rating of pain intensity (none, mild, moderate, severe) in circumstances in which numerical ratings may be problematic

Physical functioning (either one of two measures)
- Multidimensional Pain Inventory Interference Scale
- Brief Pain Inventory interference items

Emotional functioning (at least 1 of 2 measures)
- Beck Depression Inventory
- Profile of Mood States

Participant ratings of global improvement and satisfaction with treatment
- Patient Global Impression of Change

Symptoms and adverse events
- Passive capture of spontaneously reported adverse events and symptoms and use of open-ended prompts

Participant disposition
- Detailed information regarding participant recruitment and progress through the trial, including all information specified in the CONSORT guidelines

From Dworkin RH, Turk DC, Farrar JT, et al. Core outcome measures for chronic pain clinical trials: IMMPACT recommendations. Pain 2005;113(1-2):11; with permission.

is recommended for physical conditioning and either the Beck Depression Inventory or the Profile of Mood States for emotional functioning. For participant disposition, IMMPACT recommended a detailed information on the participant's recruitment and progress as recommended through a flow diagram.

Patient satisfaction embodies all the recommended outcome domains and its measurement is essential in pain studies, whether chronic, acute, or postoperative in nature. Health care organizations commonly use patient satisfaction in their evaluation of their departments and in their marketing to the public. In addition, it has particular significance in affecting clinical outcome, patient retention, medical reimbursement, and medical malpractice claims.

There are measurement tools for the outcome domains noted earlier that are specific for certain chronic pain syndromes, that is, low back pain, fibromyalgia, neuropathic pain, or cancer pain. It is beyond the scope of this article to discuss these tools in detail.

OUTCOME MEASUREMENT TOOLS IN ACUTE PAIN STUDIES

Similar to chronic pain, studies on acute pain should look not only at pain and its management, and adverse events from the intervention, but also at physical and emotional components and patient satisfaction.

Pain is most commonly assessed by patients' self-report with either a visual analog or a numeric rating scale. For adverse events, in addition to the usual side effects such as nausea, vomiting, sedation, and pruritus, some multidimensional measurement tools assess side effects in more detail. Most of the tools observe the degree of the patient's sedation (eg, Observer's Assessment of Alertness/Sedation Scale),[3] sleep quality or interference (Pittsburgh Sleep Quality Index),[4] or the presence of delirium.[5] The Opioid-Related Symptoms Distress Scale assesses symptoms related to opioid intake including difficulty passing urine, headache, feeling of lightheadedness, fatigue, or weakness.[6] The Mini-Mental Status examination has been used as a measure of sedation as well as the cognitive ability of the patient.[7] No single assessment tool is designed to assess all the side effects; rather, they mostly focus on a specific side effect.

The measurement tools on physical functioning include the measurement of activities of daily living, six-minute walking test,[8,9] mobilization scores, Constant Murley Score, the Disability of the Arm, Shoulder, Hand Score for surgery on the shoulder, and the International Knee Documentation Committee Activity Levels for operations on the knee.[10,11] The multidimensional tools Medical Outcomes Study Short Form-36 (SF-36),[12] SF-12,[13] and SF-8[14] also measure physical conditioning.

Emotional functioning is the least studied outcome domain in postoperative pain studies. The measurement tools include simple VAS and Likert scales as well as more detailed tools for assessing anxiety. Examples of the commonly used tools include the State Trait Anxiety Inventory[15] and Yale Preoperative Anxiety Scale[16] that measure anxiety and the Profile of Mood States. The Profile of Mood States, a tool recommended by the IMMPACT group, assesses the aspects of mood and also provides a summary measure of total mood disturbance.[17]

The popular multidimensional assessment tools include the McGill Pain Questionnaire (MPQ),[18] the SF-36[12] and its modifications SF-12[13] and SF-8,[14] the modified Brief Pain Inventory (BPI),[19] and the EuroQoL 5-D.[20] All have very good psychometric properties. Although they were not designed or validated for use in the immediate postoperative period, these tools have been used in postoperative pain studies. None of the multidimensional measurement tools assess all the 5 domains (**Table 1**).[21,22] If the

MPQ is used, then tools for physical conditioning, adverse events, and patient satisfaction are added. For the SF-36 variant, BPI, and European Quality of Life 5-Dimensions (EuroQol 5-D), a tool for satisfaction is added and adverse events noted.

The multidimensional Quality of Recovery (QoR) instruments were validated and have been used extensively in postoperative pain studies. Myles and colleagues[23] developed a series of QoR scores for postoperative pain (**Table 1**). The longer form, QoR-40, has 5 dimensions: physical comfort, emotional state, physical independence, psychological support, and pain. The shorter form, QoR-15, was developed to lighten the administrative burden.[24] Similar to the other complex tools, it does not assess patient satisfaction, so this has to be added in the evaluation of postoperative pain.

Another sophisticated measurement tool designed for postoperative studies is the International Pain Outcome (IPO) questionnaire.[25] The IPO questionnaire is a European Commission–funded project called PAIN OUT. Its subscales include pain intensity and interference, adverse effects, and perceptions of care including participation in decision-making and satisfaction with pain treatment.[25] As such, the IPO measures all the domains recommended by the IMMPACT group.[21]

MEASUREMENT TOOLS FOR PATIENT SATISFACTION IN POSTOPERATIVE PAIN RESEARCH

Studies on patient satisfaction after anesthesia used simple questions or validated measurement tools.[26] Simple measurement tools include satisfaction scores presented in the form of visual analog or Likert scale. Unfortunately, the reliability of these simple rating systems is unpredictable, because they fail to capture the manifold nature of satisfaction.[26] The Patient Global Impression of Change is commonly used in studies to signify patient satisfaction. However, it does not measure satisfaction. Rather, the patient comments on his/her overall status whether it is unchanged, improved, or worsened.

Table 1
Outcome domains covered by the sophisticated measurement tools

Tool	Pain	Physical Functioning	Emotional Functioning	Side Effects	Satisfaction
BPI	+	+	+		
MPQ	+		+		
SF-36	+	+	+		
SF-12	+	+	+		
SF-8	+	+	+		
EuroQoL 5-D	+	+	+		
QoR-40	+	+	+	+	
QoR-15	+	+	+	+	
APS-POQ-R	+	+	+	+	+
IPO	+	+	+	+	+

Abbreviations: APS-POQ-R, American Pain Society Patient Outcome Questionnaire-Revised; BPI, brief pain inventory; EuroQol 5-D, European Quality of Life 5-Dimensions; IPO, International Pain Outcome questionnaire; MPQ, McGill Pain Questionnaire; QoR, quality of recovery (QoR-40 and QoR-15 for the 40-item and 15-item questionnaire respectively); SF-36, Medical Outcomes Study Short Form-36 (SF-12 for 12 items; SF-8 for 8 items).

From Benzon HT, Mascha EJ, Wu CL. Studies on postoperative analgesic efficacy: Focusing the statistical methods and broadening outcome measures and measurement tools. Anesth Analg 2017;125(3):727; with permission.

Validated tools to measure patient satisfaction exist. One is the Iowa Satisfaction with Anesthesia Scale for monitored anesthesia care (MAC).[27] It should be noted that the tool measures patient satisfaction with their MAC anesthetic and not other aspects of the perioperative encounter.

Validated satisfaction tools are also available for patients undergoing general anesthesia. The Evaluation du Vécude l'AnesthésieGénérale (EVAN-G) questionnaire is designed for patients undergoing general anesthesia, whether ambulatory or inpatient.[28] A patient satisfaction questionnaire for anesthesia care, developed by investigators from Switzerland and Austria, contains items on information/involvement in decision-making, care in the recovery room, and pain management.[29] The Bauer questionnaire[30] consists of questions on anesthesia-discomfort and anesthesia care. The Bauer questionnaire was used in a large study on the outcome of perioperative anesthesia in the United Kingdom.[31] The EVAN-G and the patient satisfaction questionnaire from Switzerland and Austria have not been used frequently in postoperative pain studies. Similarly, the validated Leiden Perioperative Care Patient Satisfaction questionnaire[32] and the Patient Satisfaction with Perioperative Anesthetic Care questionnaire[33] are restricted by their regional applications (**Table 2**).

DETERMINANTS OF PATIENT SATISFACTION

The determinants of patient satisfaction are either patient-, provider-, and process-related.[34] Factors that are influenced by the patient include physical and psychological health, expectations, and sociodemographic factors. The social and personal characteristics encompass age, race, gender, culture and social class education, marital status, occupation, and income. Satisfaction is increased when the medical care matches up to the patient's expectations. Provider-associated considerations include competence (perceived vs observed) and verbal and nonverbal interactions with the patient. Empathy, length of the provider's visit, and the amount of information given influence patient's satisfaction. Those that are process-related include ancillary services, accessibility and convenience, cost, bureaucratic and environmental factors, and organization of health care.[34] Increased accessibility, shorter waiting times, and availability of the provider naturally improve patient satisfaction.

Table 2
Measurement tools for patient satisfaction

Measurement Tool	Comment
Visual analog or Likert scale	Simple, does not reflect complexity of satisfaction
Iowa Satisfaction with Anesthesia Scale	Appropriate for monitored anesthesia care
Evaluation du Vécude l'AnesthésieGénérale (EVAN-G)	Patients who have general anesthesia
Bauer Questionnaire	Questions on patient discomfort, preoperative visit, emergence from anesthesia, postoperative management of pain
Leiden Perioperative Care Patient Satisfaction Questionnaire	Regional application (Netherlands)
Patient Satisfaction with Perioperative Anesthetic Care Questionnaire	Regional application (Taiwan)

Patients who received epidural analgesia for labor pain expressed dissatisfaction during the following circumstances:

1. Instrument-assisted vaginal delivery;
2. Higher postepidural pain scores;
3. Replacement of the epidural catheter;
4. Placement of the epidural when the cervical dilation is more advanced; and
5. Occurrence of complications including headache, back ache, urinary retention, and neural deficit.[35]

In their study, the investigators observed that multiparous women had lower satisfaction scores than nulliparous women.

Surgical studies on patient satisfaction were related to the type of surgery. These include joint function, hip instability, leg length equality, and self-care after total joint surgery.[36,37] Range of motion, improvement in strength, and ability to perform activities of daily living were important after hand surgery.[38] Appearance after cosmetic surgery following a breast cancer operation was noted to be a major determinant.[39] In these[36–38] and other[40] surgical publications, patient education, inclusion in the decision process, and empathy of the provider significantly affected patient satisfaction.

Although surgical studies showed that the presence of complications increased patient dissatisfaction, a study by Brown and colleagues[41] noted that the occurrence of adverse intraoperative anesthetic events did not affect patient satisfaction. In their investigation, the patients who had airway management difficulties (laryngospasm, difficult intubation, dental injury, aspiration) or those who had cardiovascular events (hyper/hypotension, arrhythmia, myocardial ischemia) had the same satisfaction scores as the patients who had no adverse intraoperative anesthesia-related side effects. In their analysis, the patients' positive interactions with the medical personnel outweighed their negative concerns. Patient's communication with their physicians and care givers are just as important as adverse events and results of surgery.

Information given to the patient before surgery and their involvement in decisions regarding their care are major determinants of patient satisfaction. In the IPO and APS-POQ-R questionnaires, the patients are asked whether they were given information on options for the treatment of their pain and whether they are allowed to participate in decisions regarding their pain management. Information provided to the patient and their involvement with their care have been noted to be the most important dimensions in patient satisfaction.[29,32]

ROLE OF SOCIOECONOMIC STATUS IN PATIENT OUTCOMES AND SATISFACTION

Socioeconomic status is intimately linked with race. Hence, the effect of socioeconomic status on outcomes and patient satisfaction are discussed. Socioeconomic status has an impact on health care experience from access to care to self-rated health, with the presence of a single social problem associated with a decrease in overall health.[42] Health disparities exist particularly for low-income patients.

LaPar and colleagues[43] reviewed outcomes for patients undergoing 8 types of major surgery. Significant differences were noted in resource utilization, with Medicaid patients having the longest adjusted hospital lengths of stay and highest total costs.[43] They found that Medicaid and uninsured payer status conferred worse unadjusted and adjusted outcomes when compared with private insurance status. Medicaid and uninsured status was independently associated with increased risk of adjusted in-hospital mortality. Medicaid status was also associated with increased risk of adjusted in-hospital complications compared with private insurance. The cause for worse medical outcomes was likely multifactorial. Elective operations were more common for Medicare and private insurance patients, whereas Medicaid and uninsured patients more commonly underwent nonelective, emergent operations with less preoperative optimization.[43] Access to skilled and experienced surgeons also may have differed by insurance status. In addition, Medicaid and uninsured patients had the highest incidence of drug and alcohol abuse, and Medicaid patients had the highest incidence of AIDS, metastatic cancer, depression, liver disease, neurologic disorders, and psychoses.[43] Socioeconomic and lifestyle differences, language barriers, education, poor nutrition, and psychiatric illness likely contribute to differences in comorbid conditions, ability to seek and access to care, lack of health maintenance, and delay in diagnosis and treatment.

In a retrospective study by Maly and Vallerand,[44] lower income was associated with a greater incidence of experiencing difficulty accessing care, poor communication with health care providers, limited shared decision-making, delays in health care delivery, and poor satisfaction with care.[44] In addition, low socioeconomic status has been associated with a more negative experience of pain. Limited access to primary care, homelessness, low employment status or physically demanding jobs, increased risk of pain-related injury, and inadequate insurance coverage are all possible contributing factors. Prescription medication costs can lead to nonfilling of prescriptions and to missed medication doses or poor medication adherence in order to stretch prescription duration.[44] Pharmacies in socioeconomically depressed communities may also have limited availability of certain prescription medications.

Understanding the gaps in health care experience for low-income patients can help target strategies for improving care.[45] Factors at the patient, provider, and health system levels all affect care. Targeting health literacy may improve communication and shared decision-making and enhance patient engagement. Improving transportation or advancements in electronic communication and remote telemedicine may improve access to care. Changing the metrics used for hospital performance for reimbursement for hospitals with large low-income patient populations may improve the health care resources those hospitals are able to provide to their patient population.

ROLE OF ETHNICITY/RACIAL IDENTITY

Patients' values, ratings, and reports regarding primary care physicians' performance vary by race and ethnicity. A cross-sectional study of patients enrolled in a large health maintenance organization evaluated patient survey responses regarding physician performance in several dimensions of primary care: technical competence, communication, accessibility, prevention and health promotion, and overall satisfaction.[46] The investigators noted that Asian patients rated their physician's performance less favorably than white patients, and Hispanic patients reported less accessibility than white patients. Black enrollees rated their physician's promotion of lifestyle and psychosocial health higher than whites, whereas Pacific Islanders were noted receiving more health prevention services than whites.

In a major study from the RAND corporation, Agency for Healthcare Research and Quality, Center for Outcomes and Effectiveness Research, Henry J. Kaiser Foundation, and the Center for Medicare and Medicaid Services data collected from the Consumer Assessment of Health Plans Surveys (CAHPS) were summarized into 5 composite groups: receiving needed care, receiving care quickly, doctor communication, helpfulness of office staff, and customer service.[47] All minority groups (blacks, Hispanics, Asians) reported greater difficulty with access to and less use of health care. African American patients rated doctors and care higher than non-Hispanic white patients, whereas Asian American patients rated doctors and care lower than non-Hispanic white patients. Differences in ratings between racial and ethnic groups varied across health plans.

Because health care–related beliefs, practices, and values differ between racial/ethnic groups, Collins and colleagues[48] used data from CAHPS to look further at the relative importance of each of 5 composite domains: doctor communication, getting needed care, getting care quickly, customer service (courtesy and respect of customer service of plan, assist with information, ease of filling health care forms), and care coordination. These 5 domains varied across racial/ethnic and language subgroups. For non-Hispanic whites and English-preferring Hispanics, doctor communication correlated best with care ratings. For African Americans, doctor communication and getting care quickly had the strongest impact. Getting needed care correlated best with care ratings for Spanish language preferring Hispanics and Asian American patients.[48]

In the Veterans Administration system, black and Hispanic patients with osteoarthritis were noted to receive less analgesics and nonsteroidal antiinflammatory drugs than white patients, and they were less likely to be referred for joint replacement surgeries.[49] The reason for these disparities is multifactorial but involves factors at the patient, provider, and health system levels. Communication, language, trust, expectation of treatment outcome, patient provider rapport, access to care, and availability of medication affect the pain care experience. In a study of veterans who participated in the VA Survey of the Healthcare Experiences of Patients, Dobscha and colleagues[49] noted that male and female Hispanic veterans or non-Hispanic blacks were more likely to report receiving treatment of chronic pain compared with non-Hispanic white veterans. Among the veterans who received chronic pain treatment, non-Hispanic black men were less likely to rate their treatment as excellent or very good, compared with non-Hispanic white male veterans.[49] These differences could be because of variations in pain treatment, including procedural interventions and prescribed medications, between facilities or between ethnic groups. In addition, treatment expectations may vary between ethnic groups as well as pain-related anxiety, fear avoidance activity, and knowledge of procedures for treatment, which can all affect treatment effectiveness.[49]

A systematic literature review by Mehta and colleagues[50] also found that although osteoarthritis affects 45% of the white and African American population within the United States, a lower use of total hip arthroplasty persisted among African American patients when compared with white patients.[50] African American and white patients were equally referred for arthroplasty by a provider, so the reason for this disparity is unclear but may be partly due to patient preferences. Low expectations for arthroplasty outcome and preference for nontraditional interventions such as massage and prayer by blacks were considered possible factors in the disparity of total hip arthroplasty use.[50] Although there was no difference in complications, the African American patients reported more pain and poorer functional status than the white patients. Less satisfaction, more fear, and anxiety were also noted among African American patients following total hip arthroplasty.[50]

In addition, Goodman and colleagues[51] found that total knee arthroplasty (TKA) use is also lower among African American patients when compared with white patients who receive referrals for arthroplasty. Similarly African American patients reported worse pain and function following TKA in 4 of 7 studies, as well as less satisfaction than white patients.[51] Of note, African American patients are reported to have worse preoperative pain scores than whites and delay their TKA longer, presenting with more advanced arthritis than white patients, which may account for the differences in outcome.[51]

A 2009 review reported the persistence of racial and ethnic disparities in acute, chronic, cancer and palliative care across the life span and treatment settings.[52] The investigators noted that minorities receive lesser quality pain care than non-Hispanic whites. This is compounded by an absence of solutions to these disparities in public health agendas and health care reform plans.[52]

With a health care system increasingly focused on equitable and patient-centered care, identifying and eliminating ethnic and racial disparities has been a priority and the focus of recent research. There seems to be some positive results in these efforts. A prospective cohort study by Berlin and colleagues[53] found that following reconstructive surgery for breast cancer, African American patients reported equivalent or better outcomes in terms of psychosocial and sexual well-being than white patients.[53] Hispanic patients experienced fewer clinical complications following surgery.[53] The results were notable in that the African American women had higher body mass index (BMI) and lower levels of education, and the Latina women were less educated and reported lower income levels than the white women cohort. It should be noted, however, that in this study, African American women underwent more unilateral procedures and Hispanic women were younger than their white counterparts. Also, the non-white patients were fewer in number than the white patients: 6% blacks, 5.5% Hispanic, and 6% other minority groups compared with 83% whites.[53]

Studies similar to that of Berlin and colleagues involving other surgical and medical situations and with larger numbers are needed. Improving health care coverage and physician numbers might help to address receiving needed care and receiving care quickly. Doctor communication improvements might target encounter time, health lifestyle promotion, language, or cultural barriers.[46] Determining the relative importance of certain domains (accessibility, communication, physician competence, lifestyle health promotion) and tailoring of specific improvements to an appropriate patient population allows improvements in health care experience to be tailored to the specific patient mix being cared for.

ROLE OF GENDER

Investigations into the effect of gender solely on patient satisfaction are few. One study showed that female gender and increased age are associated with higher satisfaction.[54] With regard to outcomes, studies have noted that women report inferior patient-related outcomes related to satisfaction, health-related quality of life (HRQoL), and pain levels after both medical and surgical interventions, including vascular and orthopedic surgeries. This may be partly related to preoperative factors.

Two studies looked into the HRQoL after myocardial infarction (MI) or cardiac ischemic event. In a study from Sweden, the investigators noted that women had significantly lower self-reported QoL after MI than men.[55] This was despite similar baseline variables, including age, smoking, concomitant cardiovascular disease, revascularization rate, and hemodynamic and laboratory data. Treatment variables were also the same. The investigators were unable to explain the differences in the results between the 2 genders. In a study from Alberta, Canada, which examined HRQoL 1 year after their initial catheterization, men had significantly better QoL along 5 dimensions of the HRQoL instrument (exertional capacity, angina stability, angina frequency, QoL, and treatment satisfaction) after adjusting for patient comorbidities, demographics, and disease severity predictors of outcome.[56]

Two studies also noted differences between male and female patients who underwent treatment of atrial fibrillation (AF). A study in Europe showed that women patients were older, had more medical comorbidities, lower QoL, more often had heart failure with preserved left ventricular systolic function, and less often had heart failure with systolic dysfunction.[57] The women patients who had no or atypical symptoms were appropriately treated more conservatively with less rhythm control. Although the 1-year outcome was the same, the women patients had a higher chance for stroke than men. Another study, the Rate Control versus Electrical Cardioversion study showed that female patients had more AF-related complaints and lower QoL than their male counterparts.[57] In addition, the female patients who had rhythm control had higher incidences of heart failure, adverse events from the antiarrhythmic drugs, and thromboembolic complications than the female patients who were randomized to rate control. The QoL of the female patients was lower than that of men during their follow-up.[58]

In a study of vascular surgery patients with peripheral vascular disease, investigators from the Netherlands noted that women had worse physical health, more disability, and worse overall health status 3 years after their vascular surgery.[59] However, both genders reported similar health status levels at their 5-year follow-up. In this study, and interestingly at baseline, the male cohorts had higher prevalence of ischemic heart disease, MI, and previous revascularization and underwent more open procedures.

In a retrospective study after elective lumbar spine surgery, Elsamadicy and colleagues[60] determined whether there was a difference in 3-month and 1-year patient-reported outcomes and satisfaction between male and female patients.[60] Baseline patient demographics such as age, race, BMI, and education level; comorbidities such as diabetes, coronary artery disease, smoking status, and American Society of Anesthesiologists status, and operative variables including approach type and operative time were similar between the male and female cohorts, with the exception of a higher prevalence of coronary artery disease among the male patients. The female patients had slightly longer hospital stays compared with the male cohort. At 1-year follow-up, the male patients had a significantly greater mean change in visual analog scale for back pain and for EuroQol scores and a greater percentage of patients reported that the surgery met their expectations.[60] Some factors that may account for these differences include longer pain histories, greater leg and back pain, greater degree of disability, and lower QoL scores preoperatively, as well as greater postoperative pain scores for the women patients.[60]

The same inferior results were noted after total joint surgery. Two studies showed that women had higher rates of obesity, more preoperative pain, and consulted a physician later than men.[61,62] The reason for their delayed surgery seems to be "physician bias" wherein their doctors were less likely to recommend surgery, offered less information, and were less encouraged to participate in the decision-making process.[63] In the patients who had surgery, the female patients received more blood transfusions and had a longer hospital stay.[61] Although their outcome at 6 months, in terms of pain and function, was worse than men, the results at 12 months were the same.[62]

Regarding total hip arthroplasty, studies showed that male patients had increased risk of 30-day adverse events including return to the operating room, surgical site infection, cardiac arrest, and death.[64] However, men had lower overall adverse events because of higher risk of blood transfusion and urinary tract infection in women.[64] Similar functional improvements were noted at 5 years.[65]

In an effort to examine factors that most influence patient satisfaction among male and female patients after total hip replacement, Delanois and colleagues[66] analyzed the satisfaction scores to determine which factors are more germane for each

Table 3
Selected studies on the effect of socioeconomic status, race, and gender on patient satisfaction

	Comment
Socioeconomic status	
LaPar et al,[43] 2010	Medicaid and uninsured patients increased the risk of adjusted in-hospital mortality
Maly and Vallerand,[44] 2018	Low status associated with difficulty accessing care, poor communication with providers, limited shared decision-making, delay in health care delivery, and poor satisfaction
Ethnicity/Race	
Lurie et al,[47] 2003	Blacks, Hispanics, Asians had greater difficulty accessing and using health care
Dobscha et al,[49] 2009	Blacks and Hispanics received less analgesics and nonsteroidal antiinflammatory drugs
Mehta et al,[50] 2018	Lower use of total hip arthroplasty for blacks compared with whites
Goodman et al,[51] 2016	Blacks had worse pain and function and satisfaction after total knee replacement
Anderson et al,[52] 2009	Minorities received lesser quality pain care than whites
Gender	Studies showed female patients to have inferior health-related QoL results compared with men. This was true with medical (MI, AF) conditions and surgical (orthopedic) interventions (see text).[55–62]

gender.[66] They used the Press Ganey measures of satisfaction outcomes based on domains including communication with hospital staff, staff responsiveness, hospital environment, communication about medications, and pain management. Their analysis found that for the male cohort, pain management had the greatest influence on hospital rating, whereas staff responsiveness, followed by communication with nurses and doctors, had the greatest influence on overall hospital rating for the female cohort.[66] Based on this limited study there seem to be different motivators for male and female patients.

SUMMARY

The measurement of patient outcomes, pain, and satisfaction involve the examination of important outcome domains and the use of measurement tools with proven adequate psychometric properties. Studies noted that blacks and minorities with lower socioeconomic status have greater difficulty accessing and using good quality care, are given less information, and are less likely to be involved in the decision-making process regarding their treatment. Women have poor premedical or surgical intervention risk factors, partly explaining worse outcomes that they experience. Women are also given less information and are not as encouraged to participate in decisions regarding their care. Health policy makers should note the effects of socioeconomic status, race, and gender on patients' outcomes and make appropriate recommendations to ameliorate this solvable disparity (**Table 3**).

DISCLOSURE

Dr N. Kozlov and Dr H.T. Benzon have nothing to disclose.

REFERENCES

1. Turk DC, Dworkin RH, Allen RR, et al. Core outcome domains for chronic pain clinical trials: IMMPACT recommendations. Pain 2003;106:337–45.
2. Dworkin RH, Turk DC, Farrar JT, et al. Core outcome measures for chronic pain clinical trials: IMMPACT recommendations. Pain 2005;113:9–19.
3. Chernick DA, Gillings D, Laine H, et al. Validity and reliability of the Observer's Assessment of Alertness/Sedation Scale: study with intravenous midazolam. J ClinPsychopharmacol 1990;10:244–51.
4. Buysse DJ, Reynolds CF, Monk TH, et al. The Pittsburgh Sleep Quality Index: a new instrument for psychiatric practice and research. PsychiatryRes 1989;28:193–213.
5. Trepacz PT, Baker RW, Greenhouse J. A symptom rating scale for delirium. J Psychiatr Res 1988;23:89–97.
6. Apfelbaum JL, Gan TJ, Zhao S, et al. Reliability and validity of the perioperative opioid-related symptom distress scale. AnesthAnalg 2004;99:699–709.
7. Tombaugh TN, McIntyre NJ. The mini-mental state examination: a comprehensive review. J Am GeriatrSoc 1992;40:922–35.
8. ATS Committee on Proficiency Standards for Clinical Pulmonary Function Laboratories. ATS statement: guidelines for the six-minute walk test. Am J RespirCritCare Med 2002;166:111–7.
9. Ilfeld BM, Le LT, Meyer RS, et al. Ambulatory continuous femoral nerve block decrease time to discharge readiness after tricompartment total knee arthroplasty. Anesthesiology 2008;108:703–13.
10. Germann G, Harth A, Wind G, et al. Standardisation and validation of the German version 2.0 of the disability of arm, shoulder, hand (DASH) questionnaire. Unfallchirurg 2003;106:13–9.
11. Constant CR, Murley AH. A clinical method of functional assessment of the shoulder. ClinOrthopRelat Res 1987;(214):160–4.
12. Ware JE Jr, Snow KK, Kosinski M, et al. SF-36 health survey: manual and interpretation guide. Boston: Health Institute, New Engl Medical Center; 1993.
13. Ware J, Kosinski M, Keller SD. A 12-item short-form health survey: construction of scales and preliminary test of reliability and validity. Med Care 1996;34:220–34.
14. Ware JE, Kosinski M, Dewey JE, et al. How to score and interpret single-item health status measures: a manual for users of the SF-8 health survey. Lincoln (RI): Quality Metric Inc.; 2001.
15. Julian LJ. Measures of anxiety: state-trait anxiety inventory (STAI), beck anxiety inventory (BAI), and hospital anxiety and depression scale-anxiety (HADS-A). ArthritisCare Res (Hoboken) 2011;63(Suppl11):S467–72.
16. Kain ZN, Mayes LC, Cicchetti DV, et al. The yale preoperative anxiety scale; how does it compare with a "gold standard"? AnesthAnalg 1999;85:783–8.
17. McNair DM, Lorr M, Droppleman LF. Profile of mood states. San Diego (CA): Educational and Industrial Testing Service; 1971.
18. Melzack R. The short-form McGill pain questionnaire. Pain 1987;30:191–7.
19. Cleeland CS, Ryan KM. Pain assessment: global use of the brief pain inventory. Ann Acad Med Singapore 1994;23:129–38.
20. Brooks R. EuroQoL: the current state of play. Health Policy 1996;37:53–72.
21. Benzon HT, Mascha E, Wu C. Studies on postoperative analgesic efficacy: focusing the statistical methods and broadening outcome measures and measurement tools. AnesthAnalg 2017;125:726–8.

22. Benzon HT, Dunn L, Tran De. I can't get no (patient) satisfaction. AnesthAnalg 2019;128:393–5.
23. Myles P, Weitkamp B, Jones K, et al. Validity and reliability of a postoperative quality of recovery score: the QoR-40. Br J Anaesth 2000;84:11–5.
24. Stark PA, Myles PS, Burke JA. Development and psychometric evaluation of a postoperative quality of recovery score: the QoR-15. Anesthesiology 2013;118: 1332–40.
25. Rothaug J, Zaslansky R, Schwenkglenks M, et al. Patients' perception of postoperative pain management: validation of the International Pain Outcomes (IPO) questionnaire. J Pain 2013;14(11):1361–70.
26. Chanthong P, Abrishami A, Wong J, et al. Systematic review of questionnaires measuring patient satisfaction in ambulatory anesthesia. Anesthesiology 2009; 110:1061–7.
27. Dexter F, Aker J, Wright WA. Development of a measure of patient satisfaction with monitored anesthesia care: the Iowa Satisfaction with Anesthesia Scale. Anesthesiology 1997;87:865–73.
28. Auquier P, Pernoud N, Bruder N, et al. Development and validation of a perioperative satisfaction questionnaire. Anesthesiology 2005;102:1116–23.
29. Heidegger T, Huseman Y, Nuebling Y, et al. Patient satisfaction with anaesthesia care: development of a psychometric questionnaire and benchmarking among six hospitals in Switzerland and Austria. Br J Anaesth 2002;89:863–72.
30. Bauer M, Böhrer H, Aichele G, et al. Measuring patient satisfaction with anaesthesia: perioperative questionnaire versus standardised face-to-face interview. ActaAnaesthesiolScand 2001;45:65–72.
31. Walker EMK, Bell M, Cook TM, et al. Central SNAP-1 Organisation, National Study Groups: patient reported outcome of adult perioperative anaesthesia in the United Kingdom: a cross-sectional observational study. Br J Anaesth 2016;117: 758–66.
32. Caljouw MA, van Beuzekom M, Boer F. Patient's satisfaction with perioperative care: development, validation, and application of a questionnaire. Br J Anaesth 2008;100:637–44.
33. Miu WC, Chang CM, Cheng KF, et al. Development and validation of the questionnaire of satisfaction with perioperative anesthetic care for general and regional anesthesia in Taiwanese patients. Anesthesiology 2011;114:1064–75.
34. Wu CL, Naqibuddin M, Fleisher LA. Measurement of patient satisfaction as an outcome of regional anesthesia and analgesia: a systematic review. RegAnesth-Pain Med 2001;26:196–208.
35. Tan DJA, Sultana R, Han NLR, et al. Investigating determinants for patient satisfaction in women receiving epidural analgesia for labour pain: a retrospective cohort study. BMC Anesthesiol 2018;18:50.
36. Kahlenberg CA, Nwachukwu BU, McLawhorn AS, et al. Patient satisfaction after total knee replacement: a systematic review. HSS J 2018;14:192–201.
37. Ding L, Gao YH, Li YR, et al. Determinants of satisfaction following total hip arthroplasty in patients with ankylosing spondylitis. IntOrthop 2018;42:507–11.
38. Marks M, Herren DB, VlietVlieland TPMV, et al. Determinants of patient satisfaction after orthopedic interventions to the hand: a review of the literature. J HandTher 2011;24:303–12.
39. Ho PJ. Determinants of satisfaction with cosmetic outcome in breast cancer survivors: a cross-sectional study. PLoS One 2018;13(2):e0193099.

40. Best JT, Musgrave B, Pratt K, et al. The impact of scripted pain education on patient satisfaction in outpatient abdominal surgery patients. J PerianesthNurs 2018;33:453–60.
41. Brown DL, Warner ME, Schroeder DR, et al. Effect of intraoperative anesthetic events on postoperative patient satisfaction. MayoClinProc 1997;72:20–5.
42. Kretsoulas C, Hassan A, Subramanian SV, et al. Social disparities among youth and the impact on their health. AdolescHealth Med Ther 2015;26(6):37–45.
43. LaPar DJ, Bhamidipati CM, Mery CM, et al. Primary payer status affects mortality for major surgical operations. Ann Surg 2010;252:544–50.
44. Maly A, Vallerand AH. Neighborhood, socioeconomic, and racial influence on chronic pain. PainManagNurs 2018;19:14–22.
45. Okunrintemi V, Khera R, Spatz ES, et al. Association of income disparities with patient-reported healthcare experience. J Gen Intern Med 2019;34(6):884–92.
46. Murray-García JL, Selby JV, Schmittdiel J, et al. Racial and ethnic differences in a patient survey: patients' values, ratings, and reports regarding physician primary care performance in a large health maintenance organization. Med Care 2000;38:300–10.
47. Lurie N, Zhan C, Sangl J, et al. Variation in racial and ethnic differences in consumer assessments of health care. Am J ManagCare 2003;9:502–9.
48. Collins RL, Haas A, Haviland AM, et al. What matters most to whom: racial, ethnic, and language differences in the health care experiences most important to patients. Med Care 2017;55:940–7.
49. Dobscha SK, Soleck GD, Dickinson KC, et al. Associations between race and ethnicity and treatment for chronic pain in the VA. J Pain 2009;10:1078–87.
50. Mehta BY, Bass AR, Goto R, et al. Disparities in outcomes for blacks versus whites undergoing total hip arthroplasty: a systematic literature review. J Rheumatol 2018;45:717–22.
51. Goodman SM, Parks ML, McHugh K, et al. Disparities in outcomes for African Americans and whites undergoing total knee arthroplasty: a systematic literature review. J Rheumatol 2016;43:765–70.
52. Anderson KO, Green CR, Payne R. Racial and ethnic disparities in pain: causes and consequences of unequal care. J Pain 2009;10:1187–204.
53. Berlin NL, Momoh AO, Qi J, et al. Racial and ethnic variations in one-year clinical and patient-reported outcomes following breast reconstruction. Am J Surg 2017;214:312–7.
54. Hall JA, Feldstein M, Fretwell MD, et al. Older patients' health status and satisfaction with medical care in an HMO population. Med Care 1990;28:261–70.
55. Agewall S, Berglund M, Henareh L. Reduced quality of life after myocardial infarction in women compared with men. ClinCardiol 2004;27:271–4.
56. Norris CM, Ghali WA, Galbraith PD, et al. Women with coronary artery disease report worse health related quality of life outcomes compared to men. HealthQualLifeOutcomes 2004;2:1.
57. Dagres N, Nieuwlaat R, Vardas PE, et al. Gender-related differences in presentation, treatment, and outcome of patients with atrial fibrillation in Europe: a report from the Euro Heart Survey on Atrial Fibrillation. J Am CollCardiol 2007;49:572–7.
58. Rienstra M, Van Veldhuisen DJ, Hagens VE, et al. Gender-related differences in rhythm control treatment in persistent atrial fibrillation: data of the Rate Control Versus Electrical Cardioversion (RACE) study. J Am CollCardiol 2005;45:1298–306.

59. Mastenbroek MH, Hoeks SE, Pedersen SS, et al. Gender disparities in disease-specific health status in postoperative patients with peripheral arterial disease. Eur J VascEndovascSurg 2012;43:433–40.
60. Elsamadicy AA, Reddy GB, Nayar G, et al. Impact of gender disparities on short-term and long-term patient reported outcomes and satisfaction measures after elective lumbar spine surgery: a single institutional study of 384 patients. World-Neurosurg 2017;107:952–8.
61. Whitlock KG, Piponov HI, Shah SH, et al. Gender role in total knee arthroplasty: a retrospective analysis of perioperative outcomes in US patients. J Arthroplasty 2016;31:2736–40.
62. Mehta SP, Perruccio AV, Palaganas M, et al. Do women have poorer outcomes following total knee replacement? Osteoarthritis Cartilage 2015;23:1476–82.
63. Borkhoff CM, Hawker GA, Kreder HJ, et al. Influence of patients' gender on informed decision making regarding total knee arthroplasty. ArthritisCare Res (Hoboken) 2013;65:1281–90.
64. Basques BA, Bell JA, Sershon RA, et al. The influence of patient gender on morbidity following total hip or total knee arthroplasty. J Arthroplasty 2018;33: 345–9.
65. Cherian JJ, Jinnah AH, Robinson K, et al. Prospective, longitudinal evaluation of gender differences after total hip arthroplasty. Orthopedics 2016;39:e391–6.
66. Delanois RE, Gwam CU, Mistry JB, et al. Does gender influence how patients rate their patient experience after total hip arthroplasty? HipInt 2018;28:40–3.

Effects of Gender and Race/Ethnicity on Perioperative Team Performance

Rebecca D. Minehart, MD, MSHPEd[a,*], Erica Gabrielle Foldy, PhD[b]

KEYWORDS

• Diversity • Perioperative teams • Gender • Race/ethnicity • Psychological safety
• Speaking up • Conflict

KEY POINTS

- Team-based research on gender and race diversity has shown mixed results within organizational behavior literature.
- Current models that attempt to explain the effects of diversity on team performance take into account communication problems and interpersonal conflict, both salient to perioperative teams.
- Deliberate strategies are proposed to reduce the negative effects of diversity on communication and conflict, and to moderate hierarchy to encourage speaking up.

INTRODUCTION

By necessity, perioperative teams comprise a multiprofessional group of health care providers. It is well established that teamwork in these types of teams is directly linked to patient safety outcomes[1] and is vulnerable to coordination challenges and outright "coordination neglect," given the number of different specialists needed to care for patients.[2] The high-intensity environment of some procedural disciplines can exacerbate preexisting unhealthy teamwork dynamics, such that the American Heart Association issued a scientific statement on the potentially deadly impact of failures in communication, coordination, and conflict management resulting from poor teamwork.[3] Preexisting stereotypes can also feed into team disharmony, and although teamwork depends on a multitude of factors, the impact of demographic diversity in perioperative teams remains largely overlooked. From extensive research in organizational behavior, diversity in teams can lead to both positive and negative results.[4] This article

[a] Department of Anesthesia, Critical Care and Pain Medicine, Massachusetts General Hospital, 55 Fruit Street, GRJ 440, Boston MA 02114, USA; [b] Wagner School of Public Service, New York University, 295 Lafayette Street, New York, NY 10012, USA
* Corresponding author.
E-mail address: rminehart@mgh.harvard.edu
Twitter: @RDMinehart (R.D.M.)

Anesthesiology Clin 38 (2020) 433–447
https://doi.org/10.1016/j.anclin.2020.01.013 **anesthesiology.theclinics.com**
1932-2275/20/

considers what it means to have diversity in perioperative teams, and how to best harness the positive side of diversity while avoiding prejudice, stereotyping, and division among team members, which ultimately puts patients at risk.

Addressing coordination neglect on perioperative teams is largely a function of how team members communicate and coordinate with each other.[5] An emerging concept, "collaborative competence," which is described as a "relational phenomenon" that refers to the "distributed capacity" of a team to support each other,[6] underscores the role of interpersonal connections in teams. How team members relate to each other is determined in part by who they are, their clinical experiences and expertise, and their unique life experiences, which are shaped by many factors, including their social identities, such as gender, race and ethnicity, and age. How these characteristics influence life experiences can be subtle and complex. In addition, how team members relate to each other is also determined by how people judge each other, based on their outward characteristics and affiliation with certain groups. People react differently to each other based on whether the person they are interacting with is, for example, man or woman or nonbinary, black, white, Asian, or Hispanic, or clearly identified as part of a religious group (eg, wearing a hijab, yarmulke, nun's habit), to name a few examples.[7,8] Even now, societal norms are shifting with regard to how people define themselves, leading to emerging self-defining categories that affect people's experiences.[9]

Moreover, research has elaborated on how diversity brings with it issues of power, theorizing that certain forms of diversity, for example, racial and ethnic diversity, bring with them dynamics "driven by power imbalances related to those forms of diversity."[10] Power and hierarchy based not just on race and ethnicity but on gender and other social identities are elements traditionally embedded in the perioperative environment and deserve exploration for their strong influences on teamwork and information sharing (or "speaking up").[11]

Although there has been little research specifically on the influence of diversity on perioperative teamwork, we can look to other research in teams to glean insights, which can inform how we anticipate and work with the impacts of diversity in the perioperative setting. With this article, the authors review literature from organizational behavior, which has analyzed diversity and power dynamics in workplace teams for more than 50 years, to compare and contrast those findings with how perioperative teams work, offer solutions to best harness the benefits of diversity in teams, and share ideas on future areas of research to further the understanding of diversity and power dynamics in the perioperative environment.

DIVERSITY, POWER, AND HIERARCHY

Until 1998, there was little consensus on what constituted diversity.[4] Through their extensive review of 40 years of research, Williams Phillips and colleagues[4] took an approach to diversity, still influential today, to refer to any attributes that individuals can identify and determine as relevant or salient, in order to make distinctions between themselves and others. Research has investigated a variety of dimensions of diversity, from age, gender, and race to organizational tenure and educational or professional background[4]; a list of categories and types of diversity studied by researchers is found in **Box 1**.[12] The authors have chosen to review the literature with a focus on race/ethnicity and gender for several reasons.

First, both race/ethnicity and gender are strongly associated with power differences in medicine and health care. As seen in **Fig. 1**, the racial/ethnic and gender compositions of perioperative team members are vastly different, largely revealing that white men occupy physician roles and white women provide critical but supportive roles,

Box 1
Categories and types of diversity

Social-category differences
- Race
- Ethnicity
- Gender
- Age
- Religion
- Sexual orientation
- Physical abilities

Differences in knowledge or skills
- Education
- Functional knowledge
- Information or expertise
- Training
- Experience
- Abilities

Differences in values or beliefs
- Cultural background
- Ideological beliefs

Personality differences
- Cognitive style
- Affective disposition
- Motivational factors

Organizational- or community-status differences
- Tenure or length of service
- Title

Differences in social and network ties
- Work-related ties
- Friendship ties
- Community ties
- In-group memberships

From Mannix E, Neale MA. What differences make a difference? The Promise and Reality of Diverse Teams in Organizations. Psychol Sci Public Interest 2005;6(2):36; with permission.

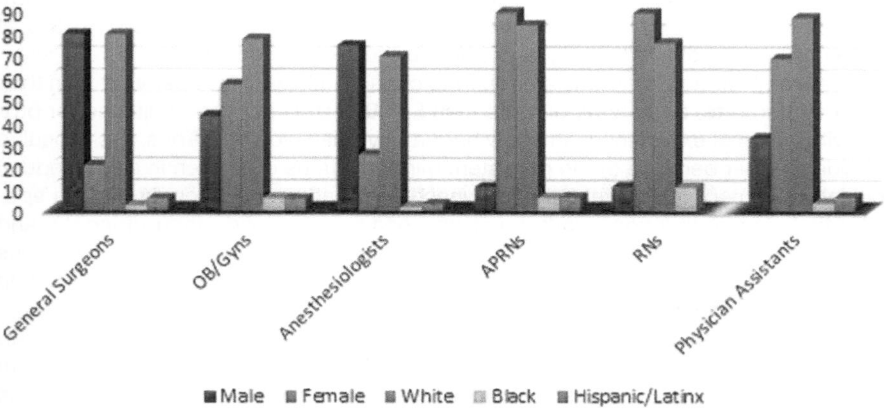

Fig. 1. Gender and racial/ethnic composition of perioperative team members. APRNs, advanced practice registered nurses; OB/Gyns, obstetricians and gynecologists; RNs, registered nurses. (*Data from* Refs.[13,15–17])

with very little representation of other races and ethnicities.[13–17] Recent reviews of clinical academic medical programs across 16 US medical specialties revealed greater underrepresentation of black and Hispanic physicians in 2016 as compared with 1990, with the sole exception of black women in obstetrics and gynecology. White female physicians were also underrepresented in many specialties.[18]

In the power structure in academic medicine, for decades researchers have demonstrated that underrepresented minority (including black, Mexican American, Puerto Rican, Native American, and Native Alaskan) academic medical school faculty are less likely to be promoted, even when adjusting for other factors,[19] and are more likely to leave the academic setting.[20] Minority faculty also report experiencing active bias and discrimination in the promotion process.[21] Bias and discrimination can have long-term impacts. A review of the Association of American Medical College's (AAMC) faculty data from 1997 to 2008 revealed that whites comprised almost 85% of professors, more than 88% of chairpersons, and more than 91% of deans of medical schools, and black physicians showed the smallest gains in career progress over this time period.[22] With titles come higher pay, and self-reported income was significantly lower for nonwhite female surgeons as compared with white female surgeons, with both groups earning less than white men and nonwhite men.[23] Diversity in health care providers matters and has the potential for great impact on health. A recent National Bureau of Economic Research working paper found black men were more likely to undergo preventative screenings when these were recommended by a black doctor, as compared with those randomized to see a non-black doctor, and their results extrapolated to a potential cardiovascular mortality benefit of 19%.[24]

Women also have discrepant rates of career progress, and even recognition for their roles, as campaigns such as the #HeforShe, #IlookLikeASurgeon, and #NYerORCoverChallenge campaigns have publicized.[25,26] In a recent study of academic medical faculty, significantly fewer women had been granted full-professor status as compared with men, and these gender differences persisted across all medical specialties.[27] This finding was upheld by Carr and colleagues[28] over a 17-year longitudinal study on women faculty's advancement, retention, and leadership, all worse than those for men. In general, there are fewer active physicians who are women, only 35.2% in 2017, and in the perioperative environment, women physicians are even less likely to be represented in most procedural specialties.[13] According to the AAMC's Physician Specialty Data Report, as of 2017, only 20.6% of women were practicing general surgeons, compared with 25.5% of anesthesiologists, 57.0% of obstetrician/gynecologists, and just 5.3% of orthopedic surgeons.[13]

Moreover, women physicians are found to consistently earn less per year than their male counterparts, to the tune of more than $18,000 USD per year (adjusted for productivity, years of experience, and how hard a physician works).[29] Thus, it is critical to consider gender because of the persistent minority status of women in all procedural specialties (except for obstetrics and gynecology, traditionally thought of as a specialty that demands longer work hours and heavier workloads than others[30]), and the discrepant financial compensation achieved by women in medicine. These gaps persist in the nursing literature as well, where male nurses average more than $6,000 USD per year than women.[31,32]

Leadership standing, such as institutional rank and high salary, are easily identified as sources of "power." The definition of "power" as used in this review is derived from Salancik and Pfeffer,[33] who described it as "...simply the ability to get things done the way one wants them to be done". Individuals in perioperative teams draw from a combination of these sources of power to exert their influence over others. Hierarchy itself has been conceptualized as "rank ordering of individuals along one or more socially important dimensions"[34] and is clearly related to power; thus, literature is included on the influence of hierarchy, whether very steep or more flattened, on team performance. The traditional hierarchy of the perioperative setting in US culture positions the attending surgeon squarely at the top of the pyramid, followed by the surgical resident or fellow, then the anesthesia provider, then the circulating nurse, and last, the "scrub person" (scrub nurse or surgical technician).[26]

Issues related to power are often the hardest for teams to address.[35] In fact, power is often the great "undiscussable" in work groups because such conversations can challenge those who decide what is discussed and what is not.[36] Adding race and gender to the mix only complicates matters.[37,38] The authors explore this issue further in later discussion, because it has serious implications for subordinates' information sharing and *speaking up*.[11,39]

TEAM PERFORMANCE AND THE ROLES OF COMMUNICATION PROBLEMS AND INTERPERSONAL CONFLICT

How do we think about overall performances of teams? In perioperative care, this could be defined in several meaningful ways, from efficiency and throughput of cases, to staff and faculty retention, to patient outcomes. One general model of work teams, suggested by Carter and Phillips,[40] denotes outcome measures like these as comprising an overall picture of "team performance." Team effectiveness as a model is influenced by group environment and group process as well as diversity and associated cognitive reactions (**Fig. 2** provides a model). The authors use this "dual-process pathway model of diversity" in order to predict the influence of diversity on perioperative work teams. It is outside the scope of this article to discuss all variables in this model, so especially salient ones are focused on for the perioperative environment under the category of group process, namely *communication problems* and *interpersonal conflict*, and how diversity influences these to inhibit team performance by limiting problem-solving and creativity is considered.

Communication errors continue to plague health care, consistently ranking within the top 3 root causes of almost all sentinel events reported to the Joint Commission (where patients suffer severe morbidity or even die because of errors).[41] A major contributor to communication errors relates to the team's psychological safety.[42] Psychological safety has been defined as a "shared belief that the team is safe for interpersonal risk-taking" and, while it is rooted in mutual respect and trust, it refers to a team-level construct rather than interpersonal relationships among individual members.[11,39] This concept is essential to team processes, particularly communication, to mitigate or avoid errors, because team members have to overcome some degree of interpersonal risk in order to *speak up*, particularly to their superiors.[42] In general, leaders influence psychological safety to a great deal, which in turn affects how team members communicate and coordinate.[11]

Robbins[43] described conflict as "any kind of opposition or antagonistic interaction between two or more parties," a definition still used today. There are generally 3 types of conflict, categorized according to the subject of the conflict: *task*, *relationship*, and *process*. *Task conflict* is focused fundamentally on the work itself, either the content or the intended outcomes. *Relationship conflict* involves issues related to people's personal characteristics and work styles. *Process conflict* deals with the process of doing the work, for example, the division of labor or free-riding (eg, putting no effort into the work but gaining benefit from it).[44] Although many theories exist regarding the role of conflict in groups, the authors adopt a "managed conflict" view, which posits that conflict may or may not be helpful to teams, but should be promptly resolved in productive

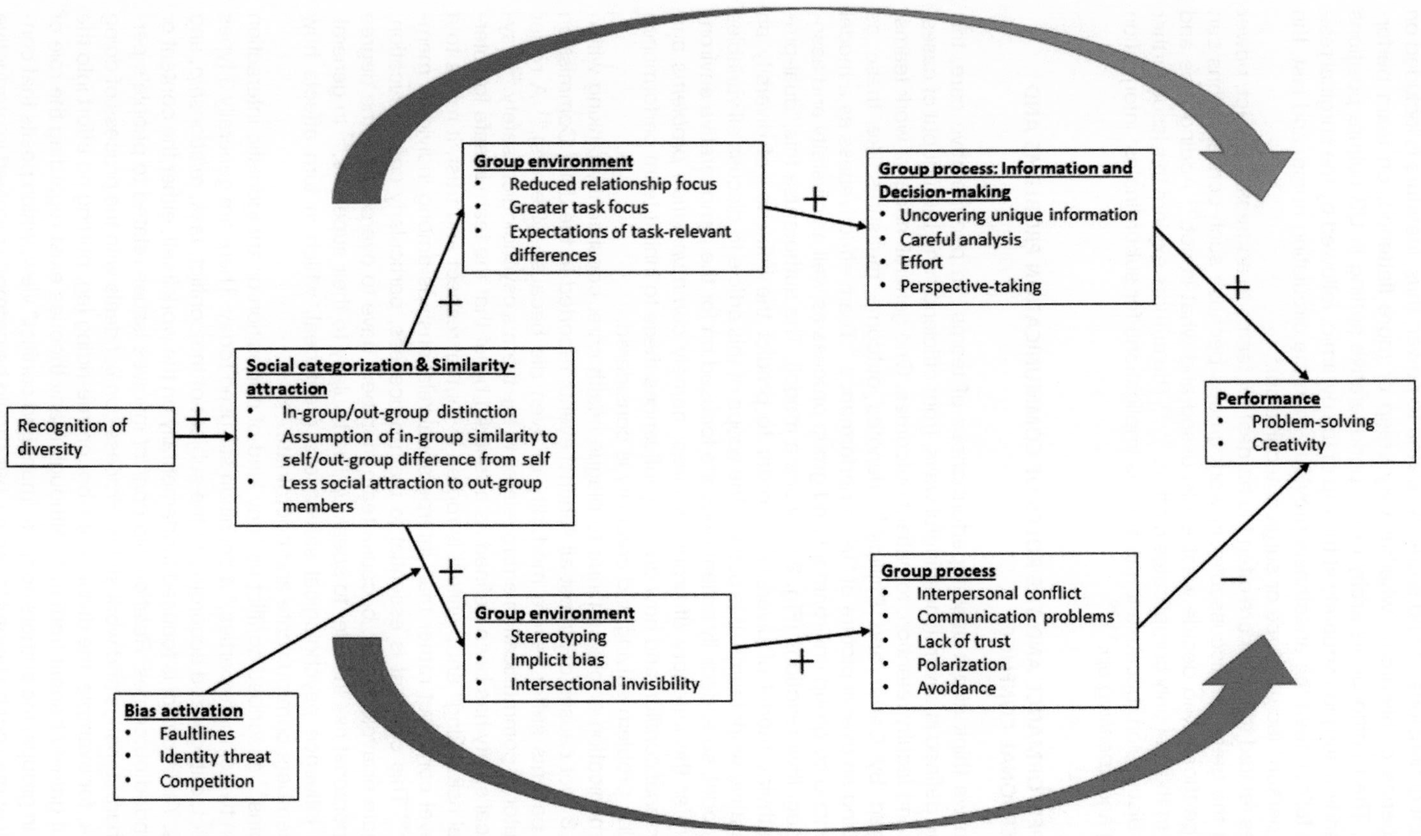

Fig. 2. A dual pathway model of diversity. (*Adapted from* Carter AB, Phillips KW. The double-edged sword of diversity: toward a dual pathway model. Soc Personal Psychol Compass 2017;11(5):e12313; with permission.)

ways to minimize negative effects (eg, taking time away from other tasks, damaging relationships over time).[44] Of the 3 types of conflict, *relationship conflict* has been most consistently linked to worsened outcomes[45] and has many implications for the perioperative environment.[46–50]

FOCUS ON THEORY: HOW DIVERSITY NEGATIVELY AFFECTS COMMUNICATION AND CONFLICT

There are several ways in which diversity may affect groups broadly, and many theories attempt to explain these effects. Three that bear mentioning, and are included in the Carter and Philips model,[40] are similarity-attraction theory, social-identity and self-categorization theories, and information-processing and problem-solving views.[12] The authors briefly summarize the salient points of each set of theories in later discussion and explain why they are applicable to thinking about diversity in perioperative teams.

Similarity-attraction theory posits that individuals who possess similar attributes, such as attitudes, values, and beliefs, will have higher rates of interpersonal attraction and conversely will avoid engaging with those who may hold differing attitudes, values, and beliefs to reduce disagreement and strain,[12] potential antecedents to conflict. When viewing gender and racial/ethnic diversity through this lens, differences in attitudes, values, and beliefs are inferred to link with visible demographic differences.[12] This theory has been upheld in empiric research on teams in many settings; for example, race predicted friendships among first-year MBA students.[51] Familiarity, friendships, and within-team ties are linked to superior team effectiveness and pursuit of team goals, as evidenced by a recent metaanalysis of 37 studies.[52] Seen through the lens of perioperative teams, this may impact team members' abilities to build friendships and exchange differing viewpoints and diverse information[2] unless specific strategies are used to invite others' viewpoints and cultivate dialogue.[33]

Self-categorization theory describes the processes by which people select characteristics according to a hierarchy (eg, which characteristics are more salient to the group, such as gender, race/ethnicity, work role), and *social-identity theory* explains how those people then identify with a specific group, which is a significant emotional connection for an individual (that is, "belonging" to a group).[12] Self-categorization theory tends to constrain nuances within categories and magnify differences between categories, ultimately leading to stereotyping,[12] which further impacts group members' behaviors.[53] Mannix and Neale[12] describe this categorization as "in-group members are characterized by high trust, support, and reward, while out-group members are characterized by low trust, support, and reward." In particular, the threat of negative stereotyping has real consequences, because people experience heightened arousal from worry and stress leading to depleted cognitive reserves for performing tasks.[54] Negative stereotyping based on various group memberships is present in the perioperative environment,[46] albeit largely unexplored in the extant literature, and may jeopardize psychological safety if left unaddressed.

In stark contrast to these more negative views on how diversity may adversely impact teams, information-processing and problem-solving approaches highlight how differences between team members may lead to better outcomes.[12] Demographic characteristics are strongly associated with experiences that shape attitudes, values, and beliefs and may impact approaches to viewing and interpreting information. Researchers adhering to information-processing approaches to studying diversity tend to avoid measuring these visible characteristics, such as gender and race/ethnicity, and instead focus on variables, such as differences in age, experience, and educational and functional background, which are thought to be more directly tied to team thinking and information processing.[12,55] Empirically, these researchers have shown that differences in perspectives create openings into deeper explorations of problems at hand.[12] The challenges lie in the group's abilities to manage coordination issues inherent in highly diverse groups to promote productive dialogue and information exchange (also known as "elaboration").[10,12,56] Under the framework of information and decision making, finding creative solutions to challenges requires 3 additional prerequisites from demographically diverse team members:

- They must bring new information to the team.
- That information must be relevant to the task.
- They must be able to communicate this effectively to other team members.[40]

It is well established that perceptual errors occur during times of high cognitive load,[57] and input from team members is valuable in these times, especially when the situation is unclear.[58] On the flip side of this, information-sharing may lead to misunderstandings and disagreements based on diversity of thought and experience,[2,56] which has been less well studied in teams. The authors posit the following refined model to attempt to explain the relationships described above as being most salient for perioperative teams (**Fig. 3**). The authors share specific strategies in later discussion and focus on how perioperative teams may enhance their abilities to manage these challenges.

EFFECTS OF GENDER AND RACIAL/ETHNIC DIVERSITY IN TEAMS: COMMUNICATION AND CONFLICT IN THE PERIOPERATIVE ENVIRONMENT

As stated previously, the effects of diversity in teams have yielded mixed results. A recent metaanalysis evaluating diversity and team performance found that race and gender diversity had small negative relationships with team performance,[59] and other research has shown more negative relationships overall between racial/ethnic diversity than other forms of diversity.[2,12] Ample research suggests that diversity has an impact on team characteristics, including receptivity to negative feedback, worsened psychological safety, and increased conflict.[38,60,61] Psychological safety has a profound influence on team communication, because team members who report low

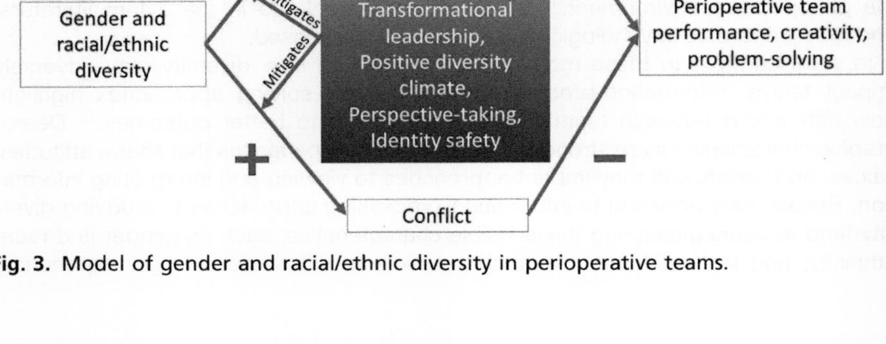

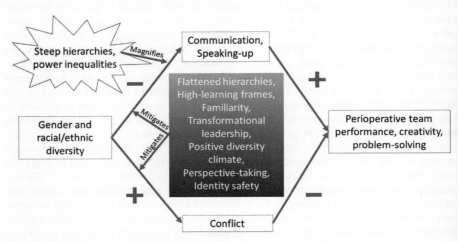

Fig. 3. Model of gender and racial/ethnic diversity in perioperative teams.

rates of psychological safety are more likely to conceal errors and stay silent,[11,39,42] dampening elaborative discourse to solve problems.

Regarding psychological safety, other forms of communication are hampered by diversity. van Knippenberg and Schippers[62] found individuals who were more dissimilar were less likely to seek information from each other, consistent with the theories of similarity attraction and self-categorization. As stated previously, stereotypes and bias may be at work here, and further research has shown that the negative effect of intergroup bias on team performance is largely due to inhibited elaboration, whereby teams did not use information creatively toward finding solutions.[56,62]

Factors involved in creating psychological safety are well known to promote speaking-up behaviors.[63] One such approach is to flatten hierarchy via a "humble leader," whose openness engenders a sense of "personal power" in subordinates, such that they feel a greater influence and are more likely to speak up.[64] To be clear, "humble leaders" still lead, although they do so in a more inclusive way.[64] Other research on speaking up shows gender may play a role, with results indicating subordinates were more likely to speak up to a female anesthesiologist than to a male anesthesiologist.[65] Hierarchy may play a role here as well; future studies may help determine the cause of this finding and whether it is consistent in other contexts and applicable to other team relationships. Given the small numbers of anesthesiologists and surgeons who are women, it is likely that gender diversity in perioperative leadership is not widespread. Although no studies in the medical literature have explored the effects of race on speaking up, research on organizational teams suggests racial minorities may choose to remain silent because of a lack of safety in the team.[10]

Several metaanalyses have shown that group diversity can be associated with increased conflict in teams, and that teams must work to mitigate social categorization processes, which can produce conflict and diminish trust and cohesion.[2,4] Task conflict may result from informational sharing differences and decrease team effectiveness.[2] Relationship conflict can arise from misattribution of team members' intentions, stereotyping, and bias, which may further worsen team effectiveness through growing hostility.[2] Explicit communication seems to be a moderating measure.[2] In the perioperative literature, a recent study by Jones and colleagues[26] looked at more than 200 surgical procedures involving 400 clinicians and analyzed their team interactions for cooperation, conflict, or neither. They found a significant influence of hierarchy and gender, with male attending surgeon and majority male team producing the most conflicts. One striking finding was that cooperation was better when most team members' gender differed from the attending surgeon's gender. The investigators determined that increased "chivalry" between team members of the opposite gender and increased competition between members of the same gender, may be the driving force for their findings.[26] If these findings hold true for more teams in the perioperative setting, then diversity here may be beneficial. However, it is important to note that given that the vast majority of attending surgeons are men, this study also signals the importance of having more women on teams as well.

MAXIMIZING THE POTENTIAL BENEFITS OF DIVERSITY IN PERIOPERATIVE TEAMS

Given the findings shared above, how do we ultimately work with diversity to harness its fullest benefits? Although diverse teams present initial challenges in the perioperative environment, there are several proactive strategies that leaders can apply to mitigate potential negative interactions of gender and racial/ethnic diversity to improve communication, specifically, by encouraging *speaking up*, and reduce nonproductive conflict (see **Fig. 3**). The authors propose the following 7 strategies to be applied proactively and deliberately within perioperative teams:

1. Modulate hierarchies toward flattening them, especially when complex problems need solving.[33,35] Minimizing the "power distance" between leaders and their subordinates can facilitate speaking up, because team members feel they have more influence within the team.[64]
2. Cultivate high-learning frames in the team (**Table 1**). Within any organization, and especially within perioperative teams, promoting a learning orientation is the key to enhancing communication by promoting psychological safety and productive approaches to failure within even a very diverse team.[10,11,66] Deliberately eliciting all team members' viewpoints and allowing for open and productive debate empowers many to speak up.[11,39]
3. Enhance familiarity. Teams who know each other better even outside of work may have better outcomes because of enhanced trust.[42,49] In addition, practicing together within the team (eg, participating in full-team simulation work) may build relational coordination, the tenets of which enhance relationships (leading to shared goals, shared knowledge, and mutual respect) to promote better communication (which is more frequent, timely, accurate, and aimed at problem-solving).[67]
4. Encourage transformational leadership styles that promote members sharing their viewpoints and combating biases.[68] Enhance the idea of "collective competence" whereby the team engages in supportive moves to help foster interdependence.[6] In addition, high cooperative interdependence may refocus the group on their shared identity, diverting their attention from thinking of team members as "other" subgroups based on demographics.[57]
5. Promote a positive diversity climate whereby team members cultivate an open-minded approach to diversity, especially where diversity can be seen as salient to the team's work.[69,70] In perioperative teams, all team members play vital roles, and their unique experiences should be recognized as valuable in order to experience the most gains from diversity.[70]

Table 1
High-learning and low-learning frames

High-Learning Frames	Low-Learning Frames
Mistakes are puzzles to be engaged.	Mistakes are crimes to be prosecuted.
Other people may have information or understanding that I lack.	I have a complete picture of this situation.
I can learn from others.	I don't have anything to learn from others in this group.
It is helpful to raise problems, even if I don't have a solution.	If I don't have a solution, I shouldn't raise the problem.
Just because I feel uncomfortable in this discussion doesn't mean I shouldn't stick with it.	If I feel uncomfortable in this discussion, something must be wrong.
I have something to say and should contribute, even though I may be criticized.	Speaking up invites criticism.
I can make a contribution here even though I don't have any formal power or authority.	I'm powerless in this group, so I will be quiet.

Adapted from Foldy EG, Rivard P, Buckley TR. Power, safety, and learning in racially diverse groups. Acad Manage Learn Educ 2009;8(1):32; with permission.

6. Imagining how others see a situation, not settling on just how you see it (perspective taking) can be helpful as well and has been shown to reduce aggression and enhance empathy and creativity.[71] One way to model this is to openly foster a sense of curiosity at how others see things.[71]
7. Enhance identity safety. Foldy and colleagues[10] developed a model for learning in racially diverse teams that proposed that psychological safety is likely to be low when diversity is high, but that this interaction could be moderated by identity safety, defined as "an individual's belief that his or her group identity—in this case racial identity—is welcome and does not incur risk as a group." This is brought to bear by fostering a respectful, inclusive climate.

FUTURE DIRECTIONS

As evidenced above, perioperative teams may benefit from more research into the dynamics of team effectiveness and how diversity impacts them. The authors put forth a streamlined model to guide research, proposing that speaking up and absence of nonproductive conflict are positively associated with team performance, as evidenced above, and that gender and racial/ethnic diversity may both have negative relationships with those. By using specific strategies to attenuate power dynamics (such as flattening hierarchies) and promoting open-mindedness and high-learning frames (see **Table 1**), these relationships between diversity and speaking up may improve, whereas diversity and nonproductive conflict can likely be attenuated (see **Fig. 3**). As diversity efforts grow in health care, we must deliberately study ways to manage diversity in our teams in order to reap the creativity and performance benefits that diversity may offer.

SUMMARY

Increased diversity in health care is a priority; yet, the impacts of diversity on perioperative team effectiveness are largely unstudied. Together, we must develop a concise research agenda and deliberately study how gender and racial/ethnic diversity influence perioperative teams, because this environment may be unique as compared with other workplace settings from which this literature base arises. With a shifting landscape of team compositions, organizations and leaders should proactively address diversity challenges by using the strategies outlined above so these highly interwoven teams can fully realize their best potential for patient care.

DISCLOSURE

The authors have nothing to disclose.

REFERENCES

1. Manser T. Teamwork and patient safety in dynamic domains of healthcare: a review of the literature. Acta Anaesthesiol Scand 2009;53:143–51.
2. Srikanth K, Harvey S, Peterson R. A dynamic perspective on diverse teams: moving from the dual-process model to a dynamic coordination-based model of diverse team performance. Acad Manag Ann 2016;10(1):453–93.
3. Wahr JA, Prager RL, Abernathy JH, et al. Patient safety in the cardiac operating room: human factors and teamwork. A scientific statement from the American Heart Association. Circulation 2013;128:1139–69.
4. Williams Phillips K, O'Reilly CA. Demography and diversity in organizations: a review of 40 years of research. Res Organ Behav 1998;20:77–140.

5. Fiscella K, Mauksch L, Bodenheimer T, et al. Improving care teams' functioning: recommendations from team science. Jt Comm J Qual Patient Saf 2017;43:361–8.
6. Lingard L. Paradoxical truths and persistent myths: reframing the team competence conversation. J Contin Educ Health Prof 2016;36(Suppl 1):S19–21.
7. Alter AL, Stern C, Granot Y, et al. The "bad is black" effect: why people believe evildoers have darker skin than do-gooders. Pers Soc Psychol Bull 2016;42(12):1653–65.
8. McConnell AR, Leibold JM. Relations among the implicit association test, discriminatory behavior, and explicit measures of racial attitudes. J Exp Social Psych 2001;37(5):435–42.
9. Bergner D. The struggles of rejecting the gender binary. Available at: https://www.nytimes.com/2019/06/04/magazine/gender-nonbinary.html. Accessed July 28, 2019.
10. Foldy EG, Rivard P, Buckley TR. Power, safety, and learning in racially diverse groups. Acad Manage Learn Educ 2009;8(1):25–41.
11. Edmondson AC. Speaking up in the operating room: how team leaders promote learning in interdisciplinary action teams. J Manage Stud 2003;40(6):1419–52.
12. Mannix E, Neale MA. What differences make a difference? Psychol Sci Public Interest 2005;6(2):31–55.
13. Association of American Medical Colleges. Physician specialty data report. 1.3. Active physicians by sex and specialty, 2017. 2018. Available at: https://www.aamc.org/data/workforce/reports/492560/1-3-chart.html. Accessed August 4, 2019.
14. Medscape I lifestyle report 2017: race and ethnicity, bias and burnout. Available at: https://www.medscape.com/sites/public/lifestyle/2017. Accessed August 4, 2019.
15. Data USA: registered nurses. Available at: https://datausa.io/profile/soc/registered-nurses#demographics. Accessed August 5, 2019.
16. Data USA: nurse practitioners & nurse midwives. Available at: https://datausa.io/profile/soc/2911XX/#demographics. Accessed August 5, 2019.
17. National Commission on Certification of Physician Assistants. Statistical profile of certified physician assistants by specialty annual report. 2018. Available at: http://prodcmsstoragesa.blob.core.windows.net/uploads/files/2018StatisticalProfileofCertifiedPAsbySpecialty1.pdf. Accessed August 5, 2019.
18. Lett LA, Orji WU, Sebro R. Declining racial and ethnic representation in clinical academic medicine: a longitudinal study of 16 US medical specialties. PLoS One 2018;13(11):e0207274.
19. Fang D, Moy E, Colburn L, et al. Racial and ethnic disparities in faculty promotion in academic medicine. JAMA 2000;284(9):1085–92.
20. Kaplan SE, Raj A, Carr PL, et al. Race/ethnicity and success in academic medicine: findings from a longitudinal multi-institutional study. Acad Med 2018;93:616–22.
21. Peterson NB, Friedman RH, Ash AS, et al. Faculty self-reported experience with racial and ethnic discrimination in academic medicine. J Gen Intern Med 2004;19:259–65.
22. Yu PT, Parsa PV, Hassanein O, et al. Minorities struggle to advance in academic medicine: a 12-year review of diversity at the highest levels of America's teaching institutions. J Surg Res 2013;182:212–8.
23. Frohman HA, Nguyen TC, Co F, et al. The nonwhite woman surgeon: a rare species. J Surg Educ 2015;72:1266–71.

24. Alsan M, Garrick O, Graziani GC. Does diversity matter for health? Experimental evidence from Oakland. Working Paper 24787, NBER working paper series. 2019. Available at: https://www.nber.org/papers/w24787. Accessed August 4, 2019.
25. Logghe HJ, Rouse T, Beekley A, et al. The evolving surgeon image. AMA J Ethics 2018;20(5):492–500.
26. Jones LK, Mowinski Jennings B, Higgins MK, et al. Ethological observations of social behavior in the operating room. Proc Nat Acad Sci U S A 2018;115(29): 7575–80.
27. Jena AB, Khullar D, Ho O, et al. Sex differences in academic rank in US medical schools in 2014. JAMA 2015;314(11):1149–58.
28. Carr PL, Raj A, Kaplan SE, et al. Gender differences in academic medicine: retention, rank, and leadership comparisons from the National Faculty Survey. Acad Med 2018;93:1694–9.
29. Desai T, Ali S, Fang X, et al. Equal work for unequal pay: the gender reimbursement gap for healthcare providers in the United States. Postgrad Med J 2016; 92(1092):571–5.
30. Rabinerson D, Kaplan B, Glezerman M. The feminization of obstetrics and gynecology. Harefuah 2010;149:729–32, 748, 747.
31. 2018 Nurse.com Nursing Salary Research Report. Available at: http://mediakit.nurse.com/wp-content/uploads/2018/06/2018-Nurse.com-Salary-Research-Report.pdf. Accessed August 4, 2019.
32. Wilson BL, Butler MJ, Butler RJ, et al. Nursing gender pay differentials in the new millennium. J Nurs Scholarsh 2018;50(1):102–8.
33. Salancik G, Pfeffer J. Who gets power. In: Thushman M, O'Reilly C, Nadler D, editors. Management of organizations. New York: Harper & Row; 1989.
34. Anderson C, Brown CE. The functions and dysfunctions of hierarchy. Res Organ Behav 2010;30:55–89.
35. Edmondson AC. The local and variegated nature of learning in organizations: a group-level perspective. Organ Sci 2002;13(2):128–46.
36. Argyris C, Putnam R, Smith DM. Action science: concepts methods and skills for research and intervention. San Francisco (CA): Jossey-Bass; 1985.
37. Avery DR, Richeson JA, Hebl MR, et al. It does not have to be uncomfortable: the role of behavioral scripts in black-white interracial interactions. J Appl Psychol 2009;94:1382–93.
38. Karakowsky L, Miller D. Teams that listen and teams that do not: exploring the role of gender in group responsiveness to negative feedback. Team Perform Management 2002;8(7/8):146–56.
39. Edmondson AC. Psychological safety and learning behavior in work teams. Administrative Sci Q 1999;44:350–83.
40. Carter AB, Phillips KW. The double-edged sword of diversity: toward a dual pathway model. Soc Personal Psychol Compass 2017;11:e12313.
41. The Joint Commission. Sentinel event data: root causes by event type, 2004-2015. Available at: https://hcupdate.files.wordpress.com/2016/02/2016-02-se-root-causes-by-event-type-2004-2015.pdf. Accessed August 15, 2019.
42. Edmondson AC. Learning from failure in health care: frequent opportunities, pervasive barriers. Qual Saf Health Care 2004;13:ii3–9.
43. Robbins SP. "Conflict management" and "conflict resolution" are not synonymous terms. Calif Manage Rev 1978;21(2):67–75.

44. Robbins SP, Judge TA. Chapter 14: conflict and negotiation. In: Robbins SP, Judge TA, editors. Organizational behavior. 15th edition. Boston: Pearson Education, Inc; 2013. p. 445–77.
45. De Dreu CKW, Weingard LR. Task versus relationship conflict, team performance, and team member satisfaction: a meta-analysis. J Appl Psychol 2003;88(4): 741–9.
46. Cooper JB. Critical role of the surgeon-anesthesiologist relationship for patient safety. Anesthesiology 2018;129:402–5.
47. Lingard L, Reznick R, DeVito I, et al. Forming professional identities on the health care team: discursive constructions of the 'other' in the operating room. Med Educ 2002;36:728–34.
48. Lingard L, Regehr G, Espin S, et al. Perceptions of operating room tension across professions: building generalizable evidence and educational resources. Acad Med 2005;80(10 Suppl):S75–9.
49. Lingard L, Vanstone M, Durrant M, et al. Conflicting messages: examining the dynamics of leadership on interprofessional teams. Acad Med 2012;87:1762–7.
50. Katz JD. Conflict and its resolution in the operating room. J Clin Anesth 2007;19: 152–8.
51. Mollica K, Gray B, Trevino L. Racial homophily and its persistence in newcomers' social networks. Organ Sci 2003;14:123–36.
52. Balkundi P, Harrison DA. Ties, leaders, and time in teams: strong inference about network structure's effects on team viability and performance. Acad Manage J 2006;49(1):49–68.
53. McGrath J, Berdahl J, Arrow H. Traits, expectations, culture, and clout. In: Jackson S, Ruderman M, editors. Diversity in workteams. Washington, DC: APA Books; 1995. p. 47–68.
54. Block CJ, Koch SM, Liberman BE, et al. Contending with stereotype threat at work: a model of long-term responses. Couns Psychol 2011;39(4):570–600.
55. Pitcher P, Smith AD. Top management team heterogeneity: personality, power, and proxies. Organ Sci 2001;12(1):1–18.
56. van Knippenberg D, De Dreu CKW, Homan AC. Work group diversity and group performance: an integrative model and research agenda. J Appl Psychol 2004; 89(6):1008–22.
57. Greig PR, Higham H, Nobre AC. Failure to perceive clinical events: an under-recognised source of error. Resuscitation 2014;85:952–6.
58. Orasanu JM. Shared problem models and flight crew performance. In: Johnston N, McDonald N, Fuller R, editors. Aviation psychology in practice. Aldershot (England): Ashgate Publishing Group; 1994.
59. Gomez LE, Bernet P. Diversity improves performance and outcomes. J Natl Med Assoc 2019. https://doi.org/10.1016/j.jnma.2019.01.006.
60. Van Dijk H, Meyer B, van Engen M, et al. Microdynamics in diverse teams: a review and integration of the diversity and stereotyping literatures. Acad Management Ann 2017;11(1):517–57.
61. Mackie DM, Smith ER. Group-based emotion in group processes and intergroup relations. Group Process Intergroup Relations 2017;20(5):658–68.
62. van Knippenberg D, Schippers MC. Work group diversity. Annu Rev Psychol 2007;58:515–41.
63. Raemer DB, Kolbe M, Minehart RD, et al. Improving anesthesiologists' ability to speak up in the operating room: a randomized controlled experiment of a simulation-based intervention and qualitative analysis of hurdles and enablers. Acad Med 2016;91(4):530–9.

64. Lin X, Chen ZX, Tse HHM, et al. Why and when employees like to speak up more under humble leaders? The roles of personal sense of power and power distance. J Bus Ethics 2019;158:937–50.
65. Pattni N, Bould MD, Hayter MA, et al. Gender, power and leadership: the effect of a superior's gender on respiratory therapists' ability to challenge leadership during a life-threatening emergency. Br J Anaesth 2017;119(4):697–702.
66. Argyris C. Overcoming organizational defenses: facilitating organizational learning. Boston: Allyn and Bacon; 1990.
67. Brazil V, Purdy E, Alexander C, et al. Improving the relational aspects of trauma care through translational simulation. Adv Simulation 2019;4:10.
68. Kearney E, Gebert D. Managing diversity and enhancing team outcomes: the promise of transformational leadership. J Appl Psychol 2009;94(1):77–89.
69. McKay PF, Avery DR, Tonidandel S, et al. Racial differences in employee retention: are diversity climate perceptions the key? Pers Psychol 2007;60(1):35–62.
70. Homan AC, Hollenbeck JR, Humphrey SE, et al. Facing differences with an open mind: openness to experience, salience of intragroup differences, and performance of diverse work groups. Acad Management J 2008;51(6):1204–22.
71. Parker SK, Axtell C. Seeing another viewpoint: antecedents and outcomes of employee perspective taking. Acad Management J 2001;44(6):1085–100.

Women and Underrepresented Minorities in Academic Anesthesiology

Paloma Toledo, MD, MPH[a,b,*], Choy R. Lewis, MD[a], Elizabeth M.S. Lange, MD[a]

KEYWORDS

- Women • Gender • Underrepresented minorities • Academic anesthesiology
- Diversity • Leadership

KEY POINTS

- The number of women in academic anesthesiology is increasing.
- The number of women and underrepresented minorities in leadership positions is still significantly less than men and non-underrepresented minorities, respectively.
- Many studies have focused on gender differences in anesthesiology. Studies on racial/ethnic differences are limited due to lack of access to information of self-identified race/ethnicity of anesthesiologists.
- A diverse workforce has been cited as 1 strategy for eliminating health care disparities.

INTRODUCTION

In 2017, there were 41,718 active physician anesthesiologists in the United States,[1] and approximately 20% of physician anesthesiologists are in academic anesthesiology.[2] Workforce diversity has been a topic of much discussion in recent years, as increasing the diversity of the physician workforce has been suggested as a potential solution for reducing health care disparities.[3–5] Gender and racial/ethnically diverse teams have been shown to perform better than less diverse teams.[6] Gender equity has been associated with improved employee engagement and better organizational

---

Author Contributions: P. Toledo, C.R. Lewis, and E.M.S. Lange drafted and approved the final version of the article.

[a] Department of Anesthesiology, Northwestern University Feinberg School of Medicine, 251 East Huron Street, F5-704, Chicago, IL 60611, USA; [b] Center for Health Services and Outcomes Research, Northwestern University Feinberg School of Medicine, Chicago, IL, USA

* Corresponding author. Department of Anesthesiology, Northwestern University Feinberg School of Medicine, 251 East Huron Street, F5-704, Chicago, IL 60611.

E-mail address: p-toledo@northwestern.edu

Anesthesiology Clin 38 (2020) 449–457
https://doi.org/10.1016/j.anclin.2020.01.004
anesthesiology.theclinics.com
1932-2275/20/

outcomes.[7,8] In medicine, increased diversity in the physician workforce has been shown to improve patient satisfaction,[9] patient-provider communication,[9] access to care,[10] and result in better patient outcomes.[4] Several studies in recent years have focused on the demographic makeup of the academic anesthesia workforce, as well as in areas in which gender or racial gaps exist within anesthesiology. In this study, we summarize the current literature and provide a framework for academic advancement.

Academic Workforce Demographics

The American Association of Medical Colleges (AAMC) maintains a master file of physicians practicing in the United States and reports demographics of all physicians in the Physician Specialty Data Report. The demographics of medical school faculty are reported annually in the US Medical School Faculty report.[11] Of the 41,718 active physician anesthesiologists in the United States,[1] there were 8835 anesthesiologists on medical school faculty in 2018.[11] The AAMC reports data on sex, not gender, and defines underrepresented minorities as racial or ethnic groups that have been historically underrepresented in medicine (ie, African American/black, Hispanic/Latino, American Indian/Alaska Native, Native Hawaiian/Pacific Islander).[12] In 2018, there were 3229 female anesthesiologists (36.6% of all anesthesiologists), and 863 URM anesthesiologists (9.8% of all anesthesiologists).[11] These numbers contrast starkly with the percentage of women and URM in the general population of the United States in 2018 (50.8% and 33.2%, respectively).[13]

Underrepresented Minorities in Academic Anesthesiology

There has been a relative paucity of studies on URM faculty in academic anesthesiology, in contrast to the number of studies on women in academic anesthesiology. This is in part because of a lack of access to publicly available data on race/ethnicity. Studies of women in anesthesiology have been benefited from using first name conventions or Internet-based searches of photographs to assign gender.[14] This methodology cannot be applied to race/ethnicity.[15,16]

Several indirect methods for assigning race/ethnicity exist. Surname analysis uses patient's last name to identify their race/ethnicity (ie, a patient with the last name Martinez would be assigned Hispanic ethnicity). Although surname analysis has been shown to be accurate for Hispanic ethnicity compared with self-identified ethnicity,[17] as well as for Asian ethnicity,[18,19] to date, it has not been used to assess non-Hispanic white, black/African American, or Native American surnames.[20] A further limitation is that surname analysis may misclassify women who assume a married name that would be attributed to their husband's racial/ethnic group, which is different than their own.[20] The use of photographs to assign race/ethnicity is similarly problematic. A study published in 2003 compared hospital staff's accuracy in assigning patient race/ethnicity based on appearance or spoken language compared with patient's self-identified race/ethnicity, the results of which were collected for another purpose (n = 15,102).[15] Hospital staff could select from 6 categories: Hispanic, American Indian, black/African American, Asian, white, and unknown/missing. Although the agreement between the assigned race/ethnicity and the self-reported race/ethnicity was best for white patients (76%), the agreement decreased for other racial/ethnic groups: 68% agreement for black/African American, 57% for Hispanics, 33% for Asians, and 1% for American Indians.[15]

Geocoding is another indirect measure of race/ethnicity, in which geographically coded data from the United States Census is to characterize people living within that zip code. Studies have shown that geocoded data may be used as a reasonable substitute for self-identified race/ethnicity data,[21] and this methodology has been recommended by the Institute of Medicine.[16] A limitation of geocoding is that many Americans may identify with more than 1 racial or ethnic group, and the categorical race options given on forms may not truly be representative of their true self-identified race or ethnicity. Geocoding is not an option for studies of demographics in medicine, as publicly available datasets do not have data on physician's zip codes. Self-identification of race/ethnicity remains the gold standard for data collection.[22]

Self-identification of race/ethnicity was used in a study published in 2017 that evaluated the proportion of women and URM anesthesiologists in the American Society of Anesthesiology (ASA) leadership, and compared that with the proportions in the general population in the United States and the general physician workforce.[23] Two hundred and ninety-nine physician anesthesiologists responded (54% response rate). A total of 21.1% (95% CI, 16.4–25.7) of respondents were women and 6.0% (95% CI, 3.3–8.7) identified as URM. The proportion of URM ASA leaders was lower than the proportion of URM in the United States ($P<.001$). Among the URM respondents, 6 were women (1.1%; 95% CI, 0.2–1.9).

Women in Academic Anesthesiology

The underrepresentation of women in medicine and in leadership positions has been the focus of significant attention.[8,24–28] In 2019, several articles focused on the issues of gender parity in anesthesiology.[29–38]

Trends for women in anesthesiology

In 2019, Bissing and colleagues[29] evaluated the current status and trends for women in academic anesthesiology. The authors compared contemporary data with data from a study published in 2008 by Wong and Stock,[14] which evaluated the status of women in academic anesthesiology over 2 decades. Data were obtained from multiple sources, including AAMC data, and for each category data were collected for the 10-year period after the dates used in the previous publication.[14]

The number of women faculty members in anesthesiology increased from 1783 in 2006 to 2945 in 2015.[29] The distribution of women anesthesiology faculty members, by rank, was not significantly different in 2015 compared with 2005 ($P = .270$)[29]; however, the number of women with the academic rank of full professor in anesthesiology nearly doubled, increasing from 109 in 2006 to 210 in 2016.[29] Although the number of women full professors increased, the percentage of women full professors was less than men full professors in anesthesiology (7.4% vs 17.3%, respectively, difference −9.9%, 95% CI of the difference −8.5 to −11.3; $P<.001$).[29]

An evaluation of anesthesiology residents revealed that there was a linear increase in the number of women residents over time, from 1570 in 2006 to 2145 in 2016, with a median yearly increase of 44.[29] In contrast, over the same time period, there was a negative linear trend in the proportion of women medical school graduates ($P = .001$).

Professional Activities of Women in Anesthesiology

Several articles have explored the representation of women in various aspects of academic anesthesiology, including authorship of manuscripts, speaking at national meetings, grant awards, and leadership in departments of anesthesiology and of national societies.

Manuscript authorship

Authorship in medical journals is often considered as a criterion for promotion in the United States. In 2006, Jagsi and colleagues[39] published an article evaluating the gender gap in authorship in the academic literature over a 35-year period. The authors reviewed 6 journals, the *New England Journal of Medicine*, the *Journal of the American Medical Association*, the *Annals of Internal Medicine*, the *Annals of Surgery*, *Obstetrics and Gynecology*, and the *Journal of Pediatrics*. The gender of the first and last author for each research article and editorial was categorized for authors who held an MD degree. From 1970 to 2004, the proportion of women first authors increased from 5.9% to 29.3% ($P<.001$), and the proportion of women senior authors also increased from 3.7% to 19.3% ($P<.001$). Several studies have since used similar methodology and had relatively consistent findings; the proportion of women authors ranges between 25% and 40% and there is an increasing trend in the number of women authors over time.[35,40,41]

In July 2019, Miller and colleagues[34] evaluated the proportion of women authors published in *Anesthesiology* and *Anesthesia & Analgesia* during the years 2002, 2007, 2012, and 2017. In addition to evaluating first and senior authorship for research articles, the authors extracted data on study type, anesthesia subspecialty topic, and the total number of authors. A total of 2600 manuscripts were included in the analysis. In 2017, 30% of first authors were women, and 23% of senior authors were women.[34] Over the 15-year time period, there was an absolute increase in the proportion of women first authors by 10%, and by 9% for senior authors.[34] In this same time period, there was an 8% absolute increase in the number of women full-time anesthesia faculty members. An interesting finding was that the percentage of women first authors with women senior authors was higher than the percentage of women first authors with men senior authors (36% vs 23.8%, $P<.01$),[34] suggesting a more positive mentor-mentee effect when the first and senior authors are of the same gender.

Grant awardees

Grant awards are similarly used as a metric for academic promotion in US institutions; however, anesthesiology as a specialty has been historically underrepresented in NIH funding.[42] Using the NIH RePORT database for funded awards, Mayes and colleagues[38] compared gender differences in K08 and K23 awards (ie, career development awards) for women versus men anesthesiologists, and also compared funding for anesthesiology versus surgery for the years 2006 to 2016. Over the 10-year period, there were 88 career development awards given to anesthesiologists, of whom 29 (33%) were women. In comparison, surgeons received nearly 3 times more career development awards (n = 261), with a similar proportion of women being funded (28%).[38] In both specialties, women were less likely to receive an award than men ($P<.03$).[38]

The Foundation for Anesthesia Education and Research (FAER) and International Anesthesia Research Society (IARS) both have grants for physician scientists in anesthesiology. In addition to evaluating the number of women FAER and IARS award recipients, Bissing and colleagues[29] evaluated trends in funding over 2 periods (1997–2007 compared with 2007–2016). The proportion of women grant recipients was 32% in 2007 to 2016, which had increased from 21% in 1997 to 2007 ($P = .02$).[29] This trend is promising in that FAER and IARS awards are often given to early-career scholars, and are often considered pre-K level awards. Therefore, it suggests an increased interest in early-career women physician scientists who will go on to receive K level and R level awards, as well as advance academically in rank.

A more recent evaluation of grants funded by the Society of Cardiovascular Anesthesiologists (SCA) between 2014 and 2019 revealed that women applicants had a lower funding success rate than men applicants (8.7% vs 22%). As part of an initiative to decrease the gender gap in cardiac anesthesiology research, the SCA plans to create a $50,000 2-year starter grant dedicated to promoting early-career women in research in 2020 (personal communication with Lindsey Baris, Operations Administrator, Society for Cardiovascular Anesthesiologists, 2019).

Speaking at national meetings

Three studies published in 2019 evaluated gender representation of speakers at national meetings.[29,30,37] Moeschler and colleagues[37] evaluated the gender representation of all speakers at the ASA annual meeting between 2011 and 2016. Of the 5167 speaker slots, 1293 were women speakers (25%). There was no difference between the proportion of women speakers and the proportion of ASA members who identify as women ($P = .15$). There was no change in the proportion of women speakers between 2011 and 2016 ($P = .062$).[37] Between 1985 and 2016, only 4 women had delivered the prestigious Rovenstine lecture.[29]

A similar proportion of women speakers (28.5% of 1256 speaker slots) was identified at the Canadian Anesthesiologists Society (CAS) annual meeting between 2007 and 2019.[30] In contrast to the ASA annual meeting, the number of women speakers is increasing at the CAS meeting over time.[30] Women were more likely to be speakers in obstetric anesthesia topics and were least likely to be speakers in cardiothoracic and transplant critical care topics.[30]

Editorial board membership

Two studies evaluated editorial board membership in anesthesiology. Bissing and colleagues[29] evaluated the editorial board composition of *Anesthesiology* (established 1940) and *Anesthesia & Analgesia* (established 1922). At present, a woman has not served as editor-in-chief for either journal. In 2017, only 1 of the 14 members of the *Anesthesiology* editorial board (executive editors and editors, combined) was a woman;[29] also only 4 of the 37 members of the *Anesthesia & Analgesia* editorial board and executive section editors were women.[29] There was no change in the proportion of women editors for either journal compared with editorial board representation in 2006.[29] Lorello and colleagues[31] evaluated the gender composition of the *Canadian Journal of Anesthesia* editorial board from its inception, in 1954, to 2018. A total of 146 editors were identified, and 10% were women. There was no correlation between women editorial board members and the proportion of women anesthesiologists in Canada (33% in 2018, $P = .93$).[31] The authors did not have access to the proportion of women in academic anesthesiology in Canada, which would have been a more appropriate comparison.

Leadership in departments of anesthesiology and national societies

Data on department chairs and residency directors was collected using the 2017 to 2018 membership list of the Association of Academic Anesthesiology Chairs and a list of residency program directors in anesthesiology from the Accreditation Council for Graduate Medical Education. Fewer than 15% of department chairs were women, and this number had not changed in the past decade ($P = .75$).[29] In contrast to department chairs, a higher percentage of women were program directors in anesthesiology residency programs (32% of 148 program directors in accredited programs).[29]

Four women have now served as president of the ASA since its inception in 1905, with terms in 1991, 2014, 2018, and 2019. The current first vice president of the ASA is also a woman. Bissing and colleagues[29] evaluated the proportion of terms served by a woman in academic and subspecialty anesthesiology societies. There were no differences in the proportion of terms served by a woman from 2008 to 2017 compared with 1998 to 2007 (20.2% vs 26.1%, respectively; $P = .29$).

Fahy and colleagues[43] evaluated the number of women American Board of Anesthesiology (ABA) diplomates, oral examiners, and directors from 1985 to 2015 using data from the ABA database. There was a steady increase in the numbers of women in each category over time, with 38% of all diplomates being women in 2015. The authors compared the percentage of oral examiners with the percentage of diplomates who were women 10 years earlier, and the percentage of directors was compared with the percentage of oral examiners 7 years earlier, to account for the typical advancement time for each position. There were comparable amounts of women examiners in 2015 (26.4%) with women diplomates in 2005 (25.8%). In contrast, there were a greater percentage of women directors than there were women oral examiners 10 years earlier (25% vs 18%, correlation coefficient 0.86, $P<.001$). This gain was attributed to the ABA's efforts to achieve diversity.

Women in leadership positions may not have achieved parity with men anesthesiologists; however, there are promising trends in almost all metrics.

Recommendations for Academic Advancement

Although there is no agreement on what the target number of women or URMs in medicine or anesthesiology should be, it is apparent that their representation is less than that of the general population. In an editorial written by Leslie and colleagues,[7] the authors suggested rules for increasing participation in leadership in our specialty (summarized in **Table 1**). Although the rules pertain to increasing the diversity of leadership in the specialty, other suggestions for academic advancement have included

Table 1
Suggested rules for increasing participation in leadership in our specialty

Recommendation	Description
1. Collect and publicly report organizational demographic data	Data on gender, race, and ethnicity should be collected and used to describe general membership and the leadership, as well as candidates for leadership positions (if applicable)
2. Develop and publicly publish relevant policies on diversity	Organizations should develop a policy regarding underrepresented groups (eg, women and minorities) and describe contingencies when insufficient numbers of apply for leadership positions
3. Include diverse stakeholders on a recruitment advisory board	For organizations that have a nominating committee, include diverse stakeholders (eg, women and minorities) on the nominations committee to increase the diversity of the candidate pool
4. Create and maintain database of diverse members who have potential for leadership	
5. Highlight the importance of diversity with members and provide mentorship for organizational officers from diverse backgrounds, if necessary	
6. Consider the timing of meetings (ie, family-friendly meeting times)	Consider the timing of meeting scheduling, particularly as it relates to parents who may have childcare responsibilities
7. Take the pledge and consider running for office to create cultural change within an organization	

Data from Leslie K, Hopf HW, Houston P, et al. Women, Minorities, and Leadership in Anesthesiology: Take the Pledge. Anesth Analg 2017;124(5):1394-1396.

increasing the number of pipeline programs and mentoring opportunities for faculty members, developing programs for retention and promotion of faculty members, ensuring successful transitions between academic levels, evaluating recruitment practices, and identifying institutional champions for diversity.[5,44–49]

SUMMARY

Women and underrepresented minorities may not have achieved parity with men or non-URM anesthesiologists; however, there are promising trends in almost all metrics. Although parity has not been achieved at the highest levels of academic achievement in our specialty, namely in department chair positions, the rank of full professor, or editorial board representation, this gap may diminish over time with the changing demographics of the specialty.

FINANCIAL DISCLOSURE

P. Toledo was supported by grants from the Agency for Healthcare Research and Quality and National Institute on Minority Health and Health Disparities (R03MD011628, R03HS025267, and R18HS026169). The content is solely the responsibility of the authors and does not necessarily represent the official views of the Agency for Healthcare Research and Quality or the National Institute on Minority Health and Health Disparities.

CONFLICTS OF INTEREST

The authors have nothing to disclose.

REFERENCES

1. Physician specialty data report: active physicians by sex and specialty, 2017. Available at: https://www.aamc.org/data-reports/workforce/interactive-data/active-physicians-sex-and-specialty-2017. Accessed November 1, 2019.
2. The state of women in academic medicine: the pipeline and pathways to leadership, 2015–2016. Available at: https://www.aamc.org/data-reports/faculty-institutions/data/state-women-academic-medicine-pipeline-and-pathways-leadership-2015-2016. Accessed November 1, 2019.
3. Institute of Medicine. Unequal treatment: confronting racial and ethnic disparities in Health care. Washington, DC: National Academy Press; 2003.
4. Cooper-Patrick L, Gallo JJ, Gonzales JJ, et al. Race, gender, and partnership in the patient-physician relationship. JAMA 1999;282(6):583–9.
5. Sullivan Commission. Missing persons: minorities in the health professions. Available at: http://www.thesullivanalliance.org/cue/research/publications.html. Accessed November 1, 2019.
6. McKinsey & Company. Women in the workplace 2016. Available at: https://womenintheworkplace.com/Women_in_the_Workplace_2016.pdf. Accessed November 1, 2019.
7. Leslie K, Hopf HW, Houston P, et al. Women, minorities, and leadership in anesthesiology: take the pledge. Anesth Analg 2017;124(5):1394–6.
8. Bickel J, Wara D, Atkinson BF, et al. Increasing women's leadership in academic medicine: report of the AAMC Project Implementation Committee. Acad Med 2002;77(10):1043–61.

9. Saha S, Komaromy M, Koepsell TD, et al. Patient-physician racial concordance and the perceived quality and use of health care. Arch Intern Med 1999; 159(9):997–1004.
10. Cantor JC, Miles EL, Baker LC, et al. Physician service to the underserved: implications for affirmative action in medical education. Inquiry 1996;33(2):167–80.
11. American Association of Mecial Colleges. Faculty Roster: U.S. Medical School Faculty. Available at: https://www.aamc.org/data-reports/faculty-institutions/report/faculty-roster-us-medical-school-faculty. Accessed November 1, 2019.
12. American Association of Mecial Colleges. Underrepresented in medicine definition. Available at: https://www.aamc.org/what-we-do/mission-areas/diversity-inclusion/underrepresented-in-medicine. Accessed November 1, 2019.
13. United States Census Bureau. Quick facts from the U.S. Census Bureau. Available at: https://www.census.gov/quickfacts/fact/table/US/PST045218. Accessed November 1, 2019.
14. Wong CA, Stock MC. The status of women in academic anesthesiology: a progress report. Anesth Analg 2008;107(1):178–84.
15. Boehmer U, Kressin NR, Berlowitz DR, et al. Self-reported vs administrative race/ethnicity data and study results. Am J Public Health 2002;92(9):1471–2.
16. Ulmer C, McFadden B, Nerenz DR, editors. Institute of Medicine: race, ethnicity, and language data: standardization for health care quality improvement. Washington, DC: National Academies Press; 2009.
17. Perkins RC. Evaluating the passel-word Spanish surname list: 1990 decennial Census post enumeration survey results. Washington, DC: Population Division, U.S. Bureau of the Census; 1993. Population Division Working Paper No. 4.
18. Lauderdale DS, Kestenbaum B. Asian American ethnic identification by surname. Popul Res Policy Rev 2000;19:283–300.
19. Nicoll A, Bassett K, Ulijaszek SJ. What's in a name? Accuracy of using surnames and forenames in ascribing Asian ethnic identity in English populations. J Epidemiol Community Health 1986;40(4):364–8.
20. Fiscella K, Fremont AM. Use of geocoding and surname analysis to estimate race and ethnicity. Health Serv Res 2006;41(4 Pt 1):1482–500.
21. Fremont AM, Bierman A, Wickstrom SL, et al. Use of geocoding in managed care settings to identify quality disparities. Health Aff (Millwood) 2005;24(2):516–26.
22. Wynia MK, Ivey SL, Hasnain-Wynia R. Collection of data on patients' race and ethnic group by physician practices. N Engl J Med 2010;362(9):846–50.
23. Toledo P, Duce L, Adams J, et al. Diversity in the American Society of Anesthesiologists Leadership. Anesth Analg 2017;124(5):1611–6.
24. Sexton KW, Hocking KM, Wise E, et al. Women in academic surgery: the pipeline is busted. J Surg Educ 2012;69(1):84–90.
25. Rochon PA, Davidoff F, Levinson W. Women in academic medicine leadership: has anything changed in 25 years? Acad Med 2016;91(8):1053–6.
26. Byington CL, Lee V. Addressing disparities in academic medicine: moving forward. JAMA 2015;314(11):1139–41.
27. Carnes M, Johnson P, Klein W, et al. Advancing women's health and women's leadership with endowed chairs in women's health. Acad Med 2017;92(2):167–74.
28. Jena AB, Khullar D, Ho O, et al. Sex differences in academic rank in US Medical Schools in 2014. JAMA 2015;314(11):1149–58.
29. Bissing MA, Lange EMS, Davila WF, et al. Status of women in academic anesthesiology: a 10-year update. Anesth Analg 2019;128(1):137–43.
30. Lorello GR, Parmar A, Flexman AM. Representation of women amongst speakers at the Canadian Anesthesiologists' Society annual meeting: a retrospective

analysis from 2007 to 2019. Can J Anaesth 2019. https://doi.org/10.1007/s12630-019-01524-3.
31. Lorello GR, Parmar A, Flexman AM. Representation of women on the editorial board of the Canadian Journal of Anesthesia: a retrospective analysis from 1954 to 2018. Can J Anaesth 2019;66(8):989–90.
32. Ellinas EH, Rebello E, Chandrabose RK, et al. Distinguished service awards in Anesthesiology Specialty Societies: analysis of gender differences. Anesth Analg 2019;129(4):e130–4.
33. Ellinas EH, Kaljo K, Patitucci TN, et al. No room to "lean in": a qualitative study on gendered barriers to promotion and leadership. J Womens Health (Larchmt) 2019;28(3):393–402.
34. Miller J, Chuba E, Deiner S, et al. Trends in authorship in anesthesiology journals. Anesth Analg 2019;129(1):306–10.
35. Gayet-Ageron A, Poncet A, Perneger T. Comparison of the contributions of female and male authors to medical research in 2000 and 2015: a cross-sectional study. BMJ Open 2019;9(2):e024436.
36. Larson AR, Sharkey KM, Poorman JA, et al. Representation of women among invited speakers at medical specialty conferences. J Womens Health (Larchmt) 2019. [Epub ahead of print].
37. Moeschler SM, Gali B, Goyal S, et al. Speaker gender representation at the American Society of Anesthesiology Annual Meeting: 2011-2016. Anesth Analg 2019; 129(1):301–5.
38. Mayes LM, Wong CA, Zimmer S, et al. Gender differences in career development awards in United States' anesthesiology and surgery departments, 2006-2016. BMC Anesthesiol 2018;18(1):95.
39. Jagsi R, Guancial EA, Worobey CC, et al. The "gender gap" in authorship of academic medical literature—a 35-year perspective. N Engl J Med 2006;355(3):281–7.
40. Kurichi JE, Kelz RR, Sonnad SS. Women authors of surgical research. Arch Surg 2005;140(11):1074–7.
41. Filardo G, da Graca B, Sass DM, et al. Trends and comparison of female first authorship in high impact medical journals: observational study (1994–2014). BMJ 2016;352:i847.
42. Schwinn DA, Balser JR. Anesthesiology physician scientists in academic medicine: a wake-up call. Anesthesiology 2006;104(1):170–8.
43. Fahy BG, Culley DJ, Sun H, et al. Gender distribution of the American Board of Anesthesiology Diplomates, Examiners, and Directors (1985–2015). Anesth Analg 2018;127(2):564–8.
44. Kenevan MR, Gali B. History, current state, and future of diversity in the anesthesia workforce. Adv Anesth 2019;37:53–63.
45. Kaplan SE, Gunn CM, Kulukulualani AK, et al. Challenges in recruiting, retaining and promoting racially and ethnically diverse faculty. J Natl Med Assoc 2018;110(1):58–64.
46. Cahn PS. Recognizing and reckoning with unconscious bias: a workshop for health professions faculty search committees. MedEdPORTAL 2017;13:10544.
47. Hannah SD, Carpenter-Song E. Patrolling your blind spots: introspection and public catharsis in a medical school faculty development course to reduce unconscious bias in medicine. Cult Med Psychiatry 2013;37(2):314–39.
48. King TE, Dickinson TA, DuBose TD, et al. The case for diversity in academic internal medicine. Am J Med 2004;116(4):284–9.
49. Merchant JL, Omary MB. Underrepresentation of underrepresented minorities in academic medicine: the need to enhance the pipeline and the pipe. Gastroenterology 2010;138(1):19–26.

Printed and bound by CPI Group (UK) Ltd, Croydon, CR0 4YY
08/05/2025
01864691-0003